Senior Editors

SALLY A. SHUMAKER, PH.D., is a Health Scientist Administrator with the Behavioral Medicine Branch of The National Heart, Lung, and Blood Institute. She received her doctoral degree in Social Psychology from The University of Michigan and postdoctoral degree in Social Psychology from The University of Michigan and postdoctoral training in Environmental and Health Psychology from The University of California (Irvine and Los Angeles). Dr. Shumaker's primary areas of interest include patient and family adjustment to chronic diseases, health policy, social support and the provision of care, and health quality of life. Dr. Shumaker has edited books and published numerous book chapters and scientific articles in these areas. Currently, she is the Project Officer for a large, multi-site study on the biobehavioral factors associated with coronary artery bypass graft surgery, and for programs on smoking cessation and relapse prevention. She also directs health quality of life assessment in several clinical trials.

ELEANOR B. SCHRON, M.S., R.N., is a Senior Research Nurse with the Clinical Trials Branch, of The National Heart, Lung, and Blood Institute. Previously she was a Health Science Analyst and Nurse consultant with the Office of Health Research, Statistics and Technology, Office of the Assistant Secretary for Health, and the Division of Peer Review of the Office of Professional Standards Review Organizations, Health Care Financing Administration, both within the Department of Health and Human Services. Her clinical experience includes the psychiatric/mental health and critical care areas. Ms. Schron currently serves as Project Director for several international, multi-center clinical trials. Her professional interests include quality of life evaluation, adherence in clinical trials and practice, informed consent, clinical trials methodology and administration, and dissemination of research findings. Ms. Schron is a Commissioned Officer in the U.S. Public Health Service.

JUDITH OCKENE, PH.D., is Professor of Medicine and Director of the division of Preventive and Behavioral Medicine at the University of Massachusetts Medical School. Her Ph.D. is in Counseling Psychology from Boston College. Dr. Ockene's major research has been in the investigation of factors which affect lifestyle behavior change and the relationship of lifestyle behaviors to disease. Her clinical work has involved interventions for cigarette smoking, nutritional behavior, exercise, stress, coping with disease, and the management of other disease related behaviors. Dr. Ockene is a past member of Surgeon General Koop's National Interagency Advisory Committee on Smoking and Health, and was a scientific editor of the 25th anniversary and the 1990 General's Reports on Smoking and Health. She has over 50 publications in preventive and behavioral medicine.

Co-Editors

CHRISTINE T. PARKER, PH.D., is a Policy Analyst with the National Institute of Mental Health. She was previously a Health Program Specialist with The National Heart, Lung, and Blood Institute where she was the program manager for all biobehavioral research on blood diseases and transfusion medicine in the Division of Blood Diseases and Resources.

JEFFREY L. PROBSTFIELD, M.D., is a board-certified internist and a formally trained clinical pharmacologist, as well as a Scientific Project Officer at The National Heart, Lung, and Blood Institute. He has been involved in the conduct and management of clinical trials for 20 years, including Coronary Primary Prevention Trial of the Lipid Research Clinics (LRC) Program for which he and his colleagues at the Baylor-Methodist Clinic of the LRC were the first to publish a systematized approach to the recovery of drop outs and long-term follow-up.

JOAN M. WOLLE, PH.D., M.P.H., Health Scientist Administrator with The National Heart, Lung, and Blood Institute, is the Program manager of the demonstration and education research grants and programs in the Division of Lung Diseases. A Certified Health Education Specialist, Dr. Wolle was previously chief of the Health Education Center, Maryland State Department of Health and Mental Hygiene.

The Handbook of Health Behavior Change

Sally A. Shumaker, Ph.D.
Eleanor B. Schron, R.N., M.S.
Judith K. Ockene, Ph.D.

Senior Editors

Christine T. Parker, Ph.D.
Jeffrey L. Probstfield, M.D.
Joan M. Wolle, Ph.D., M.P.H.

Co-Editors

SPRINGER PUBLISHING COMPANY
New York

Springer Publishing Company, Inc.
536 Broadway
New York, NY 10012

92 93 94 / 5 4 3 2

Library of Congress Cataloging-in-Publication Data

The Handbook of health behavior change / Sally A. Shumaker, Eleanor B.
  Schron, Judith K. Ockene, senior editors ; Christine T. Parker, Jeffrey L.
  Probstfield, Joan M. Wolle, co-editors.
      p.   cm.
  Includes bibliographical references.
  ISBN 0-8261-6780-2
  1. Health behavior. 2. Health attitudes. 3. Self-care, Health.
  4. Behavior modification. I. Shumaker, Sally A. II. Schron,
  Eleanor B. III. Ockene, Judith K.
  [DNLM: 1. Behavior Therapy. 2. Health Behavior. 3. Health
  Promotion. 4. Patient Compliance. WA 590 H2356]
  RA776.9.H36   1990
  613—dc 20
  DNLM/DLC
  for Library of Congress   89-26295
                                                               CIP

Printed in the United States of America

Contents

Contributors

David P. Agle, M.D.
Department of Psychiatry
Case Western Reserve University School of
    Medicine
Cleveland, OH

Louis M. Aledort, M.D.
Department of Medicine
Mount Sinai Medical Center
New York, NY

David G. Altman, Ph.D.
Stanford Center for Research in Disease
    Prevention
Stanford University School of Medicine
Palo Alto, CA

Catherine J. Atkins, Ph.D.
Center for Behavioral Medicine
San Diego State University
San Diego, CA

Andrew Baum, Ph.D.
Department of Medical Psychology
Uniformed Services University of the Health
    Sciences
Bethesda, MD

Marshall H. Becker, Ph.D., M.P.H.
School of Public Health
The University of Michigan
Ann Arbor, MI

Faye Z. Belgrave, Ph.D.
Department of Psychology
George Washington University
Washington, DC

Margaret A. Chesney, Ph.D.
Department of Epidemiology and Biostatistics
School of Medicine
University of California, San Francisco
San Francisco, CA

Noreen M. Clark, Ph.D.
Department of Health Education and Health
    Behavior
The University of Michigan
Ann Arbor, MI

Thomas J. Coates, Ph.D.
Division of General Internal Medicine,
    Department of Medicine
University of California, San Francisco
San Francisco, CA

Steven R. Cummings, M.D.
Division of General Internal Medicine,
    Department of Medicine
University of California, San Francisco
San Francisco, CA

Susan M. Czajkowski, Ph.D.
Behavioral Medicine Branch
National Heart, Lung, and Blood Institute
Bethesda, MD

C. Edward Davis, Ph.D.
Department of Biostatistics
School of Public Health
University of North Carolina
Chapel Hill, NC

M. Robin DiMatteo, Ph.D.
Department of Psychology
University of California, Riverside
Riverside, CA

Jacqueline Dunbar, Ph.D., R.N.
Departments of Nursing and Epidemiology
University of Pittsburgh
Pittsburgh, PA

David Evans, Ph.D.
Department of Pediatrics
Columbia University College of Physicians and
  Surgeons
New York, NY

Craig K. Ewart, Ph.D.
School of Hygiene and Public Health
The Johns Hopkins University
Baltimore, MD

Ruth R. Faden, Ph.D.
Department of Psychology, Faculty Arts and
  Sciences
The Johns Hopkins University
Baltimore, MD

Charles H. Feldman, M.D.
Department of Pediatrics
Columbia University College of Physicians and
  Surgeons
New York, NY

Michael J. Follick, Ph.D.
Institute for Behavioral Medicine
Providence, RI

Howard S. Friedman, Ph.D.
Department of Psychology
University of California, Riverside
Riverside, CA

William H. George, Ph.D.
Department of Psychology
State University of New York, Buffalo
Buffalo, NY

Barbara Gerbert, Ph.D.
Department of Dental Public Health and
  Hygiene, School of Dentistry
University of California, San Francisco
San Francisco, CA

Michael G. Goldstein, M.D.
Department of Psychiatry
The Miriam Hospital
Providence, RI

Dwight L. Goodwin, Ph.D.
Department of Psychology
San Jose State University
San Jose, California

Larry Gorkin, Ph.D.
Clinical Trials Applications
Institute for Behavioral Medicine
Providence, RI

Lawrence W. Green, Dr.P.H.
Health Promotion Program
Henry T. Kaiser Family Foundation
Menlo Park, CA

Merwyn R. Greenlick, Ph.D.
Center for Health Research
Kaiser Permanente
Portland, OR

Neil E. Grunberg, Ph.D.
Department of Medical Psychology
Uniformed Services University of the Health
  Sciences
Bethesda, MD

Donald B. Hunninghake, M.D.
Departments of Medicine and Pharmacology
University of Minnesota
Minneapolis, MI

William Insull, M.D.
Department of Medicine
Baylor College of Medicine
Houston, TX

Jeffrey V. Johnson, Ph.D.
Divisions of Occupational Health and
  Behavioral Sciences
School of Public Health
The Johns Hopkins University
Baltimore, MD

Robert M. Kaplan, Ph.D.
Division of Health Care Sciences
School of Medicine
University of California, San Diego
San Diego, CA

Robert H. Knopp, M.D.
Department of Medicine
University of Washington School of Medicine
Seattle, WA

R. Craig Lefebvre
Pawtucket Heart Health Program
Brown University Program in Medicine
Providence, RI

Judith R. Levi, ACSW
Department of Social Work Services
Mount Sinai Medical Center
New York, NY

Bruce Levin, Ph.D.
Division of Biostatistics
Columbia University School of Public Health
New York, NY

Moshe J. Levison, Ph.D.
Department of Pediatrics
Columbia University College of Physicians and
  Surgeons
New York, NY

Diana Lord
Department of Medical Psychology
Uniformed Services University of the Health
  Sciences
Bethesda, MD

G. Alan Marlatt, Ph.D.
Department of Psychology
University of Washington
Seattle, WA

Barbara S. McCann, Ph.D.
Northwest Lipid Research Clinic and
  Department of Psychiatry and Behavioral
  Sciences
University of Washington School of Medicine
Seattle, WA

Robert B. Mellins, M.D.
Department of Pediatrics
Columbia University College of Physicians and
  Surgeons
New York, NY

Deborah Lewis, M.S.W., Ph.D.
Department of Psychology
National Rehabilitation Hospital
Washington, DC

Patricia D. Mullen, Dr.P.H.
School of Public Health and Department of
  Family Practice and Community Medicine
University of Texas Health Science Center
Houston, TX

Judith K. Ockene, Ph.D.
Division of Preventive and Behavioral
  Medicine
University of Massachusetts Medical Center
Worcester, MA

Christine T. Parker, Ph.D.
National Institute of Mental Health
Rockville, MD

Jeffrey L. Probstfield, M.D.
Clinical Trials Branch
Division of Epidemiology and Clinical
  Applications
National Heart, Lung and Blood Institute
Bethesda, MD

Cynthia S. Rand, Ph.D.
Lung Health Study
Francis Scott Key Medical Center
Johns Hopkins School of Medicine
Baltimore, MD

Barbara M. Retzlaff, R.D., M.S., Ph.D.
Department of Medicine
Northwest Lipid Research Clinic
University of Washington School of Medicine
Seattle, WA

Robert R. Richard, M.A.
Division of General Internal Medicine,
  Department of Medicine
University of California, San Francisco
San Francisco, CA

Andrew L. Ries, M.D.
Division of Pulmonary and Critical Care
  Medicine
Northwest Lipid Research Clinic and
  Department of Medicine
University of California, San Diego
San Diego, CA

Irwin M. Rosenstock, Ph.D.
Center for Health Behavior Studies
California State University, Long Beach
Long Beach, CA

Harold P. Roth, M.D.
Epidemiology and Data Systems Program
National Institute of Diabetes and Digestive
  and Kidney Diseases
Bethesda, MD

Michael L. Russell, Ph.D.
Deceased

Eleanor B. Schron, R.N., M.S.
Clinical Trials Branch
Division of Epidemiology and Clinical
  Applications
National Heart, Lung, and Blood Institute
Bethesda, MD

Beth Schucker, M.A.
Lipid Metabolism- Atherogenesis Branch
National Heart, Lung, and Blood Institute
Bethesda, MD

Roland B. Scott, M.D.
Center for Sickle Cell Disease
Howard University
Washington, DC

Roger Secker-Walker, M.D.
Department of Medicine
University of Vermont
Burlington, VT

Sally A. Shumaker, Ph.D.
Behavioral Medicine Branch
Division of Epidemiology and Clinical
    Applications
National Heart, Lung, and Blood Institute
Bethesda, MD

Robert Simon, M.D.
RR 1 Box 405-C
Norwich, CT

Michelle Toshima
SDSU/UCSD Doctoral Program in Clinical
    Psychology
San Diego State University and University of
    California, San Diego
San Diego, CA

Rachel Vander Martin, M.S.
Division of General Internal Medicine,
    Department of Medicine
University of California, San Francisco
San Francisco, CA

Carolyn E. Walden, M.S.
Northwest Lipid Research Clinic
Department of Medicine
University of Washington School of Medicine
Seattle, WA

Graham W. Ward, M.P.H.
Cardiovascular Institute
Boston University School of Medicine
Boston, MA

Yvonne Wasilewski, Ph.D.
Department of Pediatrics
Columbia University College of Physicians and
    Surgeons
New York, NY

Howard Weiss, Ph.D.
Ackerman Institute for Family Therapy
New York, NY

Joan M. Wolle, Ph.D., M.P.H.
Prevention, Education, and Research Training
    Branch
Division of Lung Diseases
Bethesda, MD

Salim Yusuf, M.B., D. Phil., MRCP
Clinical Trials Branch
Division of Epidemiology and Clinical
    Applications
National Heart, Lung, and Blood Institute
Bethesda, MD

Barry J. Zimmerman, Ph.D.
Department of Educational Psychology
City University of New York
New York, NY

The Adoption and Maintenance of Behaviors for Optimal Health: An Introduction

Judith K. Ockene, Sally A. Shumaker, Eleanor B. Schron

There has been a growing recognition in medicine and public health that many acute and chronic diseases of the heart, lungs, and blood can be prevented or at least have their impact lessened by increased attention to the adoption and maintenance of behaviors for optimal health. This recognition grows out of the many epidemiologic investigations that demonstrate the existence of a strong relationship among the onset, progression, and exacerbation of disease and alterable life-styles such as stopping smoking, changing diets, taking medications, or practicing safe sex. There is also an increasing awareness that for the adoption and maintenance of behaviors for optimal health to take place there are not only demands and responsibilities placed on the individual at risk; there are also demands placed on the health care system and its providers; on other channels within the community such as schools, worksites, and churches; and on the social and political context in which change occurs. This book represents a detailed review of the theoretical and empirical literature on the factors that influence the adoption of healthy behaviors, and the individual, interpersonal, social, and cultural factors that can inhibit or promote behavior change.

Chapters in the first section of the book review past and current models in behavior change and relapse prevention and the maintenance of new behaviors, and a recent model of adherence behaviors is described. A detailed discussion of research on the importance of the health provider and patient relationship is addressed, and finally, methodological problems and measurement issues in the area of adherence behaviors are described.

The chapters in Section Two focus on a broad range of life-style interventions among diverse patient populations. The chapter authors discuss health behaviors relevant to HIV-positive hemophiliac patients, patients with chronic obstructive pulmonary disease, asthmatic children, and heart patients. Methods for developing health behaviors and obstacles to behavior change are considered for each of these populations.

In Section Three the authors focus on factors that can inhibit people's ability to change their behaviors and maintain a healthier behavior pattern. Biologically based, health-provider-based, and contextually based obstacles to the successful adoption of health behaviors are considered.

The chapters in Section Four of the book consider the unique issues associated with maintained behavior change within specific populations. Adherence among minority groups, young people, and the elderly is considered.

Medical regimen adherence is a major problem in clinical research, and in Section Five the authors provide a detailed discussion of the relevant issues. Recruitment, precompliance screening, postrandomization predictors of adherence, adherence enhancement strategies, and dropout recovery methods are considered and provide a thorough examination of adherence throughout the clinical trial process.

The final section of the book places the issue of health behavior change in a broader context. The first chapter addresses the subtle interaction between placebo effects and adherence and the implications of this interaction for any behavior change believed by an individual to be health-enhancing. In the second chapter the issue of personal responsibility of self-care is contrasted with the role of the public policy domain in health promotion: the rights of the individual versus the social good. In the last chapter the ethics of interventions and behavior change are discussed. Careful consideration is given to the thin line between adherence and coercion and fully and inadequately informed consent.

In total, this book represents the first thorough examination of the factors that influence people's choices to change their behaviors in order to enhance their health, and the intrapersonal, interpersonal, and sociocultural factors that can both positively and negatively affect the choices made and one's ability to achieve a desired behavior. The content of this book will be informative to clinical investigators, behavioral and social scientists, and practitioners who grapple with the issues confronting individuals who must make well-informed decisions regarding their health-related behaviors and change many difficult health habits and adopt new behaviors.

SECTION I

Behavior Change and Maintenance: Theory and Measurement

Judith K. Ockene, Editor

Even the most cynical health practitioner has a theory of behavior change; so has the rankest empiricist. The cynic views patients or clients as perverse; the empiricist views them as unpredictable. These theories—or antitheories—are no less influential on the behavior of those who believe them than the more reasoned and formally tested theories of behavioral scientists. The point is that everyone has a theory guiding his or her repetitious behavior. When found consistently in professional practitioners, we usually refer to the theories as principles and standards. When found or suspected in patients and clients, the theories guiding their behavior are referred to variously as beliefs, attitudes, values, predispositions, expected rewards, prejudices, self-efficacy, self-attribution, and other such terms proposed in the chapters to follow.

Measurement is what distinguishes the formal from the more informal and often unconscious theories on which people base most of their decisions and actions. Measurement distinguishes the generalizable theories about personal theories from the personal theories themselves. Our task in this section is to separate the measurable and tested theories from the ephemeral and untested— the concrete from the fluff.

We must be cautious, however, in accepting measurability as the sole criterion of a useful theory. Kurt Lewin's theory that there is nothing so practical as a good theory has served us well, but it has never been measured or systematically tested, as far as I know. The problem with measurement and controlled experimental testing of theories as criteria of their relative worth is that these criteria bias the selection toward the more simplistic or mechanistic slices of reality, the more concrete and observable variables, and the theories for which measurement instruments with known psychometric or sociometric properties are at hand. Reductionism becomes rampant; empiricism becomes empirical; technology becomes technocracy.

Rand states in the final sentence of this section, "No technology now or in the future will replace the good listening and sincere concern of a first-rate therapeutic relationship." Theory can guide what a therapist or other health professional listens for and how to interpret what he or she hears. But if the theory is limited in scope (as virtually any behavioral theory must be), then listening is limited in range. The health professional reading these chapters should seek to assimilate all the theories presented rather than to select a favorite. Each is an approximation of a different slice of reality, or a different perspective on the same slice.

What the health practitioner needs is not a single theory that would explain all that he or she hears, but rather a framework with meaningful hooks or rubrics on which to hang the new variables and insights offered by different theories. With this customized metatheory or framework, the practitioner can triage new ideas into categories that have personal utility in his or her practice. The framework should emerge inductively from personal experience in practice. Theories and their variables can then be attached to the practitioner's personal framework deductively by asking of each theory how it fits, what it adds, or what it explains among the cause–effect relationships one presumes to be operating in one's practice.

A health practitioner's personal theoretical framework should contain at a minimum: (1) the major categories of intervention he or she might use to influence health behavior, on one side; (2) intended health outcomes, on the opposite side; and somewhere close to these, (3) categories of behavior related to the intended health outcomes. The theories and variables discussed in the next few chapters can then be drawn upon to flesh out the space between the interventions and the categories of behavior.

Reviews of the theoretical literature such as these need not be approached as a contest between theories, but rather as a source of ideas and insights on some of the more generalizable causes of behavior. Such insights and ideas can guide the health practitioner in listening well, caring better, and in the end transferring insights to the patient to enable better self-care.

LAWRENCE W. GREEN

Theoretical Models of Adherence and Strategies for Improving Adherence

Marshall H. Becker

It is apparent that the ultimate success of efficacious preventive and curative regimens is usually dependent upon individuals' willingness to undertake and/or maintain the required behaviors. Unfortunately, data indicate that poor adherence to professional advice often occurs wherever some form of discretionary action or self-administration is involved. One reviewer (Podell, 1975) estimates that, on average, only one third of patients correctly follow physicians' directions. Sackett (1976) points out that scheduled appointments for treatment are missed 20 to 50% of the time; about 50% of patients do not take prescribed medications in accordance with instructions; and recommended changes in habitual behaviors are even less frequently adhered to (e.g., smoking cessation programs are considered to be unusually effective if more than one third of the entrants have reduced their smoking by the end of 6 months; dietary restrictions are often not observed; and large percentages drop out of weight-control programs).

Given the extensive documentation of suboptimal public participation in screening, immunization, and other preventive health efforts, as well as low levels of individual adherence to prescribed medical therapies (Becker & Maiman, 1975; Sackett & Snow, 1979), it is not surprising that behavioral scientists devote extensive conceptual and empirical effort toward the explanation and prediction of individuals' health-related decisions. This chapter reviews 10 of the major theoretical frameworks that have been advanced to elucidate the nonadherence phenomenon and subsequently identifies some of the major approaches and techniques that have been advanced to ameliorate the problem.

MODELS OF ADHERENCE

Individuals voluntarily elect to engage in health-directed activities for three major classes of reasons (Kasl & Cobb, 1966): (1) to prevent illness or to detect it at an asymptomatic stage ("health behavior"); (2) in the presence of symptoms, to obtain diagnosis and to discover suitable treatment ("illness behavior"); and (3) in the presence of defined illness, to undertake/receive treatment aimed at restoration of health or at halting disease progression ("sick-role behavior"). As will be apparent from later discussion, different investigators focus their models and studies upon different kinds of health-related behavior; however, they appear to contain similar classes of variables.

Family Use of Health Services

From a mainly sociological perspective, Andersen (1968) developed a behavioral model to identify determinants of family utilization of health services. In this framework, behavior is seen as dependent upon (1) the predisposition of the family to use services; (2) their ability to secure services; and (3) their need for such services. Each of the three components includes several dimensions or "subcomponents" that provide the theoretical and operational definitions of the model.

The "predisposing" component of the model includes family characteristics existing prior to the onset of illness that result in differences in propensity to use health services, including demographic variables (e.g., age, sex, marital status); social structure variables (e.g., education and occupation of the family head, ethnicity); and health beliefs and attitudes about medical care, physicians, and disease (including health-related anxiety and stress). These predisposing variables are not seen as directly responsible for use of health services but rather as determinants of variation in "inclination" toward use; thus, Andersen suggests that patterns of utilization are affected by individuals in various age groups having different types and amounts of illness, by families with different social-structural characteristics having different life-styles (in terms of physical and social environment and behavior patterns), and by variations of belief in the efficacy of medical care (i.e., families with relatively stronger beliefs in the efficacy of medical treatment might seek care sooner and use more services).

The second model component refers to conditions that permit the use of health services, or that make them available. Andersen (1968) notes that "even though families may be predisposed to use health services, some means must be available for them to do so" (p. 16). "Enabling" conditions include both family resources (e.g., family income and savings, health insurance or other source of third-party coverage, including use of welfare care, and whether or not the family has a regular source of care) and community resources (e.g., availability of health services and health personnel, travel times, waiting times).

When appropriate predisposing and enabling conditions are present, variations in perception of illness (or the probability of its occurrence) and the manner of response to illness (or potential illness) will determine the use of health services. The first subcomponent, perceived "need," is measured by (1) *subjective* perceptions of illness (including reported disability days, number of symptoms experienced, and self-reported general state of health) and (2) *clinical* evaluation of illness (usually based on the weighing of reported symptoms for probability of need for care by age group) (Andersen & Newman, 1973). Finally, reaction to illness is measured by the pattern of seeing a doctor for symptoms (on a continuum from "doctor not seen for any symptoms" to "doctor seen for all symptoms") and by receipt of regular physical examinations.

In specifying hypotheses generated by the model, Andersen (1968) states that "the amount of health services used by a family will be a function of the predisposing and enabling characteristics of the family and its need for medical care" (p. 19). The components of the model are hypothesized to contribute independently to the understanding of differential utilization of health services—and need, which represents factors most directly related to use, is expected to be more important than either predisposing or enabling components.

The model has been employed with varying degrees of explanatory success in several surveys of large national samples. In Andersen's (1968) original study, based on a 1964 national survey of 2,367 families, the model explains 43% of the variance in use of health services.

Subsequent trials of the model were conducted in two national studies of determinants of health behavior, fielded in 1971 (Andersen, Kravits, & Anderson, 1975) and in late 1975 through early 1976 (Andersen & Anderson, 1979). In the 1971 study of 3,880 families comprising 11,822 individuals, need variables were the most powerful predictors, accounting for 16% of the variance in physician contacts and 23% of the volume of physician visits. In the case of physician contacts, three indicators of perceptions of illness (disability days, number of symptoms experienced, and worry about health) accounted for 14% of the variance, and all but a negligible amount of the resulting variance in volume of physician visits was due to both perceptions of illness (9%) and clinical evaluation of illness (11%). The second survey, based on a probability sample of 7,787 individuals, substantiated the findings of the previous studies concerning relationships of the predictive components of the model to physician utilization: the 22% of the variance explained by the model resulted mainly from perceptions of illness, with self-reported general state of health and number of symptoms experienced yielding standardized partial regression coefficients of .19 and .32, respectively. A number of studies have focused on the influence of enabling and predisposing conditions, and the recent work of Dutton (1978) presents empirical evidence for remedying the various barriers and structural impediments of health care systems in addition to eliminating enabling constraints and inadequate levels of predispositions to use health services in order to improve utilization.

Health Belief Model

The Health Belief Model (HBM) was developed in the early 1950s by a group of social psychologists at the U.S. Public Health Service (Rosenstock, 1974) in an attempt to understand "the widespread failure of people to accept disease preventives or screening tests for the early detection of asymptomatic disease" (p. 328); it was later applied to patients' responses to symptoms (Kirscht, 1974) and to following prescribed medical regimens (Becker, 1974).

The basic components of the HBM are derived from a well-established body of psychological and behavioral theory whose various models hypothesize that behavior depends mainly upon two variables: (1) the value placed by an individual on a particular goal and (2) the individual's estimate of the likelihood that a given action will achieve that goal (Maiman & Becker, 1974). When these variables were conceptualized in the context of health-related behavior, the correspondences were: (1) the desire to avoid illness (or if ill, to get well) and (2) the belief that a specific health action will prevent (or ameliorate) illness (i.e., the individual's estimate of the threat of illness and of the likelihood of being able, through personal action, to reduce that threat).

Specifically, the HBM consists of the following dimensions (Figure 1.1):

Perceived Susceptibility

Individuals vary widely in their feeling of personal vulnerability to a condition (in the case of medically established illness, this dimension has been reformulated to include such questions as estimates of resusceptibility, belief in the diagnosis, and susceptibility to illness in general). Thus, this dimension refers to one's subjective perception of the risk of contracting a condition.

Perceived Severity

Feelings concerning the seriousness of contracting an illness (or of leaving it untreated) also vary from person to person. This dimension includes evaluations of both medical/clinical consequences (e.g., death, disability, and pain) and

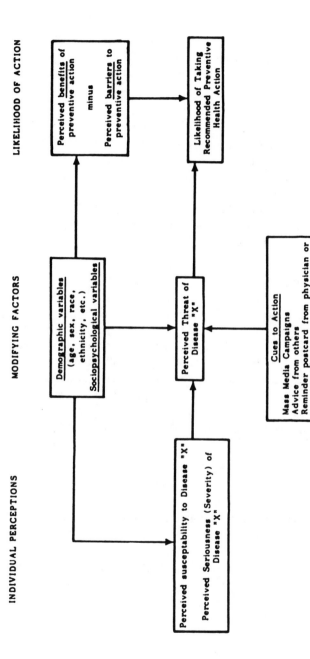

INDIVIDUAL PERCEPTIONS   MODIFYING FACTORS   LIKELIHOOD OF ACTION

Perceived benefits of preventive action

minus

Perceived barriers to preventive action

Likelihood of Taking Recommended Preventive Health Action

Demographic variables (age, sex, race, ethnicity, etc.) Sociopsychological variables

Perceived Threat of Disease "X"

Cues to Action

Mass Media Campaigns
Advice from others
Reminder postcard from physician or dentist
Illness of family member or friend
Newspaper or magazine article

Perceived susceptability to Disease "X"

Perceived Seriousness (Severity) of Disease "X"

FIGURE 1.1 The health belief model (M. H. Becker, R. H. Drachman, J. P. Kirsoht, 1974).

9

possible social consequences (e.g., effects of the conditions on work, family life, and social relations). While low perceptions of seriousness might provide insufficient motivation for behavior, very high perceived severity might inhibit action.

Perceived Benefits

While acceptance of personal susceptibility to a condition also believed to be serious was held to produce a force leading to behavior, it did not define the particular course of action that was likely to be taken; this was hypothesized to depend upon beliefs regarding the effectiveness of the various actions available in reducing the disease threat. Thus, a "sufficiently threatened" individual would not be expected to accept the recommended health action unless it was perceived as feasible and efficacious.

Perceived Barriers

The potential negative aspects of a particular health action may act as impediments to undertaking the recommended behavior. A kind of cost–benefit analysis is thought to occur wherein the individual weighs the action's effectiveness against perceptions that it may be expensive, dangerous (e.g., side effects, iatrogenic outcomes), unpleasant (e.g., painful, difficult, upsetting), inconvenient, time-consuming, and so forth. Thus, as Rosenstock (1974) notes, "the combined levels of susceptibility and severity provided the energy or force to act and the perception of benefits (less barriers) provided a preferred path of action" (p. 332).

Cues to Action

However, it was also felt that some stimulus was necessary to trigger the decision-making process. This so-called "cue to action" might be internal (i.e., symptoms) or external (e.g., mass media communications, interpersonal interactions, reminder postcards from health care providers). Unfortunately, few HBM studies have attempted to assess the contributions of "cues" to predicting health actions.

Other Variables

In the HBM context, it is understood that diverse demographic, personal, structural, and social factors are capable of influencing health behaviors. However, these variables are believed to work through their effects on the individual's health motivations and subjective perceptions rather than functioning as direct causes of health action (Becker et al., 1977).

Of all the existing models of health-related behaviors, the HBM has received the most extensive research attention, having been applied to a wide diversity of populations, settings, health conditions (acute and chronic), and recommended behaviors. A large body of evidence has accumulated in support of the HBM's ability to account for the undertaking of preventive health actions, seeking diagnoses, and following prescribed medical advice (i.e., adherence to regimens). A recent review (Janz & Becker, 1984) summarized findings from 46 HBM-related investigations (18 prospective, 28 retrospective). Twenty-four studies examined preventive health behaviors (PHB), 19 explored sick-role behaviors (SRB), and 3 addressed clinic utilization. A "significance ratio" was constructed that divides the number of positive, statistically significant findings for an HBM dimension by the total number of studies reporting significance levels for that dimension.

In the preponderance of cases, each HBM dimension was found to be significantly associated with the health-related behaviors under study; overall, the significance ratio orderings (in descending order) were: "barriers" (89%); "susceptibility" (81%); "benefits" (78%); and "severity" (65%). Findings from prospective studies were at least as favorable as those obtained from retrospective research. For PHB, "barriers" was most productive, but "susceptibility" was a close second. Only 50% of the PHB studies reporting significance levels for "severity" had obtained positive, significant results, suggesting that perceptions of seriousness may be a concept of relatively low relevance in the area of PHB but of greater salience to individuals with diagnosed illness (a notion supported by the finding of a significance ratio of 88% for "severity" in the case of SRB). The somewhat poorer results produced for SRB by "susceptibility" (77%) may be due to difficulties in operationalizing this dimension of the HBM for cases where an illness has already been diagnosed.

Despite the body of findings linking HBM dimensions to health actions, Janz and Becker (1984) note that the HBM is a *psychosocial* model; as such, it is limited to accounting for as much of the variance in individuals' health-related behaviors as can be explained by their attitudes and beliefs. It is clear that other forces influence health actions as well; for example: (1) some behaviors (e.g., cigarette smoking, tooth brushing) have a substantial habitual component obviating any ongoing psychosocial decision-making process; (2) many health-related behaviors are undertaken for what are ostensibly *non-health* reasons (e.g., dieting to appear more attractive; stopping smoking or jogging to attain social approval); and (3) where economic or environmental factors prevent the individual from undertaking a preferred course of action (e.g., a worker in a hazardous environment; a resident in a city with high levels of air pollution). Furthermore, the model is predicated on the premise that "health" is a highly valued concern or goal for most individuals, and also that "cues to action" are widely prevalent; where these conditions are not satisfied, the model is not likely to be useful in, or relevant to, explaining behavior.

Theory of Reasoned Action

In the approach taken by Ajzen and Fishbein (1980), *intention* to perform a behavior can be accounted for by a combination of attitudes about an action and perceptions of likely normative reactions to that action. More specifically, this Theory of Reasoned Action (Figure 1.2) focuses on the individual's attitude toward the behavior (i.e., the person's beliefs that the behavior leads to certain outcomes) and his or her evaluations of these outcomes and on the subjective norm (i.e., the person's beliefs that certain individuals or groups think he or she should or should not undertake the behavior weighted by the person's desire to comply with their wishes). As with the HBM, sociodemographic factors operate only through their influences on the determinants of behavioral intention. Intention will result in behavior if there is an opportunity to act. This model also emphasizes normative influences that might affect intention for *any* reason, health-related or otherwise, thus adding a strong cultural component to the prediction of behavior.

This model has been successfully applied in the areas of smoking (Jaccard, 1975) and intentions to engage in family planning (Fishbein & Jaccard, 1973)

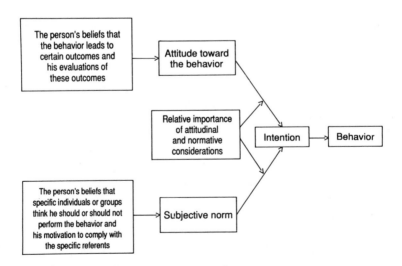

FIGURE 1.2 Theory of reasoned action (I. Ajzen, M. Fishbein).

and obtain Pap tests for cervical cancer (Seibold & Roper, 1979). However, much of this research used college students as subjects, and it would be useful to attempt replication of these studies with other adult populations.

Theory of Planning Behavior

The Theory of Planned Behavior is an extension of Ajzen and Fishbein's Theory of Reasoned Action and is appropriate for both volitional and nonvolitional behaviors. Here, performance of a behavior is a function of the strength of a person's attempt to perform a behavior and the degree of control the person has over that behavior. Control includes both personal and external factors that influence the behavior, such as having a workable plan, skills, knowledge, time, money, willpower, opportunity, etc. (Figure 1.3). The harder the person tries, and the greater his or her control over personal and external factors that may interfere with the behavior, the greater the likelihood that the behavior will be performed (Ajzen, 1985).

Intention to try to perform the behavior is the immediate determinant of an attempt to perform the behavior. In the strictest sense, then, intentions can be used only to predict a person's *attempt* to perform a behavior and not the *actual* performance of the behavior. When intentions fail to predict attempts, it may be due to a change in intention after it was measured. When intentions predict attempts but fail to predict actual performance, it may be due to factors beyond the individual's control that interfered with the completion of intentions.

Intention is seen as a function of an individual's attitude toward trying and his or her subjective norm with regard to trying. Consistent with the Theory of Reasoned Action, the relative influence of attitude and subjective norm on intention is dependent on the behavioral goal. For some behaviors, the attitudinal component will be the major determinant of intention, while for others the importance of social pressure will be the primary influence. In general, the more favorable an individual's attitude toward attempting a behavior, and the more he or she believes that significant others are in favor of his or her trying, the stronger will be his or her intention to try.

The Theory of Planned Behavior goes beyond the Theory of Reasoned Action in identifying determinants of attitude toward trying to perform a behavior. If failure to perform a behavior is a possibility, attitude toward trying will be determined both by attitude toward successful performance of the behavior as well as the individual's attitude toward a failed attempt at performance. The person's overall attitude toward trying a behavior is weighted by the person's subjective estimate of the likelihood of success or failure of performance and depends on the behavioral goal. Subjective estimate of likelihood of success or failure is a function of beliefs about the presence or absence of personal and external factors that may facilitate or inhibit performance. Attitudes toward trying

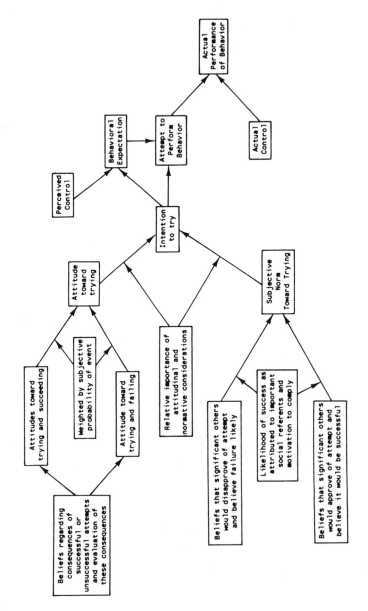

FIGURE 1.3   Theory of planned behavior (I. Ajzen).

14

and succeeding or failing are a function of the individual's beliefs about the consequences of successful or unsuccessful attempts and his or her evaluation of these consequences.

Subjective norm, the second major determinant of intention to try, is defined as the person's beliefs regarding what significant others think he or she should or should not do. Subjective norm concerning a behavioral goal is viewed as a recommendation by significant others that is based on their approval of the behavior and their belief that the attempt is likely to succeed. Here, too, the relative importance of approval or disapproval of social referents is dependent on the behavioral goal, the specific referent, and the individual's motivation to comply with this referent.

Other attempts to expand the Theory of Reasoned Action are incorporated in Ajzen's present description of the Theory of Planned Behavior (these are included in Figure 1.3). The author stresses the distinction between intention to try and what an individual really expects to do ("behavioral expectations"). According to Ajzen (1985), behavioral expectation is seen as a "person's estimate of the likelihood that he actually will perform a certain behavior" (p. 33). Behavioral expectation is viewed as a function of intention to try and the individual's belief in his or her ability to control a behavior. Factors influential in perception of behavioral control include past experience, confidence in subjective judgement of control, availability of a detailed plan of action, and general self-knowledge. Ajzen states that behavioral expectation and intention will differ whenever subjects suspect their intentions might change or when they believe that performance of a behavior is not totally under their control.

In summary, the Theory of Planned Behavior states that variables important in determining an attempt to perform a behavior "include beliefs about the likely consequences of success and failure, the perceived probabilities of success and failure, normative beliefs regarding important referents, and motivation to comply with these referents" (p. 36). In general, individuals will try to perform a behavior if they believe that the benefits of success are outweighed by the benefits of failure, and if they feel that significant others (with whom they want to comply) believe they should attempt to perform the behavior. Successful performance of the behavior will be the end result if individuals have sufficient control over internal and external factors that influence such performance.

The Theory of Reasoned Action is described as a "special case" of the Theory of Planned Behavior. "The two theories are identical when the subjective probability of success and the degree of control over internal and external factors reach their maximal values" (p. 36). When this occurs, the behavior is purely volitional and the Theory of Reasoned Action can be applied. The Theory of Planned Behavior is more appropriate when the probability of success and actual control over performance of a behavior are less than perfect.

Schifter and Ajzen (1985) tested a simplified model of the Theory of Planned Behavior using 83 college females who stated an intention to lose weight over a 6-week period. In this study, intention to lose weight was viewed as determined by three conceptually independent variables: attitude toward losing weight (favorable and unfavorable evaluation of the goal); subjective norm (perceived social pressure to lose or not lose weight); and perceived control over body weight. Perceived control was defined as referring to perceived ease or difficulty in losing weight and was assumed to reflect past experience as well as other obstacles. Intention was described as one immediate determinant of actual weight loss. Nonmotivational factors (such as time, money, willpower, skills, etc.) were also seen as influencing performance of behavior. Schifter and Ajzen state that "to the extent that a person has the required opportunities and resources, and intends to lose weight, he or she should succeed in doing so" (p. 844). Results of the study were reported as supporting the Theory of Planned Behavior.

Health Decision Model

Proposed as "a third generation model of patient behavior that focuses more specifically on health decisions" (Eraker, Kirscht, & Becker, 1984, p. 260), the Health Decision Model (Figure 1.4) attempts to combine decision analysis, behavioral decision theory, and health beliefs to yield a unifying model of health decisions and resultant behavior. The model includes recent contributions from the "patient preferences" literature (Eraker & Politser, 1982). Decision analysis provides a quantitative means for patients to express their preferences about critical trade-offs between benefits and risk—and at times, between quantity and quality of life (McNeil, Keeler, & Adelstein, 1975; Weinstein & Fineberg, 1980). Behavioral decision theory extends this quantitative emphasis by identifying a number of general inferential rules that patients use to reduce difficult mental tasks to simpler ones (Eraker & Sox, Jr., 1981; Tversky & Kahneman, 1974).

The relationships among health beliefs, decision analysis, and behavioral decision theory were demonstrated in a recent study on patient preferences of variations in the way information is presented to patients. McNeil, Pauker, Sox, Jr., and Tversky (1982) examined the results of surgery and radiation treatment for lung cancer and found that preferences for alternative therapies shifted when the outcomes were framed in terms of probability of living or the probability of dying. The investigators also found that people relied more on preexisting beliefs regarding the treatments than on statistical data presented to them. These preexisting beliefs may help to explain why some patients, based on decision–analysis criteria, are treated in a manner not reflecting their underlying preferences.

The Health Decision Model also recognizes the importance of other factors affecting health decisions and behavior, such as knowledge, experience, and social and demographic variables. The bidirectional arrows and feedback loops

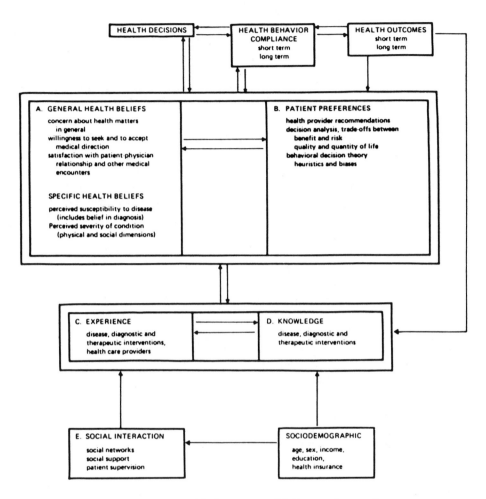

FIGURE 1.4   Health decision model (S. A. Eraker et al).

reflect the notion that adherence behavior can change health beliefs. The model also includes concepts related to the efficacy of the prescribed regimen, motivational variables involving the person's assessment of the importance of good health, and "cues to action" that refer specifically to the patient-physician interaction (Eraker, Becker, Strecher, & Kirscht, 1985).

Model of Illness Behavior

A decision-theoretic, anthropological approach to understanding illness behavior, which focuses on "the information that a person might be expected to process during an occurrence of illness," provides the framework for Fabrega's (1973, p. 473) model. ("Illness" refers to the *culturally* defined state that forms the basis of decisions about medical treatment; thus, the model has cross-cultural application.) This model tries to order and categorize the stages an individual passes through in recognizing and responding to illness by concentrating on (1) the information to be evaluated and acted upon; (2) the time ordering of events in the decision process; and (3) reducing variation in processes and events of the health illness–medical treatment cycle by providing constant and repetitive structure for channeling and processing medically relevant information.

Fabrega (1973) posits that the individual has four systems that provide "coding units . . . [or] norms or experienced levels of variations" (p. 473), which permit continuous monitoring of health-related happenings and processes. Put another way, the four systems are involved in information processing: coding, classifying, and ordering events related to symptoms and to feelings of illness. The systems are both open and interjoined, each contributing to illness behavior: (1) the *biological system*, which focuses on chemical and physiologic processes; (2) the *social system*, which executes relationships with other individuals, groups, and institutions; (3) the *phenomenologic system*, which is concerned with the individual's state of awareness and self-definition; and (4) the *memory system*, which includes earlier illness occurrences and accompanying medical attitudes and beliefs and which serves as a continual influence on the other three systems.

The model provides an abstract definition of illness behavior outlined in nine stages describing the sequence of decisions people make during illness (Figure 1.5). The first two stages reflect the individual's recognition and evaluation of symptoms. During the initial stage, "illness recognition and labeling," internal cues (biological system conjoined with phenomenological system) or external cues (appraisal of others, i.e., social system) lead the individual to realize the presence of illness and/or deviant changes and to undertake action to alleviate the perceived changes. (Recognition of illness is a subjective judgment rather than the result of objective medical diagnosis.) Illnesses are subjected to an evaluation cycle that produces constant monitoring and relabeling and that incorporates memories of past experiences with similar disease occurrences (e.g., a condition originally defined as a headache will be relabeled with the appearance of additional symptoms such as fatigue or nausea).

At the second stage of the decision-making trajectory, the negative components of the illness are evaluated on the bases of present situation and past experiences (personal, or those of others in the individual's social group). This assessment of the problem attaches an "illness disvalue" to the condition, which reflects the danger, disability, discomfort, social stigma, and sociopsychological disruption associated with the illness.

At the third stage, the individual considers a variety of mutually exclusive "treatment plans" that might be implemented; these actions, which are learned

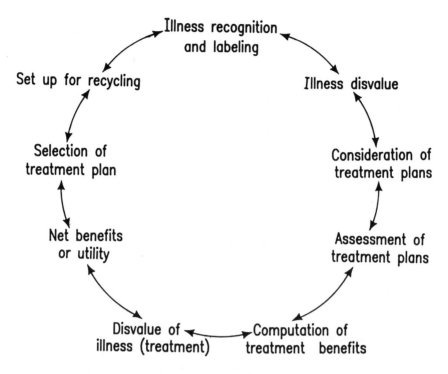

FIGURE 1.5 Model to explain illness behavior (H. Fabrega).

and evolve from the individual's prior experience with illness, include options
ranging from self-care (e.g., use of home remedies and patent medicines or
modification of dietary intake) to consulting the referral system (i.e., advice of
significant others) to obtaining formal medical care.

In stages four through seven, the individual undertakes a series of comparisons concerning alternative treatment plans: (1) "assessment of treatment plans"
(the estimation of the probability that each alternative action will reduce the
"disvalue" or threat of the illness); (2) computation of "treatment benefits" (the
amount of illness reduction that might potentially be derived from each treatment
plan); (3) computation of "disvalues of illness" (the costs, both personal and
economic, of undertaking each action); and (4) determination of the utility of
each alternative treatment plan by subtracting treatment costs from treatment
benefits, thus obtaining a "net benefits or utility" for each plan. Information from
the preceding comparisons leads to the eighth stage, "selection of treatment
plan." In choosing the treatment plan to be implemented, the individual applies
personal decision rules (e.g., to select the plan that is least costly, that has the
highest net utility, etc.).

At the final (ninth) stage, new information resulting from the outcome of the treatment plan selected in stage eight provides an updated history for the individual, which is learned and stored in the memory system. Thus, at stage nine, the individual is defined as "set up for recycling," which entails an evaluation of the illness in terms of both the treatment plan selected and the remaining manifestations. If, after a suitable lapse of time, the illness is relabeled, or if there is onset of new disease, the initial stage of the sequence is reentered.

In order for this model of illness behavior to operate, Fabrega specifies three assumptions. First, illness must be recognized as undesirable; that is, the model is not applicable to individuals who favor or who deny disease states and thus would not be motivated to undertake remedial action. Second, illness must be perceived as a discrete occurrence rather than an undifferentiated and constant state managed by habitual behaviors (which do not require decisions of illness definition and treatment selection). Finally, individuals must make their illness decisions based on rational evaluations of optimal treatment actions (rather than on random or irrational bases).

In summary, Fabrega (1974) has developed a behavioral framework to study how social and cultural behavior influences the individual's processing of information about illness and decisions about medical treatment; he suggests that the model be used in cross-cultural comparisons of the disvalues or costs of illness. Although difficulties in operationalizing the variables contained in the model are acknowledged, it is proposed that it be used as a rubric for empirical studies that would yield an "estimate" of the key variables. This approach to studying illness episodes was employed in a longitudinal study of a panel of families ($N = 174$) living in San Cristobal de las Casas, Mexico (Fabrega 1977; Fabrega & Zucker, 1977). Interviews with female heads of household (five contacts during a 1-year period) focused on actual occurrences of illness. Comparisons of two very distinct social–ethnic groups revealed important differences in perceived symptom and illness levels, as well as in the ultimate medical actions taken. However, the disparity between the illness indicators employed in the study (subjective reports of the frequency and duration of illness, and perceptions of frequency of physiological symptoms and amount of interference with work) and Fabrega's theoretical formulation illustrates the difficulties involved in assessing the elements of the nine stages of the model.

Self-Regulation Model

Leventhal and his colleagues (1980) view self-regulation as a solution to dealing with the basic problem of locus of control in adherence theory. The fundamental notion is that

the individual functions as a feedback system. He or she establishes behavioral goals, generates plans and responses to reach these goals, and establishes criteria for monitoring the effects of his/her responses on movement toward or away from the goal. This information is then used to alter coping techniques, set new criteria for evaluating response outputs, and revise goals. The individual is, therefore, an information processing system that regulates his/her relationship to the environment. (p. 34)

The analogy provided is one of the person as scientist—formulating hypotheses about physiology and the effects of illness and creating a mental picture of ability to take actions to prevent or cure illness.

The self-regulation model (Figure 1.6) contains components that depict a process not unlike Fabrega's approach: (1) extracting information from the environment; (2) generating a representation of the illness danger to oneself; and (3) planning and acting, which involves imagining response alternatives to deal with the problem and emotions it generates, then taking selected actions to achieve specific effects. Here the feedback loop is achieved by the last step: (4) monitoring or appraising how one's coping reactions affected the environmental problem and oneself. "Each component is a set of processes, each operates within its own set of rules, each has its own potentials" (p. 35).

Fundamental to component 3 above are the notions of self-effectance and learned helplessness, and Leventhal, Meyer, and Gutmann (1980) review the social learning theory literature (to be discussed in greater detail below) in support of the importance of these concepts in the overall scheme of coping responses; however, the authors note a paucity of research concerning how illness representations are created and on the manner by which such representations might influence coping strategies and evaluations of outcomes that lead to self-effectance or learned helplessness.

The self-regulation model, *qua* model, does not appear to have been employed in empirical investigation at this point. However, it does seem clear that patients' adherence to a regimen is likely to be influenced by their perceptions and evaluations of the presence or absence of symptoms. Also, this model relies to a fair degree on Bandura's formulations regarding reciprocal determinism and self-regulation, and both this work and Bandura's Social Learning Theory arise from a common theoretical heritage that strongly suggests the importance of this approach to understanding adherence behaviors.

Social Learning Theory

Bandura's (1977b) Social Learning Theory, which claims at least part of its ancestry in behaviorism, attempts to explain and predict behavior using several key concepts: incentives, outcome expectations, and efficacy expectations. Bandura (1977a) outlines the roles of these concepts in the paradigm of a person engaging in a behavior that will have a consequent outcome; here, behavior

Extracting information from the environment

Generating a representation of the illness danger to oneself

Planning and acting (including imagining response alternatives to deal with the problem and the emotions it generates, then taking actions to achieve specific effects)

Monitoring or appraising how one's coping reactions affected the environmental problem and oneself.

FIGURE 1.6 Self-regulation model (H. Leventhal, D. Meyer, M. Gutmann).

change and maintenance are a function of (1) expectations about the outcomes that will result from engaging in a behavior and (2) expectations about one's ability to engage in or execute the behavior. Thus, "outcome expectations" consist of beliefs about whether a given behavior will lead to given outcomes, whereas "efficacy expectations" consist of beliefs about how *capable* one is of performing the behavior that leads to those outcomes. It should be emphasized that both outcome and efficacy expectations reflect a person's *beliefs* about capabilities and behavior–outcome links. Thus it is these perceptions, and not necessarily "true" capabilities, that influence behavior. In addition, it is important to understand that the concept of self-efficacy relates to beliefs about capabilities of performing *specific* behaviors in *particular* situations (Schunk & Carbonari, 1984); self-efficacy does not refer to a personality characteristic or to a global trait that operates independently of contextual factors (Bandura, 1977a). This means that an individual's efficacy expectations will vary greatly depending on the particular task and context that confronts him/her. It is therefore inappropriate to characterize a person as having "high" or "low" self-efficacy without reference to the specific behavior and circumstance with which the efficacy judgment is associated.

Bandura argues that perceived self-efficacy influences all aspects of behavior, including the acquisition of new behaviors (e.g., a sexually active young adult learning how to use a particular contraceptive device), inhibition of existing behaviors (e.g., decreasing or stopping cigarette smoking), and disinhibition of behaviors (e.g., resuming sexual activity after a myocardial infarction). Self-efficacy also affects people's choices of behavioral settings, the amount of effort they will expend on a task, and the length of time they will persist in the face of obstacles. Finally, self-efficacy affects people's emotional reactions, such as anxiety and distress and thought patterns. Thus, individuals with low self-efficacy about a particular task may ruminate about their personal deficiencies rather than thinking about accomplishing or attending to the task at hand; this, in turn, impedes successful performance of the task.

According to Bandura, efficacy expectations vary along dimensions of magnitude, strength, and generality. Each of these dimensions has important implications for performance, and each implies slightly different measurement procedures. "Magnitude" refers to the ordering of tasks by difficulty level. Persons having low-magnitude expectations feel capable of performing only the simpler of a graded series of tasks, while those with high-magnitude expectations feel capable of performing even the most difficult tasks in the series. "Strength" refers to a probabilistic judgment of how certain one is of one's ability to perform a specific task (Bandura, 1984). "Generality" concerns the extent to which efficacy expectations about a particular situation or experience generalize to other situations. For example, the beliefs of post-myocardial infarction patients about their endurance capabilities generated during supervised exercise testing may or may not generalize to unsupervised exercising at home.

Efficacy expectations are learned from four major sources (Bandura, 1977a, b). The first, termed "performance accomplishments," refers to learning through personal experience where one achieves mastery over a difficult or previously feared task and thereby enjoys an increase in self-efficacy. Performance accomplishments attained through personal experience are the most potent source of efficacy expectations. Successive mastery over tasks required to engage in a behavior helps the person to develop and refine skills. In addition, it fosters development of a repertoire of coping mechanisms to deal with problems encountered.

The second source is "vicarious experience," which includes learning that occurs through observation of events and/or other people. These events/people are referred to as "models" when they display a set of behaviors or stimulus array that illustrates a certain principle, rule, or response. For example, a man who feels vulnerable to a heart attack may fear the consequences of exercising after watching a television drama in which a male character has a myocardial infarction following exercise; a woman who hopes to quit smoking but observes a friend's difficulty in abstaining from cigarettes may come to believe that she herself will never be able to quit. On the other hand, observing a model master situations that have been feared or seen as difficult can enhance one's own expectations of mastery. In order for modeling to affect an observer's self-efficacy positively, however, it is important that the model can be viewed as overcoming difficulties through determined effort rather than with ease, and that the model be similar to the observer with regard to other characteristics (e.g., age, sex). Additionally, modeled behaviors presented with clear rewarding outcomes are more effective than modeling with unclear or unrewarded outcomes.

"Verbal persuasion" constitutes the third source of efficacy expectations. This method is quite familiar to all health workers who have exhorted patients to persevere in their efforts to change behavior.

Finally, one's "physiological state" provides information that can influence efficacy expectations. Bandura has noted that because high physiological arousal usually impairs performance, people are more likely to expect failure when they are very tense and viscerally agitated. For example, people who experience extremely sweaty palms, a racing heartbeat, and trembling knees prior to giving a talk find that their self-efficacy plummets; to someone just beginning an exercise program, fatigue and mild aches and pains may be mistakenly interpreted as a sign of physical inefficacy.

While this presentation of Social Learning Theory emphasizes cognitive-perceptual dimensions, it should be noted that Bandura (1977b) recognized the influence of environmental forces. Although the cognitive–motivational aspects of the theory have recently received the most attention, situational determinants are essential to the theory as well. It is important to distinguish self-efficacy from a number of other concepts with which it is sometimes linked and frequently confused. This confusion occurs in part because the personality traits, states, and processes that these concepts represent can influence efficacy expectations or be influenced by them. However, this does not mean that any of these concepts are equivalent to self-efficacy.

"Health locus of control" refers to a generalized expectation about whether one's health is controlled by one's own behavior or by forces external to oneself (Wallston & Wallston, 1984). Health is an outcome, while self-efficacy focuses on beliefs about the capacity to undertake behavior(s) that may not lead to desired outcomes (such as health). Bandura (1977a) illustrates the importance of the distinction between locus of control and self-efficacy by noting that the conviction that outcomes (e.g., good health) are determined by one's own action can have any number of effects on self-efficacy and behavior. For example, people who view their health as personally determined but who believe they lack the skills needed to carry out the behaviors that would result in good health would experience low self-efficacy and approach those activities with a sense of futility.

"Self-esteem" refers to liking and respect for oneself that has some realistic basis (Crandall, 1978). Thus self-esteem is concerned with an evaluation of self-worth, while self-efficacy relates to an evaluation of specific capabilities in specific situations. Bandura (1984) highlights the distinction between the two concepts by pointing out that people can have high self-efficacy for a task from which they derive no self-pride (e.g., being able to brush one's teeth well) or have low self-efficacy for a task but have no loss of self-worth (e.g., not being able to ride a unicycle). However, he observes that people often try to develop self-efficacy in activities that give them a sense of self-worth, so that the two concepts are frequently intertwined.

"Coping," according to Lazarus and Folkman's (1984) conceptualization, is viewed as a process; like Bandura, they downplay notions of coping that emphasize generalized dispositional concepts such as self-esteem. "Secondary appraisal" is defined as an individual's evaluation of what might and can be done in the face of a threat or challenge. During this complex process, a person takes into account (either consciously or unconsciously) (1) which coping strategies are available; (2) the likelihood that some strategy will accomplish the expected outcome; and (3) whether one can apply that strategy or strategies effectively. Clearly the second part of this process is similar to the notion of outcome expectation, while the third is equivalent to self-efficacy. Thus, within Lazarus and Folkman's framework, efficacy expectations are part of secondary appraisal.

"Learned helplessness" refers to cognitive, affective, and motivational deficits that result from exposure to uncontrollable events. The attributional reformulation of learned helplessness suggests that there are two types of helplessness: personal and universal. Personal helplessness occurs when an individual lacks the requisite controlling response in a situation but believes this response is available to others; that is, the individual believes that although he or she cannot control the outcome, others in the same situation could. In the case of universal helplessness, the individual still lacks the requisite response but believes that the outcome is independent of any response he or she or others could make. Abramson, Garber, and Seligman (1980) view this distinction between personal and universal helplessness as consistent with Bandura's distinction between efficacy and outcome expectancies. Low efficacy and high outcome expectations characterize universal helplessness.

A recent review of empirical literature (Strecher, DeVellis, Becker, & Rosenstock, 1986) focused on the self-efficacy concept as it relates to cigarette smoking cessation, weight control, contraception, alcohol abuse, and exercise. The studies examined suggest strong relationships between self-efficacy and health behavior change and maintenance. Furthermore, experimental manipulations of self-efficacy indicate that efficacy expectations can be enhanced and that this enhancement is related to subsequent changes in health practices.

Relapse Prevention

The concept of self-efficacy is a critical component in the cognitive–behavioral model of the relapse process formulated by Marlatt (1982). The relapse-prevention approach has as its goal the education of persons who are attempting to alter their behaviors concerning how to anticipate and to cope with a lapse in appropriate behavior. In the relapse-prevention model (Figure 1.7), successful adherence to the modified-behavior program leads to increased self-efficacy and a low likelihood of relapse. However, a failure in the person's attempt to modify the target behavior in a high-risk situation is held to induce lowered perceptions

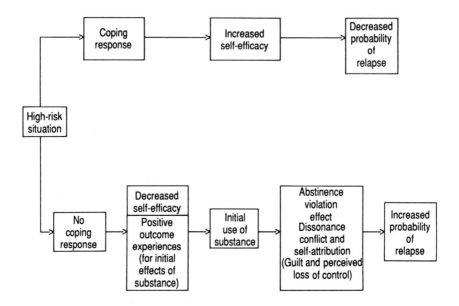

FIGURE 1.7 Cognitive-behavioral model of the relapse process (G. A. Marlatt, J. Gordon).

of self-efficacy, which, combined with the initial gratification that a return to old habits provides, leads to guilt and perceived loss of control, which, in turn, increases the probability of relapse (Marlatt & Gordon, 1985).

Behavior Modification

Finally, an approach to understanding and influencing adherence behaviors that is substantially different from the cognitive themes emphasized in the previously described models is represented by the behavior-modification approach (Figure 1.8). This framework emphasizes the roles played by habit and skill in attempts to modify undesirable personal (or "life-style") behaviors and brings to bear a wide variety of techniques (e.g., contingency contracting, self-monitoring, counter-conditioning, covert sensitization, relaxation, environmental engineering) (Matarazzo, Weiss, Herd, Miller, & Weiss, 1984; Melamed & Siegel, 1980). It would not be reasonable to suggest a single "model" for behavior modification, although the concepts of behavioral consequences and stimulus control are fairly common in these approaches. What is depicted in Figure 1.8 is the general plan that this approach frequently follows: identify the problem; describe the problem in behavioral terms; select a target behavior that is measurable; identify the ante-

1. Identify the problem
2. Describe the problem in behavioral terms
3. Select a target behavior that is measurable
4. Identify the antecedents and consequences of the behavior
5. Set behavioral objectives
6. Devise and implement a behavior change program
7. Evaluate the program

FIGURE 1.8 Behavioral intervention for habit change.

cedents and consequences of the behavior; set behavioral objectives; devise and implement a behavior-change program; and evaluate the program. Since cognitive and behavioral models and approaches both have much to offer, it seems reasonable to assume that our best bets for effective interventions to improve adherence will be strategies that combine these elements.

STRATEGIES FOR IMPROVING ADHERENCE

Much research has been devoted to identifying the "determinants" of adherence to professional recommendations (Haynes, 1976), and a smaller number of investigations have attempted to evaluate the efficacies of different strategies aimed at increasing the level of patient cooperation with suggested and prescribed therapies (Eraker et al., 1984). While no all-purpose solution to the nonadherence enigma has been discovered, enough practical knowledge and techniques have evolved to provide a foundation for programs to improve adherence. Summarized below are some of the more commonly employed (and promising) approaches to increasing client cooperation, with an emphasis on feasible interventions that could be implemented by different members of the health care team.

Providing Information

Investigations of the usefulness of providing various kinds of information have revealed a number of important considerations that influence the likelihood of patient adherence (Maiman & Becker, 1980). For example, research by Svarstad (1976) on clients of a neighborhood health center serving a low-income population revealed that 50% of the patients studied could not correctly report how long they were supposed to continue on their medication; 26% did not know the dosage prescribed; 17% could not report how often they were to take their medications; 16% believed their drugs marked "prn" were to be taken regularly; and 23% could not identify the purpose of every drug they were taking. Examining these conditions in relation to adherence showed that, while 73% of those correctly identifying their physicians' instructions followed the regimen, only 16% of those making one or more mistakes about their physicians' instructions adhered to their regimen. Of those receiving high-level instruction, 62% understood and 54% adhered; for patients who received relatively lower-level instruction, 40% understood and only 29% adhered.

Unfortunately, data regarding knowledge and adherence are, in the aggregate, neither consistent nor clear-cut; some studies have found no relationship between levels of patient information and adherence to therapy (Haynes, 1976). One approach to reconciling these seemingly conflicting results is (1) to view knowledge about certain details of the regimen as a *sine qua non* for correct adherence, but also to recognize that such information may, under particular circumstances, be insufficient to *produce* adequate patient cooperation and (2) to look at other variables that may be associated with communication of "better" information to the patient.

A study by Tagliacozzo and Ima (1970) conducted at a large urban hospital's outpatient clinic relates to the first point and concerns follow-up visit-keeping by patients with chronic conditions. Although patients with considerable disease experience showed no association between knowledge and adherence, such association became quite significant both for patients with little prior experience and for those cases where social factors interfered with making clinic visits. Thus, providing information for individuals motivated to follow advice but ignorant of the correct procedures should be beneficial; however, additional information about the regimen is less likely to enhance cooperation.

An experiment by McKenney and associates (1973) illustrates the second point. Twenty-five of 50 hypertensive patients had monthly half-hour educational visits with the pharmacist in addition to their regular physician visits. During the period of study, adherence rates for those in the "pharmacist" group increased from 25% to 79% while rates for the control group did not change. However, during the 6-month period after the special education effort was completed, cooperation in the experimental group fell back to preintervention levels. The transitory effect of the educational program suggests that the pharmacist's extra interest and exhortation probably improved adherence more than additional knowledge. While either variable yields better cooperation, the particular interpretation is important, since each explanation suggests a different focus for future attempts at intervention.

In any medical setting, some patients will not understand well what is expected of them after the visit, and these patients naturally have much higher rates of nonadherence than do others. Poor recall is part of the problem. Studies have shown that after 5 minutes patients forget about half the doctor's instructions (Ley, Bradshaw, Eaves, & Walker, 1973) and remember best the material in the first one third of the presentation (Ley, 1972). Further, they recall the diagnosis better than they do the prescribed therapy (Ley & Spelman, 1967). Such findings suggest that the provider should speak briefly and selectively, emphasizing information necessary for compliance clearly and early in the communication, and then repeat that information, both orally and through simple written instructions, to which the patient may later refer (a combination of oral and written instructions results in the highest level of patient information retention) (Dickey, Mattar, & Chudzek, 1975; Linkewich, Catalano, & Flack, 1974). Carefully organizing the information also seems important; in one study, the simple reorganization of a list of 15 medical statements into labelled categories enhanced recall by 50% (Ley et al., 1973). Specific and individualized instructions are associated with better adherence (Hulka, Cassel, Kupper, & Burdette, 1976; Korsch & Negrete, 1972).

Patients differ widely in terms of how much they know (and want to know), and they sometimes experience "information overload" (Joyce, Caple, Mason, Reynolds, & Mathews, 1969; Lasagna, 1976). This difficulty can be overcome to some degree by focusing on absolutely necessary aspects of the treatment plan and by avoiding more general discussions of the disease, the action of the medication, and so forth, since this type of information has not been shown to be related to adherence. It is remarkable how much simply modifying features of the communication often can raise patient adherence levels. For example, in an experiment conducted with female subjects on a weight-loss diet, Ley (1976) discovered that the group given a highly readable, well-organized, and repetitious leaflet experienced mean weight reductions averaging about twice those achieved by their peers (who had received the more usual type of leaflet). Patient package inserts and medication instruction sheets have been shown to be useful in improving drug knowledge (De Tullio et al., 1986).

Patients must have both knowledge and understand recommendations in order to cooperate with treatment. A considerable amount of nonadherence may be involuntary, due to a disparity in patient and provider understanding (Jette, 1982). A study of patients with diabetes mellitus or congestive heart failure found that most nonadherent patients did not deliberately choose not to comply (Hulka, Kupper, Cassel, Efrid, & Birdette, 1975). One often observes a breakdown in doctor–patient communication when the patient does not know the relevant vocabulary (Samora, Saunders, & Larson, 1961). For example, a study of communication between pediatricians and mothers demonstrated inadequate comprehension of such terms as "follow-up," "incubation period," and "workup," suggesting that even commonly used medical terms may require explanation or substitution (Korsch, Gozzi, & Francis, 1968). And, in a study of patients' interpretations of written prescription instructions, Mazullo and associates

(1974) found that 25% of the subjects interpreted the phrase "every six hours" as meaning "three times a day" (since they sleep at night); "as needed for water retention" was thought to mean that the pills would be used to cause water retention. Avoidance (or full explanation) of medical terms is therefore an obvious strategy for improving adherence.

Finally, simply reminding patients of upcoming appointments can enhance adherence. Mail and telephone reminders have been used successfully in such diverse areas as prenatal and well-child visits, medical and dental checkups, and in obtaining annual Pap smears, and have a clear, beneficial influence on appointment-keeping behavior (cf., Gates & Colburn, 1976; Nazarian, Mechaber, Charney, & Coulter, 1974; Shepard & Moseley, 1976). Foote and Erfurt (1977) achieved a considerable increase in blood pressure control among hypertensive patients through a program using mail and telephone follow-up.

Modifying Regimen Characteristics

Rates of adherence tend to be lower when the regimen is complex, of long duration, dependent on an alteration of the patient's life-style, inconvenient, or expensive (cf., Becker & Maiman, 1981; Haynes, 1976; Johannsen, Hellmuth, & Sorauf, 1966; Matthews & Hingson, 1977). For example, for patients with diabetes or congestive heart failure, medication errors were less than 15% when only one drug was prescribed; increased to 25% when two drugs were taken; and exceeded 35% when five or more drugs were taken (Hulka et al., 1975). Increasing the complexity of a regimen using digoxin by adding a diuretic agent and a potassium supplement notably decreased adherence for digoxin therapy (Weinstein, Au, & Lasagna, 1973). These (and similar) findings have led many reviewers to suggest a multiplicity of adherence-improving strategies.

The regimen can be made less complex by reducing the number of different medications required. This can be accomplished by avoiding the routine prescription of nonessential medicine and by avoiding unnecessary doses or variations in scheduling. Complexity can also be modified by emphasizing the necessity of adherence to particularly critical aspects of the treatment ("prioritizing" the regimen); by breaking the treatment plan into less complex stages that can be implemented sequentially ("graduated regimen implementation"); and by minimizing both inconvenience and forgetfulness by matching the regimen schedule to the patient's regular daily activities ("tailoring" the regimen) (Sackett et al., 1978). Frequency of dosing, in one study, was a more important factor for adherence than was the number of different medications taken at each dose interval (Porter, 1969). The importance of the duration of the regimen is highlighted by a study that found a 30% incidence rate of dosage errors in patients with diabetes who had the disease for 1 to 5 years, but an 80% dosage error rate in patients who had the disease for over 20 years (Charney, 1972). Short-term therapy, or at least the perception of it, can be accomplished by scheduling follow-up visits in quick succession when progress can be shown. This provides the patient with a feeling of accomplishment and a sense of the treatment's importance. If life-style must be altered (e.g., diet, exercise, abstinence from smoking), a target behavior should be identified (preferably by the patient), and changes should be introduced over the course of several visits ("shaping"). Cooperation that is achieved should be reinforced, and only then should the next behavioral objective be added (Matthews & Hingson, 1977).

Some pharmaceutical manufacturers have moved toward simplifying regimens by producing drug combinations, longer-acting drugs, and regimens requiring less frequent dosing. Although such approaches are often helpful when nonadherence is caused primarily by problems of regimen complexity or inconvenience, these solutions can actually create problems of their own. For example, combination and long-acting drugs hamper the physician's flexibility in prescribing and dosing, and the patient may have to pay for and receive unnecessary medications together with the essential one (Weintraub, 1976). A recent study of hypertensive treatment showed that therapeutic success relates less to the complexity of regimen than to the prescribed vigor (appropriate dosing) of the treatment (Haynes, Gibson, Taylor, Bernholz, & Sackett, 1982). Further research is needed to examine trade-offs between increased adherence and increased dangers of drug toxicity.

Modifying Health Beliefs

During the past two decades, considerable attention has been given to conceptualizing patient nonadherence as a problem in health-related decision making, wherein the individual is guided by attitudes and beliefs that may operate independently of levels of information, objective features of the condition and the regimen, and so forth (Cummings, Becker, & Maile, 1980). Beliefs that have been found most consistently to produce significant relationships with adherence to health and medical care recommendations have been the components of the Health Belief Model (Janz & Becker, 1984), social-normative variables (Ajzen, 1985), and self-efficacy (Strecher et al., 1986), concepts discussed earlier in this chapter. It is therefore recommended that more attention be paid to both monitoring and motivating the patient along these belief dimensions (e.g., does the patient care about health; agree with the diagnosis; perceive the condition as very serious or not very serious; feel the recommended therapy will work; fear medication side effects; feel the regimen will be too hard to follow; is or is not cognizant of/concerned about what others wish him/her to do about the problem?). Such an adherence-oriented history or "educational diagnosis" (Jenkins, 1979) can be viewed as a critical extension of the usual medical history and be made a routine part of the examination process.

The degree to which a provider can modify health beliefs is more difficult to assess than the extent to which more (and better) information can be transmitted or characteristics of the regimen changed. Nonetheless, research has demonstrated that these attitudes and perceptions can be altered (cf., Becker, Maiman, Kirscht, Haefner, & Drachman, 1977; Haefner & Kirscht, 1970; Strecher et al., 1986; Sutton & Eiser, 1984). Thus, by knowing which of these beliefs is below a level presumed necessary for good adherence, the provider might tailor interventions to suit the unique needs of each client. An encouraging example of the positive effects that such physician awareness has on patient adherence may be found in a controlled trial by Inui and associates (1976) in which one of two groups of physicians was given special tutorials (1 to 2 hours in length) whose content emphasized both compliance difficulties of patients with hypertension and possible strategies for altering patient beliefs and behaviors (based on the belief dimensions described above). After only a single session, physicians in the experimental group were observed to spend a greater proportion of clinic visit time on patient teaching, and their patients later exhibited higher levels of knowledge and appropriate beliefs about hypertension and its treatment; moreover, the patients of tutored physicians were subsequently more adherent to the treatment regimen and demonstrated better blood pressure control than did other patients.

Of course, knowing why many patients do not follow their regimens does not imply any particular strategy for changing their behavior. Sometimes merely providing corrective actual information will prove sufficient; in other cases, motive-arousing appeals (e.g., fear, parental or family responsibility, pride), recommendations from other sources of information that have greater credibility to the patient (e.g., another patient for whom the same treatment was successful), and other interventions will be necessary. The powerful influence that physicians' recommendations can have on adherence have been well-documented (cf., Janz et al., 1987; Ockene, 1987).

It is perhaps worth noting that attempts to change health-related attitudes and behaviors have most frequently employed fear-arousal techniques, which often do have a positive influence on adherence (Sutton, 1982). However, while low levels of concern about the threat of some illness or condition are not likely to motivate action, too much fear can serve to inhibit undertaking the appropriate behavior—as, for example, is often the case in delay in seeking care for cancer symptoms. In general, the literature suggests that fear appeals work best with persons initially little concerned about the disease and who are already convinced of the benefits the recommended action would provide. Also, fear appeals are more likely to affect adherence positively when they are used at the beginning of the effort to influence the patient and when they are accompanied by specific behavioral recommendations that the patient can easily and quickly undertake to reduce the threat.

Influencing the Treatment Experience

Modifying current experience with respect to therapeutic regimen and health care providers influences adherence. One way to alter the treatment experience is the contingency contract, wherein both parties set forth a treatment goal, the specific obligations of each party in attempting to accomplish that goal, and a time limit for its achievement. Data are now available supporting the provider-client contract as a tool for improving patient adherence (Janz, Becker, & Hartman, 1984). Contracts offer a written outline of expected behavior, the involvement of the patient in the decision-making process concerning the regimen and the opportunity to discuss potential problems and solutions with the physician, a formal commitment to the program from the patient, and rewards, such as additional time spent with the provider or lottery tickets, that create incentives for achieving compliance goals.

Experiences with health care providers can also be modified by involving other personnel in the provision of instruction, clarification, and reinforcement. Nurses, by virtue of their numbers and amount of patient contact, have great potential for exerting an impact on patient health behavior (Marston, 1977). Recent studies provide strong empirical support for the value of involving pharmacists in attempts to increase patient cooperation with prescribed therapies (cf., Schwartz, 1976; Sharpe, 1977). For example, consultation with the pharmacist before a patient left the hospital led to a 75% reduction in the previous high rate of deviation from prescribed drug regimens (Canada, 1976). Similarly, pharmacist counseling of outpatients has been successful in increasing the percentage of prescriptions refilled on time and decreasing the proportion of missed refills (Schwartz, 1976).

Influencing the Provider–Patient Relationship

In recent years, much attention has been given to developing adherence-enhancing strategies that depend upon altering the attitudes and behaviors of health care *providers*. It is in the crucial communication between physician and patient that the patient develops an understanding of the disease and its treatment (Stiles, Putnam, Wolf, & James, 1979); patient satisfaction and adherence to regimen are two outcomes with clearly documented relationships to this verbal exchange (Strecher, 1983).

Coe and Wessen (1965) have suggested that numerous aspects of the physician–patient interaction, such as impersonality and brevity of encounter, negatively affect patient behavior, and more recent reviews support their conclusion. Lack of communication—particularly communication of an emotional nature—is usually seen as the problem. Davis (1968) found that particular communication patterns are associated with patients' failure to follow doctors' advice. Such patterns include circumstances in which tension in the interaction is not released and in which the physician is formal, rejecting, or controlling, disagrees completely with the patient, or interviews the patient at length without later providing feedback. Francis and others (1969) report that a mother's cooperation with a regimen prescribed for her child is better when she is satisfied with the initial contact, regards the physician as friendly, and feels that the doctor understood the complaint. Further, they found that key factors in nonadherence included the extent to which patients' expectations from the medical visits were left unmet, lack of warmth in the doctor–patient relationship, and failure to receive an explanation of diagnosis and cause of the child's illness.

Many other investigations have also shown positive correlations between adherence and patient satisfaction with the visit, the therapist, or the clinic, including perceptions of convenience and of waiting times before and during appointments (cf., Linn, Linn, & Stein, 1982). In general, the literature indicates that adherence is greater when patients feel their expectations have been fulfilled, when the physician elicits and respects patients' concerns and provides responsive information about their condition and progress, and when sincere concern and sympathy are shown.

The provider's orientation toward the patient and desire to influence patient cooperation are important factors. Schulman (1979) found, for instance, that hypertensive patients who received medical care oriented to consider patients as active participants in the treatment process ("active patient orientation") were significantly more likely than other patients to have their blood pressures under control and to display more favorable cognitive and behavioral responses to the management of their illnesses. (Her data also imply that this productive orientation can be substantially increased by effecting incremental alteration in the system for delivering ambulatory clinic care.) Glanz (1979) was able to show that dietitians with relatively greater predispositions toward actively influencing their patients ("orientation to social influence") tended to employ more influence strategies, to involve patients in the counseling sessions, and to have patients with more appropriate health attitudes and adherence behaviors.

Although the patient–provider relationship clearly affects adherence, the actual mechanisms by which these influences occur remain obscure (Gillum & Barsky, 1974) and therefore a reasonable target for future research. One consistent finding is that the likelihood of adherence is increased when the patient's expectations of the encounter are matched by what actually occurs (Davis & von der Lippe, 1968; Francis et al., 1969; Greenwald, Becker, & Nevitt, 1978).

Enlisting Family and Social Support

Evidence is growing that social support (particularly support provided by the patient's family) plays an important role in influencing adherence. The family can enhance supervision of the patient, as well as provide assistance and encouragement. Social support seems to be especially important in long-term treatment plans that require continuous action on the part of the patient. For example, studies of weight control have shown that those persons who received assistance from another family member in cueing or in reinforcement of proper eating behavior were more likely to lose weight and to maintain their weight loss (Stuart & Davis, 1972). Similar outcomes have been described for the family's influence in adherence in taking medications (Willcox, Gillan, & Hare, 1965). A family's own health beliefs and its evaluation of the patient's illness and treatment may influence adherence. Success is greatest when the family's normal roles and patterns are compatible with the illness of the patient or when the family members are willing to make accommodating changes in their lives and in the family environment.

In a review of six studies that examined the relationship between patient adherence and family influence, Haynes (1976) concluded that "the influence of the family appears to be considerable" (p. 36), with supportive families being associated with greater adherence in five of the six investigations. Becker and Green (1975) summarized an extensive empirical literature on the multidimensional role played by the family in the extent to which the patient cooperates with medical treatment; relationships were documented between adherence and (1) assumption of responsibility for the sick member's care; (2) evaluation of the illness and the recommended treatment (including appraisal of symptoms and need for care); (3) existing patterns of illness behavior; (4) health beliefs; (5) sympathy, support, and encouragement; (6) willingness to engage in "environmental control"; (7) compatibility of normal roles and patterns with the patient's sick role or regimen; and (8) interspouse communication and attitudinal concordance.

In light of our current heightened concern with chronic conditions and the concomitant shift in emphasis from direct medical care to continuous patient self-management, the effect of the family (and other social support systems) on patients' adherence to regimens is likely to be of tremendous importance, with many possibilities for substantial positive or negative impacts. It remains a task for future research efforts to investigate potential interactions between family influence and such variables as health beliefs, knowledge, regimen characteristics, relationship with provider, and so forth.

A SYNTHESIZED MODEL

Much of the research on improving adherence is only loosely tied to the theories and models of adherence behavior described earlier in this chapter. Moreover, considerable confusion has existed among researchers with regard to the selection of a particular model of health behavior for study. Some investigators (cf.,

Becker et al., 1977), noting at the least a superficial similarity across the classes of factors included in these models, have felt that the actual number of truly distinct concepts relevant to explaining health-related behaviors was probably smaller than the large number of variables that have been described in this chapter thus far. Thus, on a "face validity" basis, Fabrega's (1973) "computation of treatment benefits" appears quite similar to the Theory of Reasoned Action's "the person's beliefs that the behavior leads to certain outcomes"; to Social Learning Theory's "outcome expectations"; to the Health Belief Model's "perceived benefits of action"; to Leventhal's "appraising how one's coping reactions affected the problem"; and so forth.

In 1979, Cummings and his colleagues (1980) abstracted a total of 109 variables from 14 existing models that had been advanced to account for people's health actions. These variables were put on separate index cards and sent to eight major developers of such models; these experts were asked to sort the cards (variables) into conceptually similar piles and return them to the investigators. Using Smallest Space Analysis, Cummings et al. identified six summary categories: (1) items pertaining to *accessibility of health services*, such as the individual's ability to pay for health care and awareness of health services, and availability of health services; (2) items dealing with the individual's *attitudes toward health care*, such as beliefs in the benefits of treatment and beliefs about the quality of medical care provided; (3) items concerning the *threat of illness*, such as the individual's perception of symptoms and beliefs about susceptibility to, and consequences of, disease; (4) items pertaining to *knowledge about disease*; (5) items dealing with the individual's *social interactions* and with *social norms and social structure*; and (6) items on *demographic characteristics* (social status, income, and education). It should be noted that, because Bandura's model was not included in this study, "self-efficacy" does not appear as a category; had it been included, it would very likely have emerged from the analysis as a distinct and important concept.

The many basic similarities among the variables contained in the different models examined by Cummings, Becker, and Maile (1980) suggest that these models are far from independent; rather, despite differences in the labeling and defining of variables, there is apparently substantial overlap among the variables *as judged by the model builders themselves*. Combining the variables provides a more complete representation of the factors that are thought to influence health-related actions and lays the groundwork for further model-testing by presenting a general framework for describing adherence behavior. Further research is needed to address questions about the possible causal associations that may exist between these dimensions and factors and about why certain factors are important in one situation (or disease, or regimen) but not in another. Combined with population-specific data, such information is prerequisite to the development of effective strategies for enhancing adherence to recommended and prescribed therapies.

SUMMARY

Patient nonadherence remains a substantial threat to the efficacy of recommended and prescribed preventive and therapeutic regimens. This chapter has summarized and depicted the major elements of a number of well-known and widely employed psychological, sociological, and anthropological models of health-related decision making and has summarized some of the major strategies advanced in the empirical literature for increasing adherence. The interventions discussed do not begin to exhaust the list of possible techniques for improving adherence; for example, much of the very extensive repertoire of behavior modification approaches (cf., Matarazzo et al., 1984; Taylor, 1986) has not been addressed. However, the strategies reviewed represent feasible and practical approaches for which substantial research support is available.

Major interventions presented included raising information and skill levels, altering characteristics of the regimen, assessing and modifying health-related attitudes and beliefs, improving various aspects of the relationship between provider and patient, altering the treatment experience (including the use of client–provider contracts), enlisting family and other social support, and utilizing all members of the health care team. While further theoretical conceptualization and empirical investigation regarding determinants of (and strategies for influencing) patient adherence are certainly still needed, the variables identified and suggestions offered in this chapter provide the foundation for a rational program that can be implemented by health care providers and public health planners wishing to improve levels of patient cooperation with health-related recommendations.

REFERENCES

Abramson, L. Y., Garber, J., & Seligman, M. E. P. (1980). Learned helplessness in humans: An attributional analysis. In J. Garber & M. E. P. Seligman (Eds.), *Human helplessness: Theory and applications* (pp. 49–74). New York: Academic Press.

Ajzen, I. (1985). From intentions to actions: A theory of planned behavior. In J. Kuhl & J. Beckman (Eds.), *Action control: From cognition to behavior* (pp. 11–39). New York: Springer-Verlag.

Ajzen, I., & Fishbein, M. (1980). *Understanding attitudes and predicting social behavior.* Englewood Cliffs, NJ: Prentice-Hall.

Andersen, R. (1968). *A behavioral model of families' use of health services.* Chicago: University of Chicago, Center for Health Administration Studies.

Andersen, R., & Anderson, O. W. (1979). Trends in the use of health services. In H. E. Freeman, S. Levine, & L. G. Reeder (Eds.), *Handbook of medical sociology* (pp. 371–391). Englewood Cliffs, NJ: Prentice-Hall.

Andersen, R., Kravits, J., & Anderson, O. W. (Eds.). (1975). *Equity in health services: Empirical analyses in social policy.* Cambridge, MA: Ballinger.

Andersen, R., & Newman, J. F. (1973). Societal and individual determinants of medical care utilization in the United States. *Milbank Memorial Fund Quarterly/Health and Society, 51,* 95–124.

Bandura, A. (1977a). Self-efficacy: Toward a unifying theory of behavioral change. *Psychological Review, 84,* 191–215.

Bandura, A. (1977b). *Social learning theory.* Englewood Cliffs, NJ: Prentice-Hall.

Bandura, A. (1984). Recycling misconceptions of perceived self-efficacy. *Cognitive Therapy and Research, 8,* 231–255.

Becker, M. H. (1974). The health belief model and sick role behavior. *Health Educaiton Monographs, 2,* 409–419.

Becker, M. H., Drachman, R. H., & Kirscht, J. P. (1974). A new approach to explaining sick-role behavior in low-income populations. *American Journal of Public Health, 64,* 205–216.

Becker, M. H., & Green, L. W. (1975). A family approach to compliance with medical treatment: A selective review of the literature. *International Journal of Health Education, 18,* 173–182.

Becker, M. H., Haefner, D. P., Kasl, S. V., Kirscht, J. P., Maiman, L. A., & Rosenstock, I. M. (1977). Selected psychosocial models and correlates of individual health-related behaviors. *Medical Care, 15* (Suppl.), 27–46.

Becker, M. H., & Maiman, L. A. (1975). Sociobehavioral determinants of compliance with health and medical care recommendations. *Medical Care, 13,* 10–24.

Becker, M. H., & Maiman, L. A. (1981). Patient compliance. In K. L. Melmon (Ed.), *Drug therapeutics: Concepts for physicians* (pp. 65–79). New York: Elsevier.

Becker, M. H., Maiman, L. A., Kirscht, J. P., Haefner, D. P., & Drachman, R. H. (1977). The health belief model and dietary compliance: A field experiment. *Journal of Health and Social Behavior, 18,* 348–366.

Canada, A. T. (1976). The pharmacist and drug compliance. In D. L. Sackett & R. B. Haynes (Eds.), *Compliance with therapeutic regimens* (pp. 129–134). Baltimore: Johns Hopkins University Press.

Charney, E. (1972). Patient–doctor communication. *Pediatric Clinics of North America, 19,* 263–279.

Coe, R. M., & Wessen, A. (1965). Social–psychological factors influencing the use of community health resources. *American Journal of Public Health, 55,* 1024–1031.

Crandall, R. (1978). The measurement of self-esteem and related constructs. In J. P. Robinson & P. R. Shaver (Eds.), *Measures of social psychological attitudes* (pp. 87–94). Ann Arbor, MI: Institute of Social Research, University of Michigan.

Cummings, K. M., Becker, M. H., & Maile, M. C. (1980). Bringing the models together: An empirical approach to combining variables used to explain health actions. *Journal of Behavioral Medicine, 3,* 123–145.

Davis, M. S. (1968). Variations in patients' compliance with doctors' advice: An empirical analysis of patterns of communication. *American Journal of Public Health, 58,* 274–288.

Davis, M. S., & von der Lippe, R. P. (1968). Discharge from hospital against medical advice: A study of reciprocity in the doctor–patient relationship. *Social Science and Medicine, 1,* 336–344.

De Tullio, P. L., Eraker, S. A., Jepson, C., Becker, M. H., Fujimoto, E., Diaz, C. L., Loveland, R. B., & Strecher, V. J. (1986). Patient medication instruction and provider interactions: Effects on knowledge and attitudes. *Health Education Quarterly, 13*, 51–60.

Dickey, F. F., Mattar, R. M., & Chudzek, G. M. (1975). Pharmacist counseling increasing drug regimen compliance. *Hospitals, 49*, 85–88.

Dutton, D. B. (1978). Explaining low use of health services by the poor: Costs, attitudes or delivery systems? *American Sociological Review, 43*, 348–368.

Eraker, S. A., Becker, M. H., Strecher, V. J., & Kirscht, J. P. (1985). Smoking behavior, cessation techniques, and the health decision model. *American Journal of Medicine, 78*, 817–825.

Eraker, S. A., Kirscht, J. P., & Becker, M. H. (1984). Understanding and improving patient compliance. *Annals of Internal Medicine, 100*, 258–268.

Eraker, S. A., & Politser, P. (1982). How decisions are reached: Physician and patient. *Annals of Internal Medicine, 97*, 262–268.

Eraker, S. A., & Sox, H. C., Jr. (1981). Assessment of patients' preferences for therapeutic outcomes. *Medical Decision Making, 1*, 29–39.

Fabrega, H., Jr. (1973). Toward a model of illness behavior. *Medical Care, 11*, 470–484.

Fabrega, H., Jr. (1974). *Disease and social behavior: An interdisciplinary perspective.* Cambridge, MA: Massachusetts Institute of Technology Press.

Fabrega, H., Jr. (1977). Perceived illness and its treatment: A naturalistic study in social medicine. *British Journal of Preventive and Social Medicine, 31*, 213–219.

Fabrega, H., Jr., & Zucker, M. (1977). Comparison of illness episodes in a pluralistic setting. *Psychosomatic Medicine, 39*, 325–343.

Fishbein, M., & Jaccard, J. (1973). Theoretical and methodological considerations in the prediction of family planning intentions and behavior. *Representative Research in Social Psychology, 4*, 37–51.

Foote, A., & Erfurt, J. C. (1977). Controlling hypertension: A cost-effective model. *Preventive Medicine, 6*, 319–343.

Francis, V., Korsch, B. M., & Morris, M. J. (1969). Gaps in doctor–patient communication: Patients' response to medical advice. *New England Journal of Medicine, 280*, 535–540.

Gates, S. J., & Colborn, D. K. (1976). Lowering appointment failures in a neighborhood health center. *Medical Care, 14*, 263–267.

Gillum, R. F., & Barsky, A. J. (1974). Diagnosis and management of noncompliance. *Journal of the American Medical Association, 228*, 1563–1566.

Glanz, K. (1979). Dietitians' effectiveness and patient compliance with dietary regimens. *Journal of the American Dietetic Association, 75*, 631–636.

Greenwald, H. P., Becker, S. W., & Nevitt, M. C. (1978). Delay and noncompliance in cancer detection: A behavioral perspective for health planners. *Milbank Memorial Fund Quarterly/Health and Society, 56*, 212–226.

Haefner, D. P., & Kirscht, J. P. (1970). Motivational and behavioral effects of modifying health beliefs. *Public Health Reports, 85*, 478–484.

Haynes, R. B. (1976). A critical review of the "determinants" of patient compliance with therapeutic regimens. In D. L. Sackett & R. B. Haynes (Eds.), *Compliance with therapeutic regimens* (pp. 26–39). Baltimore: Johns Hopkins University Press.

Haynes, R. B., Gibson, E. S., Taylor, D. W., Bernholz, C. D., & Sackett, D. L. (1982). Process versus outcome in hypertension: A positive result. *Circulation, 65*, 28–33.

Hulka, B. S., Cassel, J. C., Kupper, L. L., & Burdette, J. A. (1976). Communication, compliance, and concordance between physicians and patients with prescribed medication. *American Journal of Public Health, 66,* 847–853.

Hulka, B. S., Kupper, L. L., Cassel, J. C., Efird, R. L., & Birdette, J. A. (1975). Medication use and misuse: Physician–patient discrepancies. *Journal of Chronic Diseases, 28,* 7–21.

Inui, T. S., Yourtee, E. L., & Williamson, J. W. (1976). Improved outcomes in hypertension after physician tutorials: A controlled trial. *Annals of Internal Medicine, 84,* 646–651.

Jaccard, J. (1975). A theoretical analysis of selected factors important to health education strategies. *Health Education Monographs, 3,* 152–167.

Janz, N. K., & Becker, M. H. (1984). The health belief model: A decade later. *Health Education Quarterly, 11,* 1–47.

Janz, N. K., Becker, M. H., & Hartman, P. E. (1984). Contingency contracting to enhance patient compliance: A review. *Patient Education and Counseling, 5,* 65–178.

Janz, N. K., Becker, M. H., Kirscht, J. P., Eraker, S. A., Billi, J. E., & Woolliscroft, J. O. (1987). Evaluation of a minimal-contact smoking cessation intervention in an outpatient setting. *American Journal of Public Health, 77,* 805–809.

Jette, A. M. (1982). Improving patient cooperation with arthritis treatment regimens. *Arthritis and Rheumatism, 142,* 1673–1675.

Johannsen, W. J., Hellmuth, G. A., & Sorauf, T. (1966). On accepting medical recommendations. *Archives of Environmental Health, 12,* 63–69.

Joyce, C. R., Caple, G., Mason, M., Reynolds, E., & Mathews, J. A. (1969). Quantitative study of doctor–patient communication. *Quarterly Journal of Medicine, 38,* 183–194.

Kasl, S. V., & Cobb, S. (1966). Health behavior, illness behavior, and sick role behavior. I. Health and illness behavior. *Archives of Environmental Health, 12,* 246–266.

Kirscht, J. P. (1974). The health belief model and illness behavior. *Health Education Monographs, 2,* 387–408.

Korsch, B. M., Gozzi, E. K., & Francis, V. (1968). Gaps in doctor–patient communication. I. Doctor–patient interaction and patient satisfaction. *Pediatrics, 42,* 855–871.

Korsch, B. M., & Negrete, V. F. (1972). Doctor–patient communication. *Scientific American, 227,* 66–74.

Lasagna, L. (1976). The patient package insert. In L. Lasagna (Ed.), *Patient compliance* (pp. 77–82). Mount Kisco, NY: Futura.

Lazarus, R. S., & Folkman, S. (1984). *Stress, appraisal and coping.* New York: Springer Publishing Co.

Leventhal, H., Meyer, D., & Gutmann, M. (1980, October). The role of theory in the study of compliance to high blood pressure regimens. In R. B. Haynes, M. E. Mattson, & T. O. Engebretson, Jr. (Eds.), *Patient compliance to prescribed antihypertensive medication regimens: A report to the National Heart, Lung, and Blood Institute* (pp. 1–58) (NIH Publication No. 81-2102). Washington, DC: U.S. Department of Health and Human Services.

Ley, P. (1972). Primacy, rated importance, and the recall of medical statements. *Journal of Health and Social Behavior, 13,* 311–317.

Ley, P. (1976). Towards better doctor–patient communications. In A. E. Bennett (Ed.), *Communications between doctors and patients* (pp. 77–98). London: Oxford University Press.

Ley, P., Bradshaw, P. W., Eaves, D., & Walker, C. M. (1973). A method for increasing patients' recall of information presented by doctors. *Psychological Medicine, 3,* 217–220.

Ley, P., & Spelman, M. S. (1967). *Communicating with the patient.* St. Louis: Green.

Linkewich, J. A., Catalano, R. B., & Flack, H. L. (1974). The effect of packaging and instruction on outpatient compliance with medical regimens. *Drug Intelligence and Clinical Pharmacy, 8,* 10–15.

Linn, M. W., Linn, B. S., & Stein, S. R. (1982). Satisfaction with ambulatory care and compliance in older patients. *Medical Care, 20,* 606–614.

Maiman, L. A., & Becker, M. H. (1974). The health belief model: Origins and correlates in psychological theory. *Health Education Monographs, 2,* 336–353.

Maiman, L. A., & Becker, M. H. (1980). The clinician's role in patient compliance. *Trends in Pharmacological Sciences, 1,* 457–459.

Marlatt, G. A. (1982). Relapse prevention: A self-control program for the treatment of addictive behaviors. In R. B. Stuart (Ed.), *Adherence, compliance and generalization in behavioral medicine* (pp. 329–378). New York: Brunner/Mazel.

Marlatt, G. A., & Gordon, J. R. (Eds.). (1985). *Relapse prevention: Maintenance strategies in addictive behavior change.* New York: Guilford.

Marston, M. W. (1977). Nursing management of compliance with medical regimens. In I. Barofsky (Ed.), *Medication compliance: A behavioral management approach* (pp. 139–164). Thorofore, NJ: Slack.

Matarazzo, J. D., Weiss, S. M., Herd, J. A., Miller, N. E., & Weiss, S. M. (Eds.). (1984). *Behavioral health: A handbook of health enhancement and disease prevention.* New York: Wiley.

Matthews, D., & Hingson, R. (1977). Improving patient compliance: A guide for physicians. *Medical Clinics of North America, 61,* 879–889.

Mazullo, J., Lasagna, L., & Grinar, P. (1974). Variations in interpretation of prescription instructions. *Journal of the American Medical Association, 227,* 929–931.

McKenney, J. M., Slining, J. M., Henderson, H. R., Devins, D., & Barr, M. (1973). The effect of clinical pharmacy services on patients with essential hypertension. *Circulation, 48,* 1104–1111.

McNeil, B. J., Keeler, E., & Adelstein, S. J. (1975). Primer on certain elements of medical decision making. *New England Journal of Medicine, 293,* 211–215.

McNeil, B. J., Pauker, S. G., Sox, H. C., Jr., Tversky, A. (1982). On the elicitation of preferences for alternative therapies. *New England Journal of Medicine, 306,* 1259–1262.

Melamed, B. G., & Siegel, L. J. (1980). *Behavioral medicine: Practical applications in health care.* New York: Springer Publishing Co.

Nazarian, L., Mechaber, J., Charney, E., & Coulter, M. (1974). Effect of a mailed appointment reminder on appointment keeping. *Pediatrics, 53,* 349–352.

Ockene, J. K. (1987). Smoking intervention: The expanding role of the physician. *American Journal of Public Health, 77,* 782–783.

Podell, R. N. (1975). *Physician's guide to compliance in hypertension.* West Point, PA: Merck & Co.

Porter, A. M. (1969). Drug defaulting in a general practice. *British Medical Journal, 1,* 218–222.

Rosenstock, I. M. (1974). Historical origins of the health belief model. *Health Education Monographs, 2,* 328–335.

Sackett, D. L. (1976). The magnitude of compliance and noncompliance. In D. L. Sackett & R. B. Haynes (Eds.), *Compliance with therapeutic regimens* (pp. 9–25). Baltimore: Johns Hopkins University Press.

Sackett, D. L., Haynes, R. B., Gibson, E. S., Taylor, D. W., Roberts, R. S., & Johnson, A. L. (1978). Patient compliance with antihypertensive regimens. *Patient Counselling and Health Education, 1,* 18–21.

Sackett, D. L., & Snow, J. C. (1979). The magnitude of compliance and noncompliance. In R. B. Haynes, D. W. Taylor, & D. L. Sackett (Eds.), *Compliance in health care* (pp. 11–22). Baltimore: Johns Hopkins University Press.

Samora, J., Saunders, L., & Larson, R. (1961). Medical vocabulary knowledge among hospital patients. *Journal of Health and Human Behavior, 2,* 83–92.

Schifter, D. E., & Ajzen, I. (1985). Intention, perceived control, and weight loss: An application of the theory of planned behavior. *Journal of Personality and Social Psychology, 49,* 843–851.

Schulman, B. A. (1979). Active patient orientation and outcomes in hypertensive treatment: Application of a socio-organizational perspective. *Medical Care, 17,* 267–280.

Schunk, D. H., & Carbonari, J. P. (1984). Self-efficacy models. In J. D. Matarazzo, S. M. Weiss, J. A. Herd, N. E. Miller, & S. M. Weiss (Eds.), *Behavioral health: A handbook of health enhancement and disease prevention* (pp. 230–247). New York: Wiley.

Schwartz, M. A. (1976). The role of the pharmacist in the patient–health team relationship. In L. Lasagna (Ed.), *Patient compliance* (pp. 83–95). Mount Kisco, NY: Futura.

Seibold, D., & Roper, R. (1979). Psychosocial determinants of health care intentions: Test of the Triandis and Fishbein models. In D. Nimmo (Ed.), *Communication yearbook 3* (pp. 111–123). New Brunswick, NJ: Transaction Books.

Sharpe, T. R. (1977). The pharmacist's potential role as a factor in increasing compliance. In I. Barofsky (Ed.), *Medication compliance: A behavioral management approach* (pp. 133–138). Thorofare, NJ: Slack.

Shepard, D. S., & Moseley, T. A. (1976). Mailed versus telephoned appointment reminders to reduce broken appointments in a hospital outpatient department. *Medical Care, 14,* 268–273.

Stiles, W. B., Putnam, S. M., Wolf, M. H., & James, S. A. (1979). Interaction exchange structure and patient satisfaction with medical interviews. *Medical Care, 17,* 667–681.

Strecher, V. J. (1983). Improving physician–patient interactions: A review. *Patient Counselling and Health Education, 4,* 129–136.

Strecher, V. J., DeVellis, B. McE., Becker, M. H., & Rosentock, I. M. (1986). The role of self-efficacy in achieving health behavior change. *Health Education Quarterly, 13,* 73–92.

Stuart, R. B., & Davis, B. (1972). *Slim chance in a fat world.* Chicago: Research Press.

Sutton, S. R. (1982). Fear-arousing communication: A critical examination of theory and research. In J. R. Eiser (Ed.), *Social psychology and behavioral medicine* (pp. 303–337). New York: Wiley.

Sutton, S. R., & Eiser, J. R. (1984). The effect of fear-arousing communication on cigarette smoking: An expectancy-value approach. *Journal of Behavioral Medicine, 7,* 13–33.

Svarstad, B. L. (1976). Physician–patient communication and patient conformity with medical advice. In D. Mechanic (Ed.), *The growth of bureaucratic medicine: An inquiry into the dynamics of patient behavior and the organization of medical care* (pp. 220–238). New York: Wiley.

Tagliacozzo, D. M., & Ima, K. (1970). Knowledge of illness as a predictor of patient behavior. *Journal of Chronic Diseases, 22,* 765–775.

Taylor, S. E. (1986). *Health psychology.* New York: Random House.

Tversky, A., & Kahneman, D. (1974). Judgment under uncertainty: Heuristics and biases. *Science, 185,* 1124–1131.

Wallston, B. S., & Wallston, K. A. (1984). Social psychological models of health behavior: An examination and integration. In A. Baum, S. Taylor, & J. E. Singer (Eds.), *Handbook of psychology and health* (Vol. IV) (pp. 215–222). Hillsdale, NJ: Erlbaum.

Weintraub, M. (1976). Intelligent noncompliance and capricious compliance. In L. Lasagna (Ed.), *Patient compliance* (pp. 39–47). Mount Kisco, NY: Futura.

Weinstein, M. C., & Fineberg, H. V. (Eds.). (1980). *Clinical decision analysis.* Philadelphia: W. B. Saunders.

Weinstein, M., Au, W. Y., & Lasagna, L. (1973). Compliance as a determinant of serum digoxin concentration. *Journal of the American Medical Association, 224,* 481–485.

Willcox, D. R. C., Gillan, R., & Hare, E. H. (1965). Do psychiatric outpatients take their drugs? *British Medical Journal, 22,* 790–792.

2

Relapse Prevention and the Maintenance of Optimal Health

G. Alan Marlatt, William H. George

WHAT IS RELAPSE PREVENTION?

Relapse Prevention (RP) is a self-control program designed to help individuals to anticipate and cope with the problem of relapse in the habit-change process. *Relapse* refers to a breakdown or failure in a person's attempt to change or modify a particular habit pattern, such as giving up "bad habits" or developing new, optimal health behaviors. Based on the principle of social-learning theory (Bandura, 1986), RP combines behavioral skill-training procedures, cognitive therapy, and life-style rebalancing. Because the RP model combines behavioral and cognitive components, it is similar to other cognitive–behavioral approaches that have been developed in recent years as an outgrowth and extension of more traditional behavior therapy programs.

The RP model initially developed as a behavioral maintenance program for use in the treatment of addictive behaviors (Marlatt & Gordon, 1980, 1985). Goals of addiction treatment are either to refrain totally from performing a target behavior (e.g., to abstain from drug use) or to impose regulatory limits or controls over the occurrence of a behavior (e.g., to diet as a means of controlling food intake).

Relapse prevention can be applied either as a maintenance strategy to prevent relapse or as a more general approach to life-style change. The aim of maintenance strategies is to prevent or intervene in the relapse process after the initiation of behavior change (e.g., to prevent a recent ex-smoker from returning to habitual smoking). As such, RP procedures are designed to enhance the maintenance of behavior change and may be applied regardless of the theoretical orientation or intervention methods applied during the initial treatment phase. Once an alcoholic has stopped drinking, for example, RP methods can be applied toward the effective *maintenance* of abstinence, regardless of the methods used to *initiate* abstinence (e.g., attending AA meetings, pharmacotherapy, voluntary cessation, etc.).

The second application of the RP model is a more general one: to facilitate changes in personal habits to reduce the risk of physical disease or psychological stress. A balanced life-style is characterized by enhanced awareness and a harmonious balance between "want" and "should" activities. The development of "positive addictions" (Glasser, 1974) such as physical exercise and meditation is recommended as part of the life-style rebalancing program.

TREATMENT VERSUS MAINTENANCE: SEPARATE PROCESSES?

To illustrate the distinction between treatment and maintenance as separate processes or stages in the modification of addictive behaviors, consider the example of an alcoholic or problem drinker who is motivated to change. A wide variety of procedures and techniques is available that may be effective in getting an alcoholic to stop drinking; examples include comprehensive inpatient programs, pharmacotherapy, dietary management, marital or family counseling, group therapy, occupational therapy, behavior modification, religious conversions, Alcoholics Anonymous, and so forth. Some techniques are directed more toward initially getting the person to stop drinking (i.e., oriented toward the initial *cessation* of the problem behavior), whereas others are directed more toward the long-term *maintenance* of this change.

A typical response to the high relapse rate in addiction treatement has been to increase the number of initial treatment techniques, to build a more comprehensive broad-spectrum or multimodal treatment package designed to facilitate cessation of the target behavior. The underlying assumption here seems to be that if sufficient components are added to the initial treatment program, the effects on treatment outcome will somehow last longer. There are two major drawbacks to the multimodal approach to treatment. First, recent evidence suggests that the more techniques and procedures that are applied during treatment, the more difficult it becomes for the client to maintain compliance with the program requirements (e.g., Hall, 1980). Second, many if not all of the intervention techniques are directed primarily toward initial behavior change only, and not toward the long-term maintenance of this change. Frequently treatment techniques are geared primarily toward cessation of the target behavior, whether it be smoking, alcohol consumption, overeating, or the performance of other problem behaviors (e.g., sexual exhibitionism). What is often overlooked with this focus on initial cessation is that the maintenance of change, once induced, may be governed by entirely different principles than those associated with initial cessation.

One important difference between initial treatment procedures and those designed to enhance maintenance effects over time is that the former techniques are often externally administered to the client by the therapist (e.g., pharmacotherapy, assertive training, contingency contracting, etc.), whereas maintenance procedures are often left to the client to "self-administer." An exception to this distinction is the use of externally applied "booster" sessions, in which a technique such as pharmacotherapy is readministered to the client at various intervals following treatment in an attempt to bolster and reinforce the effects of the initial treatment program. The goal of teaching the client self-administered maintenance techniques, on the other hand, is to train the client to become his or her own therapist and to carry on the thrust of the intervention program after the termination of the formal therapeutic relationship. Instead of relying on willpower during the maintenance phase, a successfeul graduate of this type of program would be well-grounded in self-monitoring and self-management skills. This self-control orientation is characteristic of the RP approach.

RELAPSE: TWO OPPOSING DEFINITIONS

At a recent workshop for alcoholism and drug counselors, members of the audience were asked to share their subjective associations to the term *relapse*. Here are some of their replies: "treatment failure," "return to illness," "falling back into addiction," "failure and guilt," "breakdown," and so forth. These associations are reflected in one definition of "relapse" given in *Webster's New Collegiate Dictionary*: "A recurrence of symptoms of a disease after a period of improvement." This definition corresponds with the dichotomous view of treatment outcome fostered by the disease model: one is either "cured" (or the symptoms are in remission) or one has relapsed (recidivism). It has been standard practice in the addictions field to view *any* use of drugs following an abstinence-oriented treatment program as indicative of relapse. Relapse is thus seen as an end state: the end of the road, a dead end.

There are a number of problems with this rather pessimistic approach to relapse. If the black/white dichotomy of abstinence/relapse is assimilated by the individual while in treatment, this may set up an expectation leading to a self-fulfilling prophecy in which any violation of abstinence will send the pendulum to the other extreme of relapse.

Another problem with the traditional definition of relapse is its association with the return of the disease state. The cause of the relapse is usually attributed to internal biological factors associated with the disease condition (Brickman et al., 1982). Behaviors associated with relapse come to be equated with the emergence of symptoms signaling the reactivation of the underlying disease, much as the experience of fever and chills serves as a signal of relapse in malaria. This emphasis on internal causation carries the implicit message that there is nothing much one can do about the outbreak of symptoms—how does one prevent a fever from breaking out? This outlook tends to ignore the influence of situational and psychological factors as potential determinants in the relapse process. It also reinforces the notion that the individual who experiences a relapse is a helpless victim of circumstances beyond his or her control.

An alternative approach to the issue of relapse is reflected in Webster's second definition of relapse: "Relapse is the *act or instance* of backsliding, worsening, or subsiding." Italics are added to emphasize that a relapse can be viewed as a *single act* of falling back: a single mistake, an error, a slip. A more appropriate word to refer to the singular occurrence of the behavior in question (e.g., the first drink or cigarette following a period of abstinence) would be *lapse* (as in a "lapse" of attention). The same dictionary defines "lapse" as "a slight error or slip . . . a temporary fall esp. from a higher to a lower state." One thinks here of a skater in competition who trips and falls on the ice: whether the skater gets up again and continues to perform depends to a large extent on whether the fall is seen as a "lapse" or a "relapse"—as a single slip (mistake) or as an indication of total failure.

In the RP approach, relapse is viewed as a transitional process, a series of events that may or may not be followed by a return to pretreatment baseline levels of the target behavior. It is possible to view the alcoholic who takes a single drink after a period of abstinence as someone who has made a slight excursion over the border between abstinence and relapse. Whether this first lapse is followed by a return to abstinence depends considerably on the personal expectations of the individual involved. The RP approach attempts to provide the individual with the necessary skills and cognitive strategies to prevent the single occurrence of a lapse from snowballing into a total relapse. Rather than pessimistically looking upon a relapse as a dead end, the RP approach views it as a fork in the road, with one path returning to the former problem behavior and the other continuing in the direction of positive change.

Many new questions arise when one adopts this alternative perspective of relapse (Brownell, Marlatt, Lichtenstein, & Wilson, 1986). Are there any specific situational events that serve as precipitating triggers for relapse? Are the determinants of the first lapse the same as those assumed to govern a total relapse? Is it possible for an individual to covertly "plan" a relapse by setting up a situation in which it is virtually impossible to resist temptation? At which points in the relapse process is it possible to intervene and alter the course of events and thus prevent a return to the former habit pattern? How does the individual react to and conceptualize the events preceding and following a relapse, and how do these reactions affect the person's subsequent behavior? Is it possible to prepare persons in treatment to anticipate the likelihood of a relapse so that they may engage in preventive alternative behaviors? To borrow a term from the medical model, can we develop prevention procedures that would "inoculate" the individual against the inevitability of relapse?

To answer these and other questions, it is necessary to engage in a detailed micro-analysis of the relapse process itself. This fine-grained approach focuses upon the various determinants of relapse, including the immediate precipitating circumstances and the longer chain of events that may or may not precede the relapse episode. In addition, the role of such cognitive factors as expectation and attribution is examined in detail, particularly those related to the individual's reactions to the relapse. A micro-analysis of the relapse process is justified by the old maxim that we can learn much from our mistakes. Rather than being seen as an indication of failure, a relapse can be viewed more optimistically as a challenge, an opportunity for new learning to occur.

OVERVIEW OF THE RELAPSE MODEL

In the following overview, only the highlights of the RP model are presented. Background research and theory leading to the development of this model can be found in Cummings, Gordon, and Marlatt (1980), Marlatt (1978, 1982), Marlatt and Gordon (1980, 1985), and Shiffman and Wills (1985). The following overview draws extensively from these previously published accounts of the model and represents an updated version of the RP overview presented by Marlatt and George (1984).

To begin, we are assuming that the individual experiences a sense of perceived control while maintaining abstinence (or complying with other rules governing the target behavior). The behavior is under control so long as it does not occur during this period—the longer the period of successful abstinence, the greater the individual's perception of self-control. This perceived control will continue until the person encounters a high-risk situation. A high-risk situation is defined broadly as any situation (including emotional reactions to the situation) that poses a threat to the individual's sense of control and increases the risk of potential relapse. In an analysis of 311 initial relapse episodes obtained from clients with a variety of problem behaviors (problem drinking, smoking, heroin addiction, compulsive gambling, and overeating), we identified three primary high-risk situations that were associated with almost three quarters of all the relapses reported (see Cummings, Gordon, & Marlatt, 1980, for a description of other high-risk situations). A brief description of the three categories associated with the highest relapse rates follows.

1. *Negative emotional states* (35% of all relapses in the sample): situations in which the individual is experiencing a negative (or unpleasant) emotional state, mood, or feeling such as frustration, anger, anxiety, depression, boredom, and so forth, prior to or at the same time the first lapse occurs. For example, a smoker in the sample gave the following description of a relapse episode: "It had been raining continually all week. Saturday I walked down to the basement to do laundry and I found the basement filled with a good three inches of water. To make things worse, as I went to turn on the light to see the extent of the damage, I got shocked from the light switch. Later that same day I was feeling real low and knew I had to have a cigarette after my neighbor, who is a contractor, assessed the damage at over $4,000. I went to the store and bought a pack."

2. *Interpersonal conflict* (16% of the relapses): situations involving an ongoing or relatively recent conflict associated with any interpersonal relationship, such as marriage, friendship, family members, or employer–employee relations. Arguments and interpersonal confrontations occur frequently in this category. A gambler who had been abstaining from betting on the horses described his relapse in the following terms: "I came home late from a horrible day on the road and I hadn't stepped in the house 5 minutes before my wife started accusing me of gambling on the horses. Racetrack, hell! I told her if she didn't believe me, I'd give her a real reason to file for divorce. That night I spent $450 on the Longacres track."

3. *Social pressure* (20% of the sample): situations in which the individual is responding to the influence of another person or group of people who exert pressure on the individual to engage in the taboo behavior. Social pressure may either be direct (direct interpersonal contact with verbal persuasion) or indirect (e.g., being in the presence of others who are engaging in the same target behavior, even though no direct pressure is involved). Here is an example of direct social pressure given by a formerly abstinent problem drinker in our sample: "I went to my boss's house for a surprise birthday dinner for him. I got there late and as I came into the living room everyone had a drink in hand. I froze when the boss's wife asked me what I was drinking. Without thinking, I said, 'J&B on the rocks.'"

In our analyses of relapse episodes to date, we found more similarities than differences in relapse categories across the various addictive behaviors. These same three high-risk situations are frequently found to be associated with relapse, regardless of the particular problem involved (problem drinking, smoking, gambling, heroin use, or overeating). This pattern of findings lends support to our hypothesis that there is a common mechanism underlying the relapse process across different addictive behaviors.

If the individual is able to execute an effective coping response in the high-risk situation (e.g., is assertive in counteracting social pressures), the probability of relapse decreases significantly. The individual who copes successfully with the situation is likely to experience a sense of mastery or perception of control. Successful mastery of one problematic situation is often associated with an expectation of being able to cope successfully with the next challenging event. The expectancy of being able to cope with successive high-risk situations as they develop is closely associated with Bandura's notion of *self-efficacy* (Bandura, 1977), defined as the individual's expectation concerning the capacity to cope with an impending situation or task. A feeling of confidence in one's abilities to cope effectively with a high-risk situation is associated with an increased perception of self-efficacy, a kind of "I know I can handle it" feeling. As the duration of the abstinence (or period of controlled use) increases, and the individual is able to cope effectively with more and more high-risk situations, perception of control increases in a cumulative fashion. The probability of relapse decreases accordingly.

What happens if an individual does not cope successfully with a high-risk situation? The person may never have acquired the coping skills involved, or the appropriate response may be inhibited by fear or anxiety. Perhaps the individual fails to recognize and respond to the risk involved before it is too late. Motivational deficits may also undermine acquired coping strategies. Whatever the reason, as self-efficacy decreases in the precipitating high-risk situation, one's expectations for coping successfully with subsequent problem situations also begins to decrease. If the situation also involves the temptation to engage in the prohibited behavior as a means of attempting to cope with the stress involved, the stage is set for a probable relapse. The probability of relapse is enhanced if the individual holds *positive expectancies* about the effects of the activity of substance involved. Often the person will anticipate the immediate positive effects of the activity, an anticipation based on past experience, while ignoring or not attending to the delayed negative consequences involved. The lure of immediate gratification becomes the dominant figure in the perceptual field as the reality of the full consequences of the act recedes into the background. For many persons, smoking a cigarette or taking a drink has long been associated with coping with stress. "A drink would sure help me get through this" or "If only I could have a smoke, I would feel more relaxed" are common beliefs of this type. Positive outcome expectancies are a primary determinant of alcohol use and other forms of substance abuse (Marlatt, 1987; Marlatt & Rohsenow, 1980). Expectancies figure prominently as determinants of relapse in the RP model.

The inability to cope effectively in a high-risk situation, coupled with positive outcome expectancies for the effects of the habitual coping behavior, greatly increases the probability that an initial lapse will occur. On the one hand, the individual is faced with a high-risk situation with no coping response available; self-efficacy decreases as the person feels less able to exert control. On the other hand, there is the lure of the old coping response, the drink, the drug, or other substance. At this point, unless a last-minute coping response or a sudden change of circumstance occurs, the individual may cross over the border from abstinence (or controlled use) to relapse. Whether or not this first excursion over the line, the first lapse, is followed by a total relapse depends to a large extent on the individual's perceptions of the "cause" of the lapse and the reactions associated with its occurrence.

The requirement of abstinence is an absolute dictum. Once someone has crossed over the line, there is no going back. From this all-or-none perspective, a single drink or cigarette is sufficient to violate the rule of abstinence: once committed, the deed cannot be undone. After a lapse experience, the person is likely to experience a decrease in self-efficacy, frequently coupled with a sense of helplessness and a tendency to passively give in to the situation. "It's no use, I can't handle this" is a common reaction. To account for this reaction to the transgression of an absolute rule, we have postulated a mechanism called the *Abstinence Violation Effect* or AVE (Curry, Gordon, & Marlatt, 1987; Marlatt & Gordon, 1985). The AVE is postulated to occur under the following conditions: Prior to the first lapse, the individual is personally committed to an extended or indefinite period of abstinence. The intensity of the AVE will vary as a function of several factors, including the degree of prior commitment or effort expended to maintain abstinence, the duration of the abstinence period (the longer the period, the greater the effect), and the subjective value or importance of the prohibited behavior to the individual. We hypothesize that the AVE is characterized by two key cognitive–affective elements: cognitive dissonance (conflict and guilt), and a personal attribution effect (blaming the self as the cause of the relapse).

COVERT ANTECEDENTS AND RELAPSE SET-UPS

In the foregoing discussion of the immediate determinants and reactions to relapse, the high-risk situation is viewed as the precipitating or triggering situation associated with the initial lapse or first "slip" following a period of abstinence or controlled use. In many of the relapse episodes we have studied in our research program, the first lapse is precipitated in a high-risk situation that the individual unexpectedly encounters. In many cases the person is not expecting the high-risk situation to occur and/or is generally insufficiently prepared to cope effectively with the circumstances as they arise. Quite often, individuals will suddenly find themselves in a rapidly escalating situation that cannot be dealt with effectively. For example, one of our clients who had a serious drinking problem experienced her first lapse after several weeks of abstinence when she treated a new friend to lunch. A last-minute change of plans led them to eat at a restaurant that served alcoholic beverages. Just moments after their arrival, a cocktail waitress approached their table and asked for drink orders. Our client's friend ordered a cocktail first, and then the waitress turned to the client saying, "And you?" She too ordered a drink, the first of a series of events that culminated in a full-blown relapse. As the client said later, "I didn't plan it and I wasn't prepared for it." Suddenly confronted with a high-risk situation (a social-pressure situation, in which the client was influenced both by her friend's ordering a drink and by the waitress asking her for an order), she was unable to cope effectively.

In other relapse episodes, however, the high-risk situation appears to be the last link in a chain of events preceding the first lapse. In another case study, for example, the client was a compulsive gambler who came to us for help in controlling his habit, which had caused him numerous marital and financial problems. Although he had abstained from all gambling for about 6 months, he had had a relapse and was unable to regain abstinence. We asked the client, a resident of Seattle, to describe this last relapse episode. "There's nothing much to talk about," he began. "I was in Reno and I started gambling again." Reno, Nevada is clearly a high-risk city for any gambler trying to maintain abstinence. We then asked him to describe the events preceding his arrival in Reno (Reno is 1,000 miles from Seattle). A close analysis of this chain of events led us to the conclusion that this client had covertly set up or "planned" the relapse. Although our client strongly denied his responsibility in this covert planning process, it was clear to us that there were a number of choice points (forks in the road) preceding the relapse where the client "chose" an alternative that led him closer to the brink of relapse. He finally ended up in a downtown Reno casino where he succumbed to a slot machine, an event that triggered a weekend-long binge of costly gambling. It was as if he had placed himself in a situation that was so risky only a moral Superman could have resisted the temptation to resume gambling.

Why do some clients appear to set up their own relapse? From a cost-benefit perspective, a relapse can be seen as a very rational choice or decision for many individuals. The benefit is swift in coming: the payoff of immediate gratification (and the chance of hitting the jackpot). For many the reward of instant gratification far outweighs the cost of potential negative effects that may or may not occur sometime in the distant future (especially if one is a gambler at heart). Why not take the chance—this time it might be different, and perhaps it could be done with impunity? Cognitive distortions such as denial and rationalization make it much easier to set up one's own relapse episode: One may deny both the intent to relapse and the importance of long-range negative consequences. There are also many excuses to rationalize the act of indulgence.

One of the most tempting rationalizations is that the desire to indulge is justified. This justification is exemplified in the title of a book describing the drinking life-styles of derelict alcoholics: *You Owe Yourself a Drunk* (Spradley, 1970). Our research findings and clinical experience in working with a variety of addictive behavior problems suggest that the degree of balance in a person's daily life-style has a significant impact on the desire for indulgence or immediate gratification. Here we are defining "balance" as the degree of equilibrium that exists in one's daily life between those activities perceived as external demands (or "shoulds") and those perceived as activities the person engages in for pleasure or self-fulfillment (the "wants"). Paying household bills and performing routine chores or menial tasks at work would count highly as "shoulds" for many individuals. At the other end of the scale are the "wants"—the activities the person likes to perform and gains some immediate gratification from engaging in (e.g., going fishing, taking time off for lunch with a friend, engaging in a creative work task, etc.). Other activities represent a mixture of "wants" and "shoulds." We find that a life-style encumbered with a preponderance of perceived "shoulds" is often associated with an increased perception of self-deprivation and a corresponding desire for indulgence and gratification. It is as if the person who spends his or her entire day engaged in activities that are high in external demand (often perceived as "hassling" events) attempts to balance this disequilibrium by engaging in an excessive "want" as a means of justifying self-indulgence at the end of the day (e.g., drinking to excess in the evening).

ASSESSMENT AND INTERVENTION STRATEGIES

In this section, we present highlights of the RP assessment and intervention strategies. We first discuss strategies that are designed to teach the client how to anticipate and cope with the possibility of relapse, how to recognize and cope with high-risk situations that may precipitate a lapse, and how to modify his or her cognitions and other reactions and thus prevent a single lapse from developing into a full-blown relapse. Because these procedures are explicitly focused on the immediate precipitants of the relapse process, we refer to them collectively as *specific intervention strategies*. Second, we present strategies designed to rebalance the client's life-style and to identify and cope with covert determinants of relapse. We refer to these procedures as *global self-control strategies*.

Both specific and global RP strategies can be placed in three main categories: skill training, cognitive reframing, and life-style rebalancing. Skill-training strategies include both behavioral and cognitive responses to cope with high-risk situations. Cognitive reframing procedures are designed to provide the client with alternative cognitions concerning the nature of the habit-change process (i.e., to view it as a learning process), to introduce coping imagery to deal with urges and early warning signals, and to reframe reactions to the initial lapse (restructuring of the AVE). Finally, life-style rebalancing strategies (e.g., relaxation and exercise) are designed to strengthen the client's overall coping capacity and to reduce the frequency and intensity of urges and craving that are often the product of an unbalanced life-style.

Which of the various intervention techniques should be applied with a particular client? It is possible to combine techniques into a standardized "package," with each subject receiving identical components, if the purpose is to evaluate the effectiveness of a package program. Most readers, however, will be applying the RP model with clients in an applied clinical setting. In contrast to the demands of treatment outcome research, clinicians typically prefer to develop an individualized program of techniques for each client. The individualized approach is the one we recommend for most clients. Specific techniques should be selected based on a carefully conducted assessment program (Donovan & Marlatt, 1988). Therapists are encouraged to select intervention techniques based on their initial evaluation and assessment of the client's problem and general life-style pattern. The overall goal of the specific intervention procedures is to teach the client to anticipate and cope with the possibility of relapse: to recognize and cope with high-risk situations that may precipitate a slip, and to modify cognitions and other reactions so as to prevent a single lapse from developing into a full-blown relapse.

The first step in the prevention of relapse is to teach the client to recognize high-risk situations that may precipitate or trigger a relapse. Here, the sooner one become aware that one is involved in a chain of events that increases the probability of a slip or lapse, the sooner one can intervene by performing an appropriate coping skill and/or recognize and respond to the discriminative stimuli associated with entering a high-risk situation, using these cues both as warning signals and as reminders to engage in alternative or remedial action.

To introduce a metaphor that we use with our clients, imagine that the client involved in a self-control program is a driver setting out on a highway journey. The trip itinerary (i.e., moving from excessive drug use to abstinence) includes both "easy" and "hard" stretches of road (from the plains to mountain passes). From this metaphorical perspective, the high-risk situations are equivalent to those dangerous parts of the trip where the driver must use extra caution and driving skills to keep the car on the road and prevent an accident. The discriminative stimuli that signal a high-risk situation can be thought of as highway signs providing the driver with information about upcoming dangers and risks on the road (e.g., "Icy patches ahead: SLOW to 25"). The responsible, alert driver is trained to keep an eye out for these signs and to take appropriate action to prevent a mishap. Similarly, the person attempting to refrain from engaging in a particular target behavior (smoking, drinking, overindulging, etc.) must be on the lookout for cues that signal the proximity of potentially troublesome situations. These cues are early warning signals that remind the individual to "Stop, Look, and Listen" and to engage in an appropriate coping response. The sooner these signs are noticed, the easier it is to anticipate what lies around the next bend and to take appropriate steps for effectively dealing with the situation.

An essential aspect of teaching clients to handle high-risk situations more effectively is to first enable them to identify and anticipate these situations. Earlier we discussed prototypic kinds of high-risk situations. However, ultimately the identification of high-risk situations is an individualized question requiring idiographic assessment procedures. Whenever it is possible to have clients keep a record of their addictive behaviors for a baseline period prior to treatment, self-monitoring procedures offer an effective method for assessing high-risk situations. As little as 2 weeks of self-monitoring data can often highlight the situational influences and skill deficits that underlie an addictive behavior pattern.

In the assessment of self-efficacy, the client is presented with a list of potential relapse situations. For each situation the client uses a rating scale to estimate his or her subjective expectation of successful coping. Ratings across a wide range of situations enable the individual to identify both problematic situations and skill deficits in need of remedial training. Results from these types of assessment can later dictate the focus of skill-training procedures. Self-efficacy scales have been developed for addictive behavior problems such as smoking (Condiotte & Lichtenstein, 1981) and alcoholism (Annis, 1986).

Determining the adequacy of preexisting coping abilities is a critical assessment target. In a treatment outcome investigation aimed at teaching alcoholics to handle situational temptations, Chaney, O'Leary, and Marlatt (1978) devised the Situational Competency Test to measure coping ability. In this technique, the client is presented with a series of written or audiotaped descriptions of potential relapse situations. Each description ends with a prompt for the client to respond. Later, the client's responses to the scenes are scored on a number of dimensions, including response duration and latency, degree of compliance, and specification of alternative behaviors.

Carefully executed assessment procedures will enable the individual to identify many high-risk situations. The client must then learn an alternative approach for responding to these situations. A first step in this new approach is to recognize that high-risk situations are best perceived as discriminative stimuli signaling the need for behavior change in the same way that road signs signal the need for alternative action. When viewed in this way, these situations can be seen as junctures where choices are made rather than as inevitable and uncontrollable challenges that must be endured. In this light, the choice to simply avoid or take a detour around risky situations becomes more available to the individual. However, routine avoidance of particular high-risk situations is unrealistic.

Therefore, clients must acquire coping skills that enable them to cope with these situations.

Remedial skill training necessitated by identification of coping skill deficits is the cornerstone of the RP treatment program. When the individual lacks coping skills, a variety of remedial skills can be taught. The content of the skill-training program is variable and will depend on the needs of the individual. Possible content areas include assertiveness, stress management, relaxation training, anger management, communication skills, and general social and/or dating skills. In addition to these specific content areas, the RP approach routinely includes training in more general problem-solving skills (Goldfried & Davison, 1976). The advantage of this latter feature is that it provides the client with a set of highly flexible skills that are generalizable across situations and problem areas. Equipping the client with general problem-solving skills obviates the need for overreliance on rote memorization and execution of the relatively mechanized behavioral prescriptions that often typify content-focused skill-training programs. In skill training, the actual teaching procedures are based on the work of McFall (1976) and other investigators. The range of methods includes behavior rehearsal, instruction, coaching, evaluative feedback, modeling, and role playing. In addition, Meichenbaum's (1977) work on cognitive self-instruction has proven especially valuable for teaching clients constructive self-statements. For troubleshooting and consolidating the newly acquired skills, regular homework assignments are an essential ingredient in skill training.

To reiterate, implementation of a specific skill-training program will be dictated by the client's unique profile of high-risk situations. If the individual typically drinks or overdrinks after arguments with a spouse or significant other, then communication or anger-management skills are indicated. If risky encounters revolve around contact with the opposite sex, then dating and social skills may be recommended. To illustrate with a specific example, suppose that the client's drinking routinely follows interpersonal interactions where he or she passively submits to unreasonable demands from others. The clear indication here is for assertiveness training. To accomplish this, a therapist would begin by advising the client of his or her personal rights in the situation and proceed with instruction on the principles of assertion, modeling of an assertive response, role-playing the interaction with the client, providing coaching and corrective feedback, and encouragement to rehearse and implement the new behaviors.

In some instances, it will be impractical to rehearse the new coping skills in real-life situations. This problem can be surmounted through *relapse rehearsal*. In this procedure, the client is instructed to imagine being in actual high-risk situations, but performing more adaptive behaviors and thinking more adaptive thoughts. The emphasis here is on *coping* rather than *mastery* imagery. That is, the individual is encouraged to visualize that he or she is successfully handling the difficult situation through some effortful struggle rather than through easy mastery. To emphasize self-efficacy enhancement, the client may be instructed to imagine that the rehearsed experience is accompanied by mounting feelings of competence and confidence. As a consequence, the person experiences heightened expectations of successful coping in future real-life situations, thereby reducing the probability of relapse. We have found that the relapse rehearsal procedure can be readily carried out as an intersession homework assignment.

That the client may fail to effectively employ these coping strategies and experience a slip must be anticipated. The client's postslip reaction is a pivotal intervention point in the RP model because it determines the degree of escalation from a single isolated slip to a full-blown relapse. The first step in anticipating and dealing with this reaction is to devise an explicit therapeutic contract to limit the extent of substance use if a slip occurs. The contract specifications should be worked out individually with the client. However, the fundamental method of intervention after a slip is to use cognitive restructuring to counter the cognitive and affective components of the AVE. The main objective here is to enable the client to construe the slip as a unique occurrence, a mistake. If instead he or she views the slip as an irreversible failure and succumbs to the conflict, guilt, and personal attribution that characterize the AVE, then a full-blown relapse is more likely to occur. A highly useful technique here is to have the client carry a wallet-sized reminder card with instructions to read and follow in the event of a slip. The text of this card should include the name and phone number of a therapist or treatment center to be called, as well as a cognitive reframing antidote to the AVE.

The final thrust in the RP self-management program is the global intervention procedure of life-style rebalancing. It is insufficient to teach clients mechanistic skills for handling high-risk situations and regulating consumption. A comprehensive self-management program must also improve the client's overall life-style and thus increase his or her capacity to cope with more pervasive stress factors, antecedents to the occurrence of high-risk situations. To accomplish this training, a number of treatment strategies have been devised to short-circuit the covert antecedents to relapse and promote mental and physical wellness.

In an unbalanced life-style, a persistent and continuing disequilibrium between shoulds and wants can pave the way for relapse by producing a chronic sense of deprivation. To reiterate, when the individual perceives his or her life-style as predominated by duties and obligations and as lacking commensurate indulgence in gratifying activities, then a sense of deprivation begins to accrue. As these feelings mount, the person may experience a growing desire to treat himself or herself to an immediately gratifying indulgence. For most clients, drug use is a source of immediate gratification and a method for restoring balance to an "unfairly" lopsided equation. This desire for indulgence translates into urges, cravings, and cognitive distortions that lead clients "unintentionally" closer to the brink of relapse.

An effective method to induce clients to view the disequilibrium of wants and shoulds as a precursor of relapse is to have them self-monitor the number of wants and shoulds that prevail in their lives. By keeping a daily record of duties and obligations on one hand and indulgences on the other, clients can soon become acutely aware of the discrepancy between shoulds and wants. Next, the client should be encouraged to seek a restoration of balance by making time each day to engage in worthwhile indulgences, including more positive addictions. Glasser (1974) described negative addictions (e.g., excessive drinking) as activities that initially feel good but produce long-term harm. Conversely, positive addictions (e.g., running) produce short-term discomfort while yielding long-range benefits. After short-range disincentives have been surmounted, a positive addiction acquires a great deal of attraction value for the individual and comes to be perceived as a want. At this point, the person feels deprived if prevented from engaging in the activity. Furthermore, positive addictions contribute toward the person's long-term health and well-being while also providing an adaptive coping response for life stressors and relapse-risk situations. As long-range health benefits accrue, the person begins to develop more self-confidence and self-efficacy.

Activities having potential for positive addiction include meditation, relaxation procedures, and aerobic exercise. Meditation and other relaxation techniques (Marlatt & Marques, 1977) offer an easily learnable and readily available method for achieving a constructive "high" experience. Jogging and regular exercise regimes require more physical exertion and perhaps more attention to scheduling (particularly if done with others), but also provide sources of constructive personal indulgence. Recent research in our laboratory has shown that a regular program of aerobic exercise (running) is associated with a significant reduction in drinking behavior among heavy drinkers (Murphy, Pagano, & Marlatt, 1986).

Despite the efficacy of these techniques for counteracting feelings of deprivation that would otherwise predispose the individual toward relapse, occasional urges and cravings may still surface from time to time. For this reason, various urge-control procedures are recommended. Sometimes urges and cravings are directly triggered by external cues like the sight of one's favorite beer mug or wine goblet in the kitchen cabinet, or meeting an old friend who is a heavy smoker. The frequency of these externally triggered urges can be substantially reduced by employing simple stimulus control techniques aimed at minimizing exposure to these cues. In some instances, avoidance strategies offer the most effective way of reducing the frequency of externally triggered urges. Certain events or situations like the biweekly poker games or the wine section of the local grocery may just have to be avoided temporarily while the individual develops more coping skills. Generally, avoidance strategies can often come in handy for dealing with unexpected high-risk situations that emerge. A selection of viable avoidance strategies can enhance the individual's sense of choice when confronted with dangerous situations.

In teaching clients to cope with urge and craving experiences, it is important to emphasize that the discomfort associated with these internal events is natural. Often the person undergoing cravings has a tendency to feel as though the discomfort will continue to mount precipitously until resistance collapses under the overwhelming weight of a ballooning urge. In working with this concern, we stress that urges and cravings are often triggered by environmental cues; they rise in intensity, reach a peak, and then subside. In this respect, urges can be likened to waves in the sea: they rise, crest, and fall. Using this metaphor, we encourage the client to wait out the urge, to look forward to the downside, and to endure that time when the urge discomfort is peaking.

Recall that urges and cravings may not always operate at a conscious level but may become masked by cognitive distortions and defense mechanisms. As such they can still exert a potent influence by allowing for "apparently irrelevant decisions" that inch the person closer to relapse. To counter this, we train the client to see through these self-deceptions by recognizing their true meanings. Explicit self-talk can help in making apparently irrelevant decisions seem more relevant. By acknowledging to oneself that certain "minidecisions" (e.g., keeping wine at home in case friends drop over) actually represent urges and cravings, one becomes able to use these experiences as early warning signals. An important objective in these urge-control techniques is to enable the individual to externalize urges and cravings and to view them with detachment. Another way to achieve this detachment is to encourage the client to deliberately label the urge as soon as it registers into consciousness. Urges should be viewed as natural occurrences that happen in response to environmental and life-style forces rather than as signs of being a failure and indicators of future relapse.

EMPIRICAL SUPPORT AND FUTURE DIRECTIONS

The RP model discussed in this chapter is still in the formative stages of development. The empirical underpinnings of this approach have been reviewed by Marlatt and Gordon (1985). As for treatment efficacy, only a few outcome studies have appeared in the literature that have compared the RP model with other approaches to the treatment of addiction or the prevention of relapse, although research is currently under way on this issue. The few outcome studies that have appeared, along with research on the role of expectancies (self-efficacy and outcome expectancies) and coping skills in the habit-change process, have provided general support for the model (Abrams, Niaura, Carey, Monti, & Binkoff, 1986; Brownell et al., 1986; Shiffman & Wills, 1985).

Most research has been conducted in the areas of alcohol dependency and smoking, although work is under way applying the RP model to other addictive behaviors. In the alcohol field, the pioneering work of Litman and her colleagues at the Addiction Research Unit at the Maudsley Hospital has provided valuable insight into the role of coping with high-risk situations as a factor that discriminates between alcoholics who relapse after treatment and those who "survive" or show a good treatment outcome. Litman and her co-workers have provided extensive documentation of relapse situations and associated coping responses related to treatment outcome (Litman, 1980; Litman, Eiser, Rawson, & Oppenheim, 1977, 1979; Litman, Eiser, & Taylor, 1979).

Similar research on the role of coping as a factor reducing relapse risk among ex-smokers has been described by Shiffman and his colleagues (Shiffman, 1982, 1984; Shiffman, Read, Maltese, Rapkin, & Jarvik, 1985). Related studies in the smoking area have shown that self-efficacy ratings are valid predictors of subsequent treatment outcome (Baer & Lichtenstein, 1988; Condiotte & Lichtenstein, 1981; DiClemente, 1981).

Skill-training approaches have also received some attention in the treatment-outcome literature. To take a specific example from our own skill-training research with alcoholic clients (Chaney, O'Leary, & Marlatt, 1978), the client's responses to the Situational Competency Test are first considered in planning the specific skill-training program. For one particular client, the problem may involve an inability to resist social pressure to indulge; for another, the problem may involve a deficit in coping with feelings of loneliness or depression. In the skill-training program described in the Chaney et al. study, alcoholics in treatment met together in a small group for a series of treatment sessions. Each group was led by two therapists, who began by describing a particular high-risk situation. The group members then discussed the situation and generated various ways of responding to it. The therapists then modeled an appropriate coping response and practiced it in front of the group. During this procedure, each client received individualized feedback from group members and specific coaching and instructions from the therapists. The client was then required to repeat the coping response until it matched the therapists' criteria for adequacy. This particular skill-training program was evaluated in a year-long follow-up study in comparison with two control groups: a group that spent an equivalent amount of time discussing their emotional reactions to the same high-risk situations (as in psychodynamic group therapy), and a no-treatment control condition (regular hospital program only). The skill-training condition proved to be more successful than either control group, showing a significant improvement at the 1-year follow-up period for such variables as amount of posttreatment drinking, duration of time spent drinking before regaining abstinence, and frequency of periods of intoxication. Similar positive results for skill training with alcoholics have been reported in recent studies by Jones and Lanyon (1981) and Oei and Jackson (1982).

A final question concerns the range of application of the RP model. The primary focus is on the application of RP principles to the modification of addictive behaviors in the usual sense of the term: excessive use of alcohol, tobacco, food, or other substance abuse problems. The model does, however, seem to have applications in areas other than addictive behavior or substance abuse. One such area is sexual aggression. In the treatment of the sexual aggressor (e.g., pedophiles and rapists), the overall goal is the same as it often is in the treatment of addiction: to abstain from engaging in the taboo behavior. A recent chapter by Pithers, Marques, Gibat, and Marlatt (1983) explores the application of the RP model in the treatment of sexual aggression. Despite emerging empirical support, many basic tenets of the RP model and the effectiveness of its approach with various addictive behaviors have yet to be firmly established. Based on future research, refinement of the basic assumptions and clinical applications of the relapse prevention model will undoubtedly occur.

REFERENCES

Abrams, D. B., Niaura, R. S., Carey, K. B., Monti, P. M., & Binkoff, J. A. (1986). Understanding relapse and recovery in alcohol abuse. *Annals of Behavioral Medicine, 8,* 27-32.

Annis, H. M. (1986). A relapse prevention model for treatment of alcoholics. In W. R. Miller & N. Heather (Eds.), *Treating addictive behaviors* (pp. 407-421). New York: Plenum.

Baer, J. S., & Lichtenstein, E. (1988). Classification and prediction of smoking relapse episodes: An exploration of individual differences. *Journal of Consulting and Clinical Psychology, 56,* 104-110.

Bandura, A. (1977). *Social learning theory.* Englewood Cliffs, NJ: Prentice-Hall.

Bandura, A. (1986). *Social foundations of thought and action: A social cognitive theory.* Englewood Cliffs, NJ: Prentice-Hall.

Brickman, P., Rabinowitz, V. C., Karuza, J., Coates, D., Cohn, E., & Kidder, L. (1982). Models of helping and coping. *American Psychologist, 37,* 368-384.

Brownell, K. D., Marlatt, G. A., Lichtenstein, E., & Wilson, G. T. (1986). Understanding and preventing relapse. *American Psychologist, 41,* 765-782.

Chaney, E. F., O'Leary, M. R., & Marlatt, G. A. (1978). Skill training with alcoholics. *Journal of Consulting and Clinical Psychology, 46,* 1092-1104.

Condiotte, M. M., & Lichtenstein, E. (1981). Self-efficacy and relapse in smoking cessation programs. *Journal of Consulting and Clinical Psychology, 49,* 648-658.

Cummings, C., Gordon, J. R., & Marlatt, G. A. (1980). Relapse: Strategies of prevention and prediction. In W. R. Miller (Ed.), *The addictive behaviors: Treatment of alcoholism, drug abuse, smoking, and obesity* (pp. 291-321). Oxford, England: Pergamon Press.

Curry, S. G., Gordon, J. R., & Marlatt, G. A. (1987). Abstinence violation effect: Validation of an attributional construct with smoking cessation. *Journal of Consulting and Clinical Psychology, 55,* 145-149.

DiClemente, C. C. (1981). Self-efficacy and smoking cessation maintenance. *Cognitive Research and Therapy, 5,* 175-187.

Donovan, D. M., & Marlatt, G. A. (1988). *Assessment of addictive behaviors: Behavioral, cognitive, and physiological processes.* New York: Guilford Press.

Glasser, W. (1974). *Positive addiction.* New York: Harper & Row.

Goldfried, M. R., & Davison, G. C. (1976). *Clinical behavior therapy.* New York: Holt, Rinehart & Winston.

Hall, S. (1980). Self-management and therapeutic maintenance: Theory and research. In P. Karoly & J. J. Steffen (Eds.), *Toward a psychology of therapeutic maintenance: Widening perspectives* (pp. 263–300). New York: Gardner Press.

Jones, S. L., & Lanyon, R. I. (1981). Relationship between adaptive skills and sustained improvement following alcoholism treatment. *Journal of Studies on Alcohol, 42,* 521–525.

Litman, A. (1980). Relapse in alcoholism: Traditional and current approaches. In G. Edwards & M. Grant (Eds.), *Alcoholism treatment in transition* (pp. 294–303). Baltimore: University Park Press.

Litman, G. K., Eiser, J. R., Rawson, N. S. B., & Oppenheim, A. N. (1977). Towards a typology of relapse: A preliminary report. *Drug and Alcohol Dependence, 2,* 157–162.

Litman, G. K., Eiser, J. R., Rawson, N. S. B., & Oppenheim, A. N. (1979). Differences in relapse precipitants and coping behaviours between alcoholic relapsers and survivors. *Behaviour Research and Therapy, 17,* 89–94.

Litman, G. K., Eiser, J. R., & Taylor, C. (1979). Dependence, relapse and extinction: A theoretical critique and behavioral examination. *Journal of Clinical Psychology, 35,* 192–199.

Marlatt, G. A. (1978). Craving for alcohol, loss of control, and relapse: A cognitive-behavioral analysis. In P. E. Nathan, G. A. Marlatt, & T. Loberg (Eds.), *Alcoholism: New directions in behavioral research and treatment* (pp. 271–314). New York: Plenum.

Marlatt, G. A. (1982). Relapse prevention: A self-control program for the treatment of addictive behaviors. In R. B. Stuart (Ed.), *Adherence, compliance, and generalization in behavioral medicine* (pp. 329–378). New York: Brunner/Mazel.

Marlatt, G. A. (1987). Alcohol, the magic elixir: Stress, expectancy, and the transformation of emotional states. In E. Gottheil, K. A. Druly, S. Pashko, & S. P. Weinstein (Eds.), *Stress and addiction* (pp. 302–322). New York: Brunner/Mazel.

Marlatt, G. A., & George, W. H. (1984). Relapse prevention: Introduction and overview of the model. *British Journal of Addiction, 79,* 261–273.

Marlatt, G. A., & Gordon, J. R. (1980). Determinants of relapse: Implications for the maintenance of behavior change. In P. O. Davidson & S. M. Davidson (Eds.), *Behavioral medicine: Changing health lifestyles* (pp. 410–452). New York: Brunner/Mazel.

Marlatt, G. A., & Gordon, J. R. (Eds.). (1985). *Relapse prevention: Maintenance strategies in the treatment of addictive behaviors.* New York: Guilford Press.

Marlatt, G. A., & Marques, J. K. (1977). Meditation, self-control, and alcohol use. In R. B. Stuart (Ed.), *Behavioral self-management: Strategies, techniques, and outcomes* (pp. 117–153). New York: Brunner/Mazel.

Marlatt, G. A., & Rohsenow, D. R. (1980). Cognitive processes in alcohol use: Expectancy and the balanced placebo design. In N. K. Mello (Ed.), *Advances in substance abuse* (Vol. 1, pp. 159–199). Greenwich, CT: JAI Press.

McFall, R. M. (1976). *Behavioral training: A skill-acquisition approach to clinical problems.* Morristown, NJ: General Learning Press.

Meichenbaum, D. (1977). *Cognitive-behavior modification.* New York: Plenum.

Murphy, T. J., Pagano, R. R., & Marlatt, G. A. (1986). Lifestyle modification with heavy alcohol drinkers: Effects of aerobic exercise and meditation. *Addictive Behaviors, 11,* 175–186.

Oei, T. P. S., & Jackson, P. R. (1982). Social skills and cognitive behavioral approaches to the treatment of problem drinking. *Journal of Studies in Alcohol, 43,* 532–547.

Pithers, W. D., Marques, J. K., Gibat, C. C., & Marlatt, G. A. (1983). Relapse prevention with sexual aggressives: A self-control model of treatment and maintenance of change. In J. G. Greer & I. R. Stuart (Eds.), *The sexual aggressor: Current perspectives on treatment* (pp. 214–239). New York: Van Nostrand Reinhold.

Shiffman, S. (1982). Relapse following smoking cessation: A situational analysis. *Journal of Consulting and Clinical Psychology, 50,* 71–86.

Shiffman, S. (1984). Coping with temptations to smoke. *Journal of Consulting and Clinical Psychology, 52,* 261–267.

Shiffman, S., Read, L., Maltese, J., Rapkin, D., & Jarvik, M. E. (1985). Preventing relapse in ex-smokers: A self-management approach. In G. A. Marlatt & J. R. Gordon (Eds.), *Relapse prevention: Maintenance strategies in the treatment of addictive behaviors* (pp. 472–520). New York: Guilford Press.

Shiffman, S., & Wills, T. A. (Eds.). (1985). *Coping and substance use.* New York: Academic Press.

Spradley, J. P. (1970). *You owe yourself a drunk.* Boston: Little, Brown.

3

Predicting Adherence to Prescribed Regimens Using the Health Perceptions Questionnaire (HPQ)

Dwight L. Goodwin, William Insull, Jr.,
Michael Russell, Jeffrey Probstfield

The investigation of patient nonadherence to prescribed regimens has failed to provide a clear understanding of either its etiology or treatment. While factors have been identified that demonstrate consistent associations with adherence, few have offered a sound basis for patient planning or correction. The foundation of knowledge surrounding adherence, however, is formidable and offers the

This investigation was supported in part by USPHS Senior Postdoctoral Fellowship #F33 HL6245-01,1 and grants from the Merck Sharp and Dohme Research Laboratories and the Best Foods Co. We gratefully acknowledge the volunteer men and women for their dedication to the clinical trial and the skilled assistance of Linda Hicks, M.S., R.D.; Janice Henske, M.P.H., R.D., and B. J. Whitfill-Byington, M.S. R.D.

investigator a basis for the further development of models that can extend the boundaries of direct patient care and treatment.

This chapter will report on an investigation of patient adherence that sought to identify and measure factors that would achieve three objectives: (1) provide for an improved understanding of factors influencing adherence; (2) allow for the prediction of patient adherence, and (3) provide a basis for the selection of interventions to improve adherence behaviors. A literature review, information reported by adherence counselors, and the clinical experience of these investigators confirms that adherence can be understood best as the result of several factors, each having its own independent and interactive effects on individual patient behavior. As these factors are identified, measured, and managed for optimum adherence, nonadherence may cease to continue to be a substantial barrier to the effective treatment of disease.

The theoretical foundation for this investigation was the cognitive–social learning model (Bandura & Walters, 1963; Kanfer & Phillips, 1970; Mahoney, 1974), which regards behavior as acquired, maintained, or weakened as a function of interactions between the patient and his or her environment. Thus, adherence behaviors can be understood, predicted, and modified by an assessment of ongoing events in the patient's environment and of how the patient perceives the impact of these events in daily life. The thought processes that interface between the external environment and the formation of the patient's perception of those events has been described by Bandura (1977), Mahoney (1977), and Meichenbaum (1977). While this position acknowledges the significance of such cognitive functions as beliefs, understandings, and intentions, cognitive–behavioral theory also emphasizes the contribution of the environment in providing models for behavior, incentives for performance, and an intricate array of signals and cues that ultimately determine whether a specific behavior occurs or not. The patient may be clear about his or her susceptibility to a disease and understand and believe in the steps to take to diminish its effects. Good intentions may fail to materialize into proper compliance without a vivid demonstration of the specific acts that must be performed, without suitable rehearsal to be sure he or she has learned the behavior, without the sympathetic reminders of a spouse or a cue on the bathroom mirror, and without the reinforcement of an internal cue. The cognitive–behavioral position expands the predictors or causes of behavior from an assessment of patients' beliefs and understandings to an analysis of the day-to-day events and interactions that may facilitate certain classes of behaviors and suppress others.

The purpose of the investigation reported here was to develop a questionnaire, the Health Perceptions Questionnaire (HPQ), to assess patient perceptions and attitudes toward a variety of acknowledged factors and to use the patient's responses to predict adherence to treatment regimens. These factors include patients' perceptions regarding their routines, support systems, physical well-being, self-management options, and stressors.

These adherence factors were intended to provide a prospective identification of patients at risk of nonadherence to prescribed regimens. Previous efforts to prospectively identify patients at risk of nonadherence have failed to achieve sufficient variance to warrant reliable prediction (Sackett & Snow, 1979) or were too labor-intensive to be considered for practical use by the physician. As more than half the patients on long-term regimens fall below efficacious levels of medication due to nonadherence (Haynes, Taylor, & Sackett, 1979), waiting to see which patients require modification of their regimens has been regarded as a cost-effective alternative. Although extensive work has been reported on the relationship of socioeconomic factors and cardiovascular disease (Shekelle, Ostfeld, & Paul, 1969), the present investigation did not intend to address these factors other than through an examination of variables associated with factors operating in the patient's daily circumstances and perceptions about those events. It is noteworthy that researchers in the field of adherence have devoted far greater attention to exploring methods for improving the adherence of recalcitrant patients than to predicting their identity at the outset.

METHODS

This chapter describes the initial stages in the development and testing of a new instrument for predicting adherence. The HPQ was constructed and evaluated using procedures that are conventional for *de novo* development and validation of psychosocial assessment instruments. The procedures are described in three phases: (1) the development of the questionnaire; (2) estimating the instrument's reliability; and (3) comparing predictors against endpoints to assess the questionnaire's validity.

Development of the Instrument

Selecting Adherence Factors

Potential adherence factors for assessment by the HPQ were initially selected from those identified in the literature and in the authors' clinical experience. The final selection of adherence factors was guided by four criteria: (1) the amount of influence a factor may be predicted to exert on adherence behaviors, (2) the factor's usefulness in indicating possible causes for nonadherence in individual patients, (3) the degree to which the particular factor is modifiable, and (4) whether or not the factor can be measured reliably and provide a prediction to adherence endpoints. Each of these criteria is discussed below.

First, the *amount of influence* a factor may exert on adherence behaviors was estimated by a review of previous investigations in which that specific factor's ability to predict endpoints was estimated. Haynes, Taylor, and Sackett (1979) have provided a classification of factors studied for their effect on patient adherence. They have attempted to group such factors under headings of features of the disease, the referral process, clinical setting, and characteristics of the regimen. Although few single factors demonstrated consistently high correlations with adherence, the cumulative effect of a combination of factors generally offered more promise. Investigations of the health belief model, for example, have used analyses that estimate the additive effect of several factors (Becker, Maiman, Kirscht, Haetner, & Drachman, 1977; Kirscht, 1974). Investigations of specific modifications of the patient's immediate social environment have provided a more direct estimation of conditions likely to influence adherence (Dunbar, 1979).

Second, a factor's *usefulness in indicating probable causes* for nonadherence gains its value in clinical applications where the prediction and management of regimen adherence is critical in providing effective treatment or in clinical trials management. First, a near-infinite number of factors might contribute to non-adherence. Relying upon trial and error to discover the primary causes of a patient's nonadherence would be wasteful to both provider and patient. Second, the physician's effectiveness in treating patients would be substantially improved by having available a prediction of both a patient's nonadherence and the probable causes to be explored. Third, practitioners require information regarding conditions over which they or their patients exercise control in order to design strategies to overcome barriers to regimen adherence. Factors such as the amount and kind of family support a patient may require in changing a health behavior can be influenced by direct contact with family members, specifying the type of help to be offered, etc. Fourth, variables that are defined operationally would offer more promising avenues for change strategies than those more vague or ambiguous. For example, information regarding the timing of daily work routines might be of greater use in scheduling medication regimens than the patient's scores on a measure of self-esteem.

Third, the *modifiability* of a factor has not been a primary criterion in identifying variables associated with adherence. Previous efforts to predict adherence have depended upon factors that were relatively immune from manipulation, such as demographics, personality variables, and disease characteristics. A patient's age, sex, and socioeconomic or educational level are relatively stable and not amenable to modification. Personality traits also have been regarded as fixed, although efforts are currently being made to alter selected disease-relevant lifestyles such as Type A behaviors. Although disease features such as increasing symptoms and concurrent illnesses do not offer a basis for the development of interventions, they may shed light upon understanding of noncompliance (Haynes, Taylor, & Sackett, 1979). For purposes of this investigation, however, a factor's susceptibility to modification was employed as one criterion for selection.

Efforts were made to identify factors that would be amenable to modification, were identified in previous investigations as responsive to interventions, and could be defined operationally to permit reliable measurement. Consequently, we included factors such as patients' perceptions of their daily routines, the amount of control they exert over their lives, their typical response to stressors, and the amount of support to be expected from the family.

Fourth, *ease in measurement* utilizes three factors: (1) the degree to which a factor or variable lends itself to observation; (2) the clarity of the dimension being observed; and (3) the number of items or statements needed to establish a complete and accurate estimate of the factor. For example, patients' perceptions of the amount of support that could be expected from family members might be measured more reliably than more vague concepts such as the degree to which patients regard family members as loyal or devoted.

Describing Adherence Factors

The final selection of adherence factors included five areas drawn from the patient's circumstances of daily living: the regularity of daily routines, the activity of the patient's support system, perception of physical well-being, the degree of control exerted over the environment, and response to stress events. Each of these areas is described as a separate subscale.

1. *Regularity of daily routines (RE).* This subscale was designed to measure patients' preferences for routine and orderliness, and their threshold for tolerating ambiguity. In Haynes, Taylor, and Sackett's (1979) Categorial Tables of Factors Studied in Relation to Compliance, studies are not reported that expressly examine the association between adherence (by any of the several definitions) and the regularity of daily routines of patients. Yet this very area is one in which adherence counselors report spending much of their time adjusting medication schedules and suggesting aids in improving adherence. It must be noted, though, that several aspects relating to daily schedules are reported by Sackett and Haynes (1979) in their table Reasons Given for Non-compliance (Table 10, p. 466).

2. *Support system (SS).* This subscale was designed to measure the patient's perceptions of the amount of support and encouragement from family and friends. The effect of support systems has been previously studied more as a component in interventions than as a predictor of adherence and has been related more directly to behaviors and activities of a patient's support system than to evaluate the patient's perceptions of that system (Becker, Maiman, Kirscht, Haefner, & Drachman, 1977).

3. *Well-Being (WB).* This subscale was designed to measure patients' perception of their own health and well-being. The precise effect of positive or negative

views of one's own health remains unclear. While there is evidence that patients who regard themselves as more susceptible to illness adhere better than those who do not (Averill, 1973), the question of whether those who regard themselves as healthy adhere better to regimens than those who do not has not been answered. This subscale was designed to predict adherence from the participants' view of their perceived control over their own physical well-being.

4. *Self-management (SM)*. This subscale was designed to measure the degree to which patients regard themselves as effective in achieving their goals. As several items were stated in a reverse manner to avoid response set, wording of several statements reflected a vulnerability to significant events in patients' lives. A few authors have explored the importance of self-control and found positive relationships to exist between adherence to regimens and higher levels of self-control (Averill, 1973). In addition, the demonstration of effective strategies to improve adherence has included self-management strategies. The perceptioon of self-control was assumed to reflect the existence of capabilities for self-control.

5. *Stress Management (ST)*. This subscale was designed to measure patients' estimate of difficulty in coping with situations commonly associated with stress. Numerous studies have been devoted to estimating the effect of stress on the onset of disease (Holmes, 1978; Holmes & Rahe, 1967). A conflict, however, has arisen regarding the differential effects of stress measured by the number and types of life-change events as opposed to the patient's perception of those events. Byrne and Whyte (1980) report that patients' perceptions of stress were the distinguishing feature between patients suffering chest pains and diagnosed as experiencing an infarct versus those given other diagnoses and referred to other services. Those suffering a coronary event perceived life-change events as far more stressful than did those referred to other services, even though no differences were observed between the two groups in the number or type of life-change events. The Stressor Scale was included as an adherence factor to provide an additional test of the relation between perceived response to stressors and adherence to regimens.

The total subscale score was derived by the simple addition of the patient's score on each of the five subscales without equalizing for differences in number of items per scale. The scoring was designed so that higher numbers were assumed to reflect improved adherence. Subsequent multiple regression analysis did not include a subscale total.

Designing and Constructing Questionnaire Items

Six steps were taken in the design and construction of test items for the Health Perceptions Questionnaire. First, following the selection of the subscale areas, lists of statements or "item pools" were composed. These "item pools" were designed to cover the main content of each of the subscale areas. Each item described, in a word or brief phrase, a self-perception about which the respondent would have an opinion with some degree of agreement or disagreement (see Table 3.1). Second, a Likert-type scoring system was employed that allowed patients to indicate their degree of agreement or disagreement with the questionnaire statements using a five-point scale from "agree very much" to "disagree very much." Third, the items in each subscale were distributed throughout the questionnaire in a manner so as to avoid disclosing their purpose, and several were restated in a reverse manner to control for tendencies to rate all responses as positive or negative. Fourth, the newly constructed test was given a field test to see whether a group of volunteers could understand the statements and follow the directions for recording their reactions and to learn how long it would take them to answer the questionnaire. Fifth, revisions were performed, redesigning or discarding unclear statements, improving the method for recording answers, and clarifying directions for administration. These procedures yielded an initial questionnaire composed of 68 statements, which were subsequently winnowed to 49 statements that comprised the final HPQ. Sixth, the revised instrument was prepared for administration to the cohort of an ongoing controlled clinical dietary trial. The final risk factor subscales were evaluated by pools of 4- to 17-item statements apiece, Support System and Well-Being having 4, Regularity 10, Stress Management 17 and Self-Management 14.

Each participant completed the HPQ during one of the regularly scheduled visits to the clinic and was informed that the questionnaire would provide additional information on characteristics of the participants involved in the study. The average time for administration was less than 10 minutes.

Standardization of the Instrument

Overview

The HPQ's reliability and validity were tested by evaluating the test's application during a controlled clinical trial in which assessment of diet adherence was obtained by a 5-day food diary, clinician–dietician appraisal, and biochemical tests.

Description of Clinical Trial Protocol

The clinical trial compared three common edible commercial oils, sunflower, corn, and soybean, for their effects on plasma lipid, lipoprotein, and linoleic acid levels when fed as a meal ingredient to healthy normal lipidemic adult men and women. A cohort of 22 men and 31 women who were adult working individuals consumed, at home, diets of common foods prepared centrally to have 25%

calories from fat. The test fats were substituted by random sequence and constituted 49% of fat calories. Test diets were fed for 5-week periods, which were separated by 5 weeks of ad-lib diet to prevent carryover effects. The food consumed during the test diet period was confined to the dispensed items and foods from a suggested supplementary list. These supplementary foods were basically high in carbohydrate and low in fat. Adherence to these diets was monitored by trial staff using 5-day diet diaries and biochemical parameters. Blood samples were obtained for monitoring of plasma lipids, lipoproteins, and linoleic acid levels at the fourth and fifth week of both the test and ad-lib dietary periods. Data from the study demonstrated that polyunsaturated vegetable oils consumed in diets of common foods may reduce plasma concentrations of total cholesterol and low-density and high-density lipoprotein cholesterols. The lipids and lipoprotein results of this study are reported in detail elsewhere (Insull, Silvers, Hicks, & Probstfield, 1988).

Design

The questionnaires were completed by the trial participants following randomization of participants and prior to the completion of diet records and plasma lipid assays. Ratings by clinical staff of participant adherence behaviors were completed immediately following the termination of the trial.

Analyses were confined to the second and third of three controlled feeding periods defined by the trial protocol as limited dietary information was collected at baseline. For most analyses, correlations were performed between the five subscales of the HPQ and endpoints for each feeding period separately as well as with change scores, or deltas, between the second and third feeding periods.

Subject Sample

Of the total dietary trial cohort of 65 participants, 53 were included in this questionnaire standardization, of whom 35 were females and 28 males. The mean age for males was 32.7 years and for females 36.4 years, with a range from 20 to 64 years. The loss of 12 participants from the original sample of 65 occurred due to participants failing to return questionnaires.

Data Analysis

A factor-analysis procedure was completed on outcomes of the pilot study, and a correlational matrix for each subscale was computed to provide a measure of how well each of the individual items agreed with the remaining items in each subscale. This procedure, in achieving greater factorial purity, allowed for the deletion of items showing a less than .40 correlation with the item total and a recoding of items showing inverse but significant coefficients.

Reliability

The Health Perceptions Questionnaire consists of a 49-statement test that was revised from its original 68-statement length. The 49 items in turn are sub-divided into five subscales designed to measure specific factors predictive of adherence to regimens. The reliability analysis consisted of (1) the degree of agreement or equivalence between the subscales and (2) estimates of the internal consistency for the total 49-item questionnaire and split-half estimates using Cronbach's Alpha Test.

Table 3.1 presents the final 49-statement questionnaire as it is presented to patients for their response. Individual statements belonging to a particular subscale have been distributed throughout the test, and several items have been reversed to avoid tendencies to mark all items in the same manner. The membership of each item to its subscale is indicated by an x under the appropriate subscale title.

The first analysis determined the degree of agreement between each individual subscale and the total questionnaire. Table 3.2 presents a correlational matrix of the five subscales and provides the coefficient between pairs of subscales, the number of patients whose scores made up the correlation, and the level of significance. For the purposes of this investigation, a probability of .05 or less was regarded as the criterion for rejection of the null hypothesis.

The analysis indicated that several of the subscales shared common factors and that the design goal of total independence of factors as a criterion was not met. As items were written to reflect the content of specific variables associated with adherence, some of the 49 items on the questionnaire might be expected to correlate well with each other. In summary, the subscale matrix suggested that these scales were not independent, with Self-Management showing significant commonalities with other subscales.

A second analysis determined the reliability of the questionnaire by computing alphas for the total 49-items and the split-halves. These outcomes suggest that the 49 items comprising the questionnaire, when divided randomly, yield equal and acceptably high levels of agreement and hence met criteria for internal consistency.

Validity

The validity of the HPQ was established by examining the strength and direction of relationships with three independent measures of patient adherence. The three endpoint measures selected were presumed to reflect how well participants

TABLE 3.1 Item Statements and Subscale Membership in the Health Perceptions Questionnaire (HPQ)

Item	1	2	3	4	5
1. I think before I act		X			
2. I'm healthy most of the time					X
3. Life is pretty much the same from week to week	X				
4. It's hard for me to disappoint people			X		
5. I keep wondering what will go wrong next			X		
6. I schedule my time carefully		X			
7. I enjoy routines	X				
8. I want to feel more confident about my health					X
9. Disorganization bothers me	X				
10. I envy people who are physically fit					X
11. I seldom miss a day of work					X
12. I seek variety	X				
13. I like to stir up excitement in my work	X				
14. I don't like surprises in my work	X				
15. It's easy for me to gain weight			X		
16. Breaking bad habits is very difficulty for me		X			
17. I like a job that challenges me		X			
18. My life is predictable	X				
19. Even temporary setbacks are upsetting			X		
20. I like to please others around me			X		
21. I envy people who can eat all they want and not get fat			X		
22. I envy people with strong will power		X			
23. I regard myself as capable		X			
24. I can count on my family to help me stay healthy				X	
25. It's difficult for me to admit that I've failed at something		X			
26. I generally have dinner by myself				X	
27. In our family it's everyone for himself				X	
28. When I'm in a hurry, I almost always make a mistake			X		
29. I would be surprised if my family told me to stay on a diet				X	
30. I like to work at my own pace		X			
31. If I have to eat by myself, I don't have much of an appetite			X		
32. Routines are not my cup of tea	X				
33. I enjoy new challenges		X			
34. It's hard for me to accept compliments		X			
35. Hard working		X			
36. Eager for change	X				
37. Easily upset			X		
38. Works best alone			X		
39. Long suffering			X		
40. Seldom finishes anything			X		
41. Smiles easily			X		
42. Stable			X		
43. Gets things done		X			
44. Adjusts easily to change		X			
45. Conservative	X				
46. Enthusiastic		X			
47. Good natured			X		
48. Aggressive			X		
49. Strives to please			X		

*Note. Subscales are labeled as: 1. Regularity, 2. Self Management, 3. Stressors, 4. Support System, and 5. Well Being.

TABLE 3.2 Correlational Matrix of Five Subscales Derived from the Health Perceptions Questionnaire (HPQ)

	Subscales				
	SM	WB	SS	ST	RE
Self Management (SM)	—				
Well Being (WB)	.44**	—			
Support System (SS)	−.20	.02	—		
Stressors (ST)	.31**	.22	−.04	—	
Regularity (RE)	.24*	−.05	−.37**	−.16	—

n = 53
*p < .05
**p < .01

were following protocol-defined dietary regimens: (1) ratings of adherence behaviors by clinical staff; (2) self-recorded 5-day diet records; and (3) biochemical indicators from serum assays. These three measures were selected because they represent different vantage points for assessing adherence: direct observation of adherence, self-report, and biochemical measures. Each criterion possesses limitations as well as advantages, and all require inferences regarding their pertinence to the assessment of adherence of participants to a dietary regimen. As each criterion is presumed to measure different aspects of adherence, the assumption is made that their combined application will provide a broader foundation for the estimation of the HPQ's validity and strengthen its empirical support.

Each of the criterion measures is described in the following paragraphs. The Results section presents the outcomes of each of the predictors, the theoretically derived subscales, and the three factors derived from the 49-item questionnaire when correlated with endpoints of observed adherence, diet records, and biochemical assays.

Observation of Adherence Behaviors

A rating scale was developed to permit the systematic recording of observations made by clinic personnel engaged in the conduct of the study. These clinic personnel were trained in the application of this instrument and had regular and frequent opportunities at the outset of the trial and during weekly patient visits to observe the adherence behaviors of participants. Two clinic personnel were asked to rate independently several aspects of each patient's adherence based upon their observations, which included (1) keeping or rescheduling of clinic appointments and punctuality in returning requested forms, (2) positive or negative changes in direction of adherence that occurred over the course of the trial, (3) verbal behavior indicating frequency of positive comments about their participation, characteristics of the test diet, and other matters relating to protocol requirements, (4) prior success in smoking cessation and diet regimens taken from the initial interview, and (5) predictions for adherence made following the initial interview and based upon the clinic personnel's overall impression of the patient.

Comparisons of the independent ratings of the two clinical staff members responsible for implementing the protocol yielded Spearman ρ coefficients of greater than .90 for each of the four dimensions. The Spearman formula was selected because the data collected were essentially ordinal in nature and more conservatively analyzed by nonparametric statistics (Siegel, 1956).

Self-Recorded 5-Day Diet Records

A second criterion measure was self-recorded 5-day diet records that patients were asked to keep for the final week of each of two controlled 5-week diet periods. The diet provided participants was calculated at the outset, making it possible to estimate the degree of adherence during the periods when dietary intake was prescribed. The food elements used as a basis for estimating adherence in this investigation from self-recorded diet records were the ratios of polyunsaturated to saturated fats and polyunsaturated to total fats. These variables were examined for the total cohort, males versus females, and test-feeding periods two and three and for changes occurring between the second and third controlled feedings.

Biochemical Indicators

Biochemical indicators comprised a third set of criterion variables. Blood samples taken at week five of the second and third controlled feeding periods provided a basis for serum assays of several variables that may be regarded as linked to regimen adherence. Biochemical values examined for their relationship to subscales on the HPQ were (1) the proportion of linoleic acid in cholesterol fatty acids and (2) total cholesterol levels. Comparisons were made between males and females as well as between the second and third periods of controlled feeding.

RESULTS

Clinician Ratings of Participant Adherence

Correlations were computed first with clinical observations of patient adherence behaviors. Table 3.3 presents coefficients between the subscale total, each of the subscales and the ratings by clinical staff of their observations of patient adherence behaviors. Ratings by clinicians were recorded in such a manner that

TABLE 3.3 Independent Correlations Between Clinician Ratings of Adherence and the Health Perceptions Questionnaire (HPQ)

	All ($n = 53$)	Males ($n = 22$)	Females ($n = 31$)
Self Management (SM)	.22*	.49*	.06
Well Being (WB)	.15	.30	.01
Support Systems (SS)	−.28*	−.30	−.29
Stressors (ST)	.05	.37*	.01
Regularity (RE)	.31	.20	.38*
Subscale Total	.27*	.51**	.13

*$p < .05$
**$p < .01$

higher scores were associated with higher levels of adherence. As the HPQ also was scored in a manner so that higher scores would predict higher levels of adherence, positive correlations therefore would predict higher levels of adherence while low or negative coefficients would predict poor or lower levels of adherence.

Table 3.3 presents an analysis of the relationship between subscale scores on the HPQ and ratings of observed adherence by clinical staff. Table 3.3 presents the coefficient, the number of participants included in the statistic, and the level of significance. Subscales of Self Management, Support Systems, and Regularity and the Total score were found to be significantly related to clinician ratings of patient adherence. This suggests that the HPQ is significantly predictive of ratings of adherence behaviors in three of five areas and positively associated with adherence behaviors in four of the five areas.

A multiple regression analysis was performed to determine the combined effect of the several subscales of the HPQ as a predictor of ratings of patient adherence by clinical staff. The multiple correlation coefficient was .41 ($p < .01$), indicating the degree of linear dependence of clinicians' ratings on the five subscale predictors.

Second, comparisons of clinicians' ratings of adherence for males indicate that subscales of Self Management, Stressors, and the Total Score were significant and in the direction predicted by the questionnaire. Surprisingly, most coefficients appear substantially larger for male participants versus the total cohort, although the smaller number of participants in the computation reduced the probability of achieving statistical significance.

Third, correlation coefficients for females indicated that the Regularity subscale was significantly associated with clinicians' ratings of adherence. Some factor correlations are similar for both sexes, while others suggest a differential effect according to gender. These relationships require further investigations to establish their meaning. A subsequent discussion of these differences is provided.

Overall, the subscales of Self Management, Support Systems and Regularity and the total score were found to be significantly associated with ratings of adherence behaviors by trained clinical personnel, and the adherence factors being measured may exert differential influences according to the gender of the participants.

5-Day Diet Records

The trial protocol required any diet supplements to be high in carbohydrates and low in fats. Known amounts of fats were included in the test diets, and the addition of fats from dietary supplements would result in spurious comparisons between trial groups. Deviations from adherence to the protocol were measured by the examination of the changes in dietary fats as well as the ratio of polyunsaturated to saturated fats (P/S ratio). This latter criterion was supported on the grounds that supplements to diets would be likely to contain larger amounts of saturated than polyunsaturated fats, for example, in eating foods dispensed in fast food restaurants.

Food record analyses revealed an increase in fats from the second to third controlled feeding periods, from a mean of 9.40 grams to 12.73 grams for the 5-day recorded period. Analysis of the HPQ correlations with fats for individual feeding periods 2 and 3 indicated a significant total cohort effect for Self Management ($r = .30$, $p < .05$), Well Being for males ($r = .49$, $p < .04$), and Regularity for females ($r = .37$, $p < .03$).

Examination of changes in P/S ratio from controlled feeding period 2 to 3 did not indicate any significant relationships for the total cohort. Differential effects were observed, however, according to gender of participants. An analysis of the ratio of polyunsaturated fats to saturated fats (P/S) for male for controlled feeding period 2 demonstrated a significant association with Well Being ($r = .58$, $p < .03$), and for females, a significant relationship with Stressors ($r = .42$, $p < .02$). Analysis of changes in P/Ss from the second to third controlled feeding period yielded parallel outcomes to the analysis of changes in dietary fats. That is, although the total cohort did not reveal significant differences according to HPQ subscales, changes in P/Ss for males were predicted by Well Being ($r = .76$, $p < .001$) and Self Management for females ($r = -.35$, $p < .05$). Higher scores on these subscales for males were associated with more favorable P/S ratios.

Biochemical Indicators of Adherence: Linoleic Acid Fractions

Coefficients were obtained between subscales of the HPQ and linoleic acid fraction, a biochemical indicator associated with adherence (Marston, 1970). Participants adhering to the test diets would be expected to show increases in linoleic acid fractions over the course of the trial. Differences between the second and third controlled feeding periods for linoleic acid fractions were related to

HPQ scores. For all participants, the total score ($r = .43, p < .01$) and Well Being ($r = .58, p < .01$) were significantly related to changes in linoleic acid levels. An analysis of coefficients according to gender indicate that Well Being was significantly related for males ($r = .74$, $p < .001$), and for females, both Well Being ($p = .46, p < .02$) and total score ($r = .43, p < .03$) were significantly related.

Biochemical Indicators of Adherence: Serum Cholesterol

Lower levels of cholesterol would be consistent with adherence to a diet low in animal fats and, in turn, with adherence to the protocol requirements. The subscale Well Being was significantly related to cholesterol changes for the full cohort ($r = -.29, p < .01$) and for males ($r = -.46, p < .03$).

DISCUSSION

The HPQ was designed to measure factors predictive of adherence by the assessment of patient perceptions on five different areas of the circumstances of living. These five factor-area associations were defined as separate subscales in the questionnaire and evaluated for their potential to predict adherence. In the context of this dietary trial, adherence was defined in terms of three separate criteria: (1) ratings of adherence by clinical staff, (2) estimates of dietary fats from 5-day food records, and (3) two biochemical measures, serum cholesterol and linoleic acid fractions.

Ratings of Adherence by Clinicians

Because several of the individual subscales demonstrated significant relationships with ratings of adherence, they will be discussed separately. While three of the subscales and the total score were found to be significantly associated with ratings of adherence behaviors, the subscales demonstrated differential predictions according to gender. The adherence of males was predicted by the subscales Stressors and Self Management, while the adherence of females was predicted by the Regularity subscale. The hypothesis that the participant self-perceptions regarding these factors may operate differentially according to gender must be considered.

The initial correlations between clinicians' ratings of adherence and the HPQ suggest that differential effects according to gender of participant may be more instructive of patterns of adherence in this clinical trial than coefficients pertinent to the full cohort. The exception to this observation is the Support Systems subscale, where examination of coefficients for both sexes suggests that perceptions of social support for regimen adherence may be inversely related to ratings of adherence behaviors!

Participants who perceive strong social support for their efforts at losing weight, staying healthy, and so forth, may fail to perform effectively under conditions that fail to match those typically provided by the family. At the same time, participants who report beliefs that their families might not be counted upon to support such efforts might fare better under the stringent but possibly less nurturing conditions of a clinical trial.

The contribution of age as a correlate of clinicians' ratings of adherence behaviors in this dietary trial was confirmed ($r = .52, p < .01$).

5-Day Diet Records

Two measures were selected from the 5-day diet records to evaluate participant adherence: total fats and the ratio of polyunsaturated to saturated fats. Changes from the second to third controlled feeding periods were reported, on the assumption that adherence might be understood as a function of changes over time in addition to the second versus the third feeding period.

The results indicated that only two of the five subscales were systematically associated with changes in P/S differentially for males and females, with no differences observed for Total Fats. This outcome suggested that the dietary changes from the second to the third controlled feeding periods could be predicted only marginally from the HPQ subscales. However, specific subscales did yield significant coefficients with other measures of adherence and, according to the gender of participants, certain subscales were better predictors than others. Well Being and Regularity subscales were better predictors of adherence than others according to self-recorded diet records. The hypothesis that adherence to dietary regimens as measured by changes in reported dietary intake can be predicted by subscales of the HPQ is supported by these outcomes.

Biochemical Indicators of Adherence: Linoleic Acid Fractions

Both total score and Well Being were significantly associated with changes in levels of linoleic acid fractions for the total cohort, while somewhat larger coefficients were evident for male participants in Well Being. Female participants displayed similarly elevated coefficients for Well Being ($r = .46, p < .02$) and for the total score ($r = .43, p < .03$). In view of these relationships occurring from samples of 11 and 20 respectively, their possible meaning as predictors deserves consideration.

Biochemical Indicators of Adherence: Serum Cholesterol

The subscale Well Being again demonstrated its power to predict changes in serum cholesterol over the second to third controlled feeding period. While the total cohort yielded an inverse coefficient of $-.29$ ($p < .01$), differential coefficients for males and females suggested that more of the variance was contributed by males ($r = .46$, $p < .03$) than by females ($r = -.18$, $p < .17$, ns). In general, these outcomes suggest that the subscale Well Being was a better predictor for male participants for changes in cholesterol level over these two feeding periods. In summary, the two groups were similar to each other in overall changes, but the changes were better predicted by the Well Being subscale for males than for females.

Agreement Between Measures of Adherence

Adherence to a dietary regimen was measured in this investigation by direct observation of adherence behaviors, self-recorded 5-day diet records, and two biochemical measures. Each measure was assumed to provide, from a different vantage point, a valid estimate of how well participants had adhered to protocol requirements. Whether or not these endpoints represented valid criteria would depend in part upon their association with each other. The following analysis is devoted to that issue.

Ratings of adherence by clinicians were examined for their association with self-recorded diet records and the two biochemical measures. The relationship between ratings of participant adherence and changes in P/S ratio, serum cholesterol levels, linoleic acid fractions, and dietary fats for both males and females were examined. Results indicated that for the total cohort, ratings of adherence by clinic staff were significantly associated with changes in serum cholesterol levels. A more complete picture of this relationship was observed from comparisons between male and female coefficients, which suggest that higher levels of cholesterol are predicted from adherence ratings for males than for females.

A parallel relationship pertains to linoleic acid fractions, indicating that higher levels of linoleic acid fractions are better predicted by ratings of adherence for males than for females. While higher levels of linoleic acid fractions may be regarded as a favorable indication of adherence in this investigation, elevated cholesterol does not. In general, coefficients according to gender of participants appear to yield a possibly more comprehensive picture of the complex relationship between adherence and linoleic acid levels than those for the full cohort. The association between the HPQ and the various dependent measures can be conceptualized schematically, as shown in Figure 3.1. While more substantial associations can be observed between the HPQ and ratings by clinicians, the association with lipid values drawn from diet records and those from serum analyses is relatively equal. Given the relatively small sample ($n = 53$), the number of significant associations with selected endpoints suggests that the HPQ may possess the potential for predicting adherence to a dietary regimen.

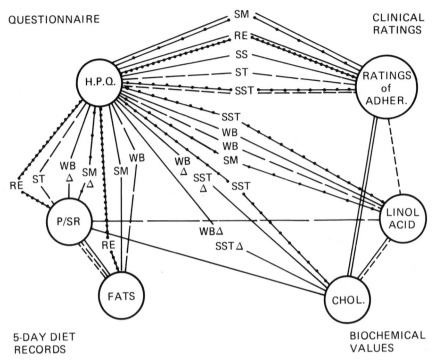

FIGURE 3.1 Schematic presentation of correlation matrix between independent and dependent variables.

The relatively large amount of variance in ratings of adherence accounted for by both subscales and total HPQ scores argues therefore that this questionnaire has direct applicability to both medication and life-style change regimens as well.

The operation of demographic variables such as the age and gender of participants contributed significantly to the prediction of adherence. In contrast to the conclusions of previous literature reviews by Haynes, Taylor, and Sackett (1979), Marston (1970), Dunbar and Stunkard (1977), and Mitchell (1974), these outcomes appear to provide support for the independent effect of these two demographic variables on the outcomes of this dietary study.

Further testing of the HPQ is needed in clinical trials of diet with other populations under the more complex conditions of totally self-administered therapeutic diets. Here the patient is responsible for meal planning, purchasing of food, meal preparation, and food consumption. The application of the HPQ to clinical trials of efficacy of drugs warrants evaluation due to the commonality of adherence factors for almost all therapies.

The performance of patients on the several subscales of the Health Perceptions Questionnaire may allow for the prediction of endpoints of significance both to clinical trials and general practice. The interaction of demographics of age and gender with performance on specific subscales suggests that predictions may be made to (1) levels of adherence to prescribed regimens; (2) the identification of specific risk factors underlying potential nonadherence; and (3) the type of interventions needed to modify or improve deficiencies or barriers to adherence revealed by the profile of risk factors. The relative effectiveness of these predictors would require validation in a large multicenter clinical trial. Combined with the assessment of significant environmental events influencing adherence, the Health Perceptions Questionnaire may be a time-saving and inexpensive method for selecting participants for clinical trials according to the likelihood of attaining desired levels of regimen adherence.

SUMMARY

An instrument termed the Health Perceptions Questionnaire (HPQ) has been developed to assess adherence to interventions in clinical trials. The instrument measures patients' perceptions of several factors shown to be associated with adherence to prescribed regimens. An analysis of the association between participants scores on the HPQ and other measures of adherence in the current investigation, a dietary trial, suggests that predictions above chance levels can be made with regard to clinician ratings of adherence behaviors, self-recorded diet records, and selected biochemical values.

These outcomes encourage further use of this instrument in the selection of participants, the monitoring of adherence in dietary trials, and the prediction of regimen adherence. The application of the HPQ with medication regimens and those requiring life-style changes appears justified by the relatively strong and consistent association found between ratings of adherence behaviors and specific subscales and total scores. Although the prediction of endpoints of biochemical measures and self-recorded dietary intake was less robust, their agreement with the ratings of adherence was demonstrated sufficiently to warrant the use of this instrument as a valid and internally consistent tool in the selection of participants for clinical trials and for identifying those participants likely to require additional support in maintaining effective adherence levels.

REFERENCES

Averill, J. (1973). Personal control over aversive stimuli and its relationship to stress. *Psychological Bulletin, 80,* 286–303.

Bandura, A. (1977). Self-efficacy: Toward a unifying theory of behavioral change. *Psychological Review, 84,* 191–202.

Bandura, A., & Walters, R. H. (1963). *Social learning and personality development.* Englewood Cliffs, NJ: Prentice-Hall

Becker, M. H., Maiman, L. A., Kirscht, J. P., Haefner, D. P., & Drachman, R. H. (1977). The health belief model and prediction of dietary compliance: A field experiment. *Journal of Health and Social Behavior, 18,* 348–365.

Byrne, D. G., & Whyte, H. M. (1980). Life events and myocardial infarction revisited: The role of measures of individual impact. *Psychosomatic Medicine, 42*(1), 1–10.

Dunbar, J. M., & Stunkard, J. A. (1977). Adherence to diet and drug regimen. In R. Levy, B. Rifkind, B. Dennis, & N. Ernst (Eds.), *Nutrition, lipids and coronary heart disease.* New York: Raven Press.

Haynes, R. B., Taylor, D. W., & Sackett, D. L. (1979). *Compliance in health care.* Baltimore: Johns Hopkins University Press.

Holmes, T. H. (1978). Life situation, emotions and disease. *Psychosomatics, 19,* 747–754.

Holmes, T. H., & Rahe, R. H. (1967). The social readjustment rating scale. *Journal of Psychosomatic Research, 11,* 213–218.

Insull, W., Jr., Silvers, A., Hicks, L., & Probstfield, J. L. (1988). *Plasma lipid effects of three common vegetable oils in reduced fat diets of free living adults.* Submitted for publication.

Kanfer, F. H., & Phillips, J. S. (1970). *Learning foundations of behavior therapy.* New York: Wiley.

Kirscht, J. P. (1974). The health belief model and illness behavior. In M. H. Becker (Ed.), The health belief model and preventive health behavior. *Health Educator Monograph, 2*(4), 387–408.

Mahoney, M. J. (1974). *Cognition and behavior modification.* Cambridge, MA: Ballinger.

Mahoney, M. J. (1977). Reflections on the cognitive-learning trend in psychotherapy. *American Psychologist, 32,* 5–13.

Marston, M. (1970). Compliance with medical regimens: A review of the literature. *Nursing Research, 19,* 312–323.

Meichenbaum, D. B. (1977). *Cognitive behavior modification: An interpretive approach.* New York: Plenum.

Mitchell, J. H. (1974). Compliance with medical regimens: An annotated bibliography. *Health Educator Monographs, 2,* 75–87.

Sackett, D. L., & Snow, J. (1979). The magnitude of compliance and non-compliance. In R. B. Haynes, D. W. Taylor, & D. L. Sackett (Eds.), *Compliance in health care* (pp. 11–22). Baltimore: Johns Hopkins University Press.

Shekelle, R. B., Ostfeld, A. M., & Paul, O. (1969). Social status and incidence of coronary heart disease. *Journal of Chronic Disease, 22,* 381–394.

Siegel, S. (1956). *Nonparametric statistics for the behavioral sciences.* New York: McGraw-Hill.

4

Patient–Physician Interactions

Howard S. Friedman, M. Robin DiMatteo

COMPLIANCE, ADHERENCE, AND COOPERATION

> You enter at the scheduled moment. You strip down to your briefs and put on a robe. You go to the weigh-in. And then you climb up onto the platform.

Is this: (a) a visit to the doctor; or (b) the beginning of a boxing match? It is curious that the two types of interactions begin in such similar ways, and it is unfortunate that sometimes they end in similar ways—with doctor and patient boxing as adversaries. If the physician and patient should not be adversaries, what should be the nature of their relationship and how will it affect the treatment?

Patients must overcome many challenges in seeking advice from their physicians. In most cases, they must make appointments, obtain transportation to their clinic, fill out forms, disclose intimate information, wait for the doctor, submit to a physical examination and diagnostic tests, and, finally, pay directly or indirectly (through insurance) for the service. After all this, many patients fail to follow their physicians' orders. About one third of all patients do not cooperate with the medical recommendations given to them for short-term treatments, and

This chapter was supported in part by intramural research grants from the University of California, Riverside.

half or more do not follow long-term treatments (Becker & Maiman, 1980; DiMatteo & DiNicola, 1982; Gillum & Barsky, 1974; Haynes, 1979; Sackett & Snow, 1979). The noncompliance of patients with medical regimens is danger-ous to patients (since they may develop serious complications from their condi-tions), and it is a costly waste of medical resources. How can we explain it and prevent it? Specifically, what is the role played by the doctor–patient relation-ship?

This question raises the issue of the term we should use in discussing the following of a medical regimen. The traditional term is patient *compliance* with treatment. This term perpetuates the image of patients as passive, submissive, and unable to make their own decisions. It implies a very one-sided relationship: The physician gives orders and the patient complies. Another term, which seems to find increasing favor, is patient *adherence*. This is a little better, but it focuses too much on the patient—the patient must "stick to it" or adhere like a fly to prescription flypaper.

Many physicians believe that lack of patient cooperation with treatment can be attributed to the "uncooperative personalities" of their patients (Davis, 1966; Haynes, Taylor, & Sackett, 1979). However, as we shall see, noncompliance usually results from particular aspects of the doctor–patient relationship and the way in which health care is delivered. When patients are simply given orders, noncompliance may result. Having the patient and practitioner work together as a team is more effective. Therefore, the best term is patient *cooperation* with treatment, because the term "cooperation" emphasizes that the physician and patient must work together, and that the patient must function in a society (Friedman & DiMatteo, 1979).

Noncooperation can take many forms. A patient may fail to cooperate with primary prevention measures (which are designed to prevent illness from devel-oping) or fail to cooperate with secondary prevention measures (such as mea-sures designed to lower blood pressure to prevent stroke). Perhaps the aspect of greatest concern to physicians is failure to cooperate with therapeutic measures that are designed to treat a diagnosed disease, such as diabetes.

Patients can fail to cooperate with therapeutic drug treatment by varying the size of the dose of medication that is taken, the number of doses taken, the spacing, or the number of days over which the therapy is continued. Such deviations point out that what is termed lack of cooperation on the part of the patient could easily involve lack of understanding (Hulka, 1979). If a patient is supposed to carry out complicated or long-term recommendations for appro-priate dosage, temporal spacing, and duration of medication ingestion, the patient needs to understand fully what is to be done and the reasons for it (Haynes, Taylor, & Sackett, 1979). Unfortunately, many times the patient does understand the treatment but is insufficiently motivated to carry it out. Patients may also fail to cooperate with important follow-up treatment, again often because their motivation is not strong enough. In short, a successful doctor-patient relationship should promote both patient understanding and patient motivation.

Models of the Doctor–Patient Relationship

Basic models of doctor–patient relations were sketched out more than 30 years ago by Szasz and Hollender (1956). The first is the Activity–Passivity model. In this type of relationship the health professional does something to the patient but the patient is totally passive. The patient has no control or responsibility; the practitioner has absolute control and absolute responsibility.

The second model is very common in medical practice and is presently accepted as the norm. It is the Guidance–Cooperation model. The patient is aware of what is happening and is capable of following instructions. The practitioner tells the patient what to do, and the patient is expected to comply. In this model the health practitioner decides what is best for the patient and makes the recommendation. The patient is expected to follow the recommendation because "the doctor knows best."

However, Szasz and Hollender pointed out the problems with models in which there is a passive patient or in which there is a "physician-as-rule-setter." Here, the physician must disidentify with the patient as a person and places the former in absolute control of the patient. They preferred a "Mutual Participation" model, in which the physician and patient are pursuing common goals of eliminating illness and preserving health. The doctor and patient have equal power and are mutually interdependent; there is shared responsibility, and mutual dignity and respect; and their behaviors must be mutually satisfying for the relationship to continue. The patient's input is continually included in medical decisions before they are made because there is an open and responsible partnership. This is the model most likely to promote cooperation and health.

This mutual participation model has not become the standard for doctor-patient relations, although elements of it are increasingly seen, such as in various "Patients' Bills of Rights." As I was reminded recently when I had a viral infection, it is only in medicine that various personnel can walk in and shoot x-rays at you, stick needles in your arm, and order you to pee in a cup without ever even introducing themselves.

The mutual participation model has been developed into related models, one of which is a health transactions model (Stone, 1979). Such later models incorporate more of the social environment. In this approach, the physician must look carefully at the question of whether the recommendations really address the client's problem adequately and whether the suggestions that are made (the doctor's "orders") are necessary and reasonable steps for the patient to follow.

In the first stage of the health care transaction the patient brings a problem to the physician. An example of this part of the transaction is the patient who describes feeling faint and dizzy and having difficulty breathing while walking outside. The physician must decide whether the patient is having heart trouble or is having an anxiety reaction. It is essential to know something about the patient's life-style, beliefs, family or other support systems, coping mechanisms, and general emotional health.

During the second stage of the health care transaction, the health professional makes a decision about the diagnosis and discusses the treatment to prescribe for the patient. The physician of course has a great deal of knowledge about the intricate details of various treatments. But a rational selection among these possible treatments demands some knowledge of the values assigned by the patient to the various complicating factors and outcomes.

The third and final stage of the health care transaction is implementing the treatment. Traditionally, total responsibility has been placed on the patient for carrying out the treatment. But if full responsibility for carrying out the treatment—say, taking medication for hypertension—is borne by the patient, both parties to the health care encounter may be reluctant to admit the patient's inability to carry out the treatment regimen. The physician is likely to avoid the fact that he or she has not explained the treatment adequately or convinced the patient to follow it. In fact, evidence suggests that physicians are not very good at recognizing noncooperation when it occurs (Charney, 1972; Kasl, 1975). The patient, on the other hand, may be reluctant to admit an embarrassing inability to carry out the regimen.

The doctor probes halfheartedly for noncooperation, and the patient hides it as much as possible. In this social game the patient fails to benefit from treatment. If, on the other hand, the entire health care transaction is considered the shared responsibility of the health professional and the patient, no fault is assigned when difficulties arise. Difficulties are expected to occur, and noncooperation is addressed together by the physician and the patient. They design or redesign a treatment program that the patient can follow successfully—a program that fits the patient's social, psychological, economic, and cultural situation.

Other Reasons for Mutual Participation

Nearly all patients recognize and acknowledge that objectively there is a risk attached to any medical procedure and that medicine is not foolproof. After a failed treatment, this objective analysis does not always occur, however. Often emotionality and anger result from a breakdown in the doctor–patient relationship, and the patient sues.

Under which conditions do patients decide to attempt to file a malpractice suit, regardless of the actual degree of "malpractice"? Analyses suggest that it is the nature of the doctor–patient relationship that determines the likelihood of litigation more than any other factor (Blum, 1960; Lander, 1978; Vaccarino, 1977). Physicians who become involved in malpractice litigation tend to be unwilling or unable to communicate with their patients. They do not listen to patients, they fail to explain treatment details and attendant risks to patients, and they do not talk to patients about their dissatisfactions. In fact, when something does go wrong, the physicians prone to being sued are unable to admit their own limitations.

In the ideal situation, the physician carefully explains the medical procedures to the patient. The attendant risks are described, the expected results considered, and a trust is built up between the physician and the patient. A joint decision is then made, and if the treatment does not go as expected, the patient is informed and takes part in the additional decision making. In this ideal case, the patient can rely on the physician for continued support and respect. The patient is an active, rather than a passive, participant. Many physicians perform high-risk procedures and are never sued.

Other problems can result from a patient's lack of cooperation. Diagnoses are often made on the basis of the responses of the patient's symptoms to a particular medication. If the patient has not actually taken the medication that was prescribed, but the physician believes that the medication is not working, a misdiagnosis might occur.

Importantly, it has long been recognized that the physician can be a therapeutic agent who is just as effective as a drug or therapeutic procedure. The manner in which care is delivered—the positive expectations that are communicated to the patient—may at least in part be responsible for the patient's getting well. It has been suggested that the history of medicine before the twentieth century is in fact the history of the communication of comfort and positive expectations from physician to patient (Shapiro, 1960, 1971). Relatedly, there is evidence that negative emotional states play a role in chronic illness (Booth-Kewley & Friedman, 1987; Friedman & Booth-Kewley, 1987). The rapport from a cooperative relationship may thus have implications far beyond the cooperation itself.

A final important consequence of the proper doctor–patient relationship involves doctor-shopping. Each time a patient changes physicians, it is an expensive and time-consuming event. The new primary care physician must repeat a medical history, conduct a physical examination and systems review, and also perform the necessary diagnostic tests. Few patients terminate the relationship with their physician because they believe the physician is incompetent technically (Ben-Sira, 1976; Bloom, 1963; DiMatteo & DiNicola, 1982; Haynes, Taylor, & Sackett, 1979); rather, it is because of the way in which health professionals have behaved toward the patients. Furthermore, if physicians do not provide the important socioemotional aspects of care and give patients both reassurance and information about what will be done for them, seriously ill patients can easily feel abandoned by their physicians. Then they are more likely to reject the medical establishment altogether and seek nonmedical cures (Cobb, 1954).

Should a patient always go along with a doctor's advice? Is compliance necessarily in the best interest of the patient? Many examples of iatrogenic illness suggest that the answer may be "no" (Illich, 1976). Although iatrogenic illness is often imagined to be the result of problems occurring in surgery (e.g., perforation of the bowel with resultant peritonitis during abdominal surgery), it is probably more often the direct result of the side effects of drugs or the dangerous interaction of two drugs or treatments. Or the patient may be unable to carry out the regimen in the safe and proper manner. However, with a mutual participation model in place, iatrogenic illness is less likely to occur in the first place (as the patient provides significant input into potential problems special to his or her case), and it is likely to be better dealt with when it does occur.

Now that a general overview of the best ways to think about the doctor–patient relationship has been sketched, we will consider some important related issues in ongoing doctor–patient relations. These remarks are directed at the common situations in which a physician would like the patient to stop smoking, modify diet, and so on. We are not considering special situations in which very complex or time-consuming regimens for treating advanced illness are involved.

ASSESSMENT STRATEGIES

In a successful doctor–patient interaction, the physician must be able to understand and communicate verbal and nonverbal information. What are the specific elements of a successful interaction?

A Historical Perspective

Although concern with the doctor–patient relationship dates from the earliest times in the history of medicine (Hippocrates [1923] in the fourth century B.C. recognized the importance of the doctor's manner and his or her delivering of care with special sensitivity), the development of a science of effective human communication began in the early part of this century. The prominent medical educator Frederick Shattuck wrote in 1907 that a serious problem in health care would occur if the gap between the science of medicine and its actual practice were to grow. Shattuck suggested that the gap could be bridged by the so-called art of medicine, noting that disease is one phenomenon whereas the diseased person is another. Shattuck wrote of the importance of sensitivity and genuine concern for patients' feelings when taking a history; much can be learned about patients from the way in which they tell their stories.

This tone of focus on the patient as a whole human being was set by Sir William Osler (1904), who in 1899 recommended that a health care professional listen to the patient, for the patient may actually reveal the diagnosis. Formal attention to the role of psychology in medicine soon began appearing in both psychological and medical circles (DiMatteo & Friedman, 1982). By 1926, Dr. Francis Peabody (1927) gave an address at the Harvard Medical School warning of the oncoming dehumanizing and isolating experiences of specialty care. This address is often read today by first-year medical students and cited by eminent physicians. The early physicians were, in sum, suggesting a special kind of sensitivity on the part of the doctor in dealing with patients.

Some have assumed that relating to patients in an artful manner involves simply good manners, respect, and compassion (Chafetz, 1970; Headlee, 1973). Physicians often see the art of medicine as "common sense." However, these behaviors are far from simple. Many factors operate to impair communication between physicians and patients. In order to practice successfully the "art" of medicine, the physician needs to understand some social science (DiMatteo, 1979; Engel, 1977a, b; Tumulty, 1970). Especially relevant here are issues of verbal and nonverbal communication.

Interviewing

The importance of clear and open verbal communication between the health care professional and the patient has been discovered again and again in research. In one important series of studies conducted in Children's Hospital in Los Angeles by Barbara Korsch and her colleagues (Francis, Korsch, & Morris, 1969; Korsch, Gozzi, & Francis, 1968), researchers tape-recorded conversations between pediatricians and the mothers of their patients. These tape recordings were analyzed and revealed that physicians whose patients were noncompliant were often vague in communicating with the mothers. They tended to use medical jargon often (e.g., "We have to watch the Coombs titre") and did not take time to answer questions thoroughly or to determine whether each mother understood what was wrong with her child and exactly how to carry out the prescribed treatment. Furthermore, the relationship was very unequal.

When a physician collects information from the patient and gives little or no information back to the patient, the patient often feels that he or she is not being treated as a valuable person (Stiles, Putnam, Wolf, & James, 1979). In fact, social psychologists have consistently found in research on human interaction that "reciprocity" (give and take) is necessary in order to maintain a relationship and to continue it in a mutually satisfying manner (Blau, 1968). Reciprocity in self-disclosure requires disclosure by the health care professional as well as the patient. Self-disclosure is important to the development of a productive physician–patient relationship (Rodin & Janis, 1982).

Cultural factors also affect communication and the ensuing cooperation with treatment. Sometimes patients fail to follow the recommendations of health care practitioners because of religious or cultural restrictions. Few patients are willing to comply with orders that go against what is prescribed by their cultural group. Only careful questioning will reveal the symbolic meaning that patients attach to various behaviors that are affected by ethnic, cultural, and religious values.

Numerous studies have documented extensive verbal communication problems between physicians and their patients. In one study over 60% of the patients actually misunderstood the oral instructions given by their physicians for taking medication; another study found that more than 50% of the patients made at least one error when they were asked to describe their physician's recommendations for their treatment only a week after their visit to the clinic (Boyd, Covington, Stanaszek, & Coussons, 1974; Svarstad, 1976). A detailed analysis of communication problems is offered by Friedman and DiMatteo (1989).

Writing instructions down for patients sometimes helps, but these written instructions must be clear and unambiguous in order to be useful. Physicians' written instructions are often so ambiguous that patients cannot understand them without a complete explanation beforehand (Stone, 1979; Svarstad, 1976). In addition, an explanation that involves giving information one-sidedly from the health professional to the patient is not sufficient to be effective. Asking patients to write down their questions before meeting with the physician has proven helpful (Roter, 1984). But there has to be a give and take of information between the doctor and patient so that the doctor can obtain continual feedback from the patient about what he or she understands and can do.

There is a large literature on proper and improper ways to conduct interviews. I will not say much here except for pointing out one key conclusion that emerges from this research: The questioning should be open-ended. The physician must let the patient talk—and often, as Sir William Osler said, the patient will provide the diagnosis. This is part of what it means to cooperate.

Nonverbal Communication

Pediatricians will often have their nurses question the parents of a child about whether the child crawls yet, walks yet, talks yet, and so on; the developmental checklist is then handed to the physician. Some internists have patients fill out questionnaires that ask about how much they drink, how much they exercise, and so on. I am sure there will soon also be pressure to have computers ask these questions. This is a de-humanizing direction in which to go.

Many times in doctor–patient interactions, the nonverbal communication is much more important than the words that are said. A tremendous amount of information is available through nonverbal communciation. This falls into three categories: (1) the detection of stress; (2) the communication of emotion; and (3) the detection of deception and inaccuracies.

It is important for the physician to continually monitor whether patients are experiencing undue stress in their personal lives, in coping with their illnesses, or in their dealings with the health care system. Patients express this stress through their facial expresssions, their vocal cues, and their body movements. I describe each nonverbal cue in detail in another chapter (Friedman, 1982). Further, careful observation can yield valid information about whether someone is likely to develop disease or indeed is already ill, often even without any physical exam or tests (Friedman, Hall, & Harris, 1985).

Patients are especially uncertain about their future and so are highly motivated to seek social definition by observing others. Most of this information is transmitted nonverbally. When anger and hostility are communicated to them by health care professionals, noncooperation results (Salzman, Shader, Scott, & Binstock, 1970). On the other hand, positive expectations for improved health are also transmitted through nonverbal cues. Nonverbally expressive physicians seem to have more satisfied patients (Friedman, Prince, Riggio, & DiMatteo, 1980).

The case of deception is especially interesting in doctor–patient interactions. Patients are often motivated to please their physician, hide embarrassing thoughts or conditions, and cover up noncompliance. At the same time, many patients believe that the physician is not telling them the whole truth or has some personal agenda regarding treatment. Thus patients and doctors carefully observe each other for signs of deception. Most of these signs are communicated or hidden nonverbally. In particular, our work indicates that physicians who are sensitive to the body movements of their patients are more likely to have satisfied (and so presumably more cooperative) patients (DiMatteo, Friedman, & Taranta, 1979). Of course, if the relationship is truly one of mutual participation, there is much less need for such interpersonal spying. Still, a skilled physician must be able to detect cues of deception while communicating the proper nonverbal feelings and expectations.

Following Up

We have considered the verbal interview and the nonverbal observation, but it is also important to say a word about following up. Patient cooperation with treatment tends to fall off over time, so it is important for the health care system to follow up. Since the self-report of the patient is an unreliable indicator of cooperation, other assessment techniques such as pill counts, performance measures, clinical testing, and spouse report have been suggested (and are sometimes successful). Close observation is again also valuable. If the physician uses the proper interpersonal orientation and the most effective influence strategies, then follow-up visits can both provide a reasonable assessment of cooperation *and* help maintain the cooperation.

INFLUENCE STRATEGIES

When a social problem like lack of healthy behavior arises, there is always a call for providing more *education* to the public. However, if there is one lesson that social science best teaches, it is that education alone is generally a poor strategy of social influence. "Let's eliminate racism through education." "Let's eliminate smoking by providing warning labels." "Let's educate people about seat belts." "Let's educate people about drug abuse." "Let's educate people about the dangers of suntanning." Well, as most drivers said to education about seat belts: "Phooey."

Education is not a sufficient condition for inducing cooperation with medical regimens (although it is sometimes a necessary condition [Eraker, Kirscht, & Becker, 1984; Janz & Becker, 1984]) because much human behavior is not perfectly rational. Among other factors, people are heavily influenced by cultural expectations, by social influence and social support, by self-concept, by pursuit of pleasure and avoidance of difficulties, and even simply by habit.

When faced with noncooperation, many physicians (if they are not aware of the complexity of the problem) usually take the following steps: First, they explain the regimen to the patient and then they try rational arguments to persuade patients. After that, physicians and other health care team members may resort to threat tactics. Finally, they withdraw from the case. Obviously, it would be better if physicians could rely upon effective influence techniques.

What influence strategies do work? Some that often work, like changes in the law (e.g., seat belt laws, restricted smoking areas), have little to do with doctor-patient interactions and so are not considered in detail here. However, three physician-related strategies that do work are physician credibility and power, motivation-serving cognitive consistency, and changes in self-concept.

Physician Credibility and Power

People sometimes change their attitudes and behavior in response to a persuasive message from a credible and powerful communicator (Janis, 1984). The physician has some special influence because of being trustworthy, expert, and powerful. Respect and power are accorded physicians for three major reasons. First, the job of a health professional requires a high degree of technical competence. Signs of this competence enhance the physician's credibility. Also, this technical competence is of a special type. The computer programmers in a bank who diagnose and repair problems in monthly bank statements are also highly competent techni-cally, but the computer programmers are dealing with problems that have limited impact on the individual. People can forget for a while that their bank statement does not match the checkbook total, but it is difficult to forget a very painful sore throat and earache when continually trying to swallow. Problems with body functions are problems central to the person; they are not easily ignored and are usually accompanied by strong emotion (Moos, 1977). The physicians who can solve these problems find themselves endowed with great respect.

Second, the power and respect accorded health professionals is hinted at by the following questions: Should physicians devote a great deal of their time to financial investments? Should physicians be involved in elaborate real estate sales deals or in owning convalescent homes? These questions illustrate the point that the health professional is expected to show a high degree of commitment to serving people. That is, the health professional is supposed to be concerned about the welfare of others and to focus primarily on helping people. Whether this assumption is realistic or not, the primary goal of the physician is *expected* to be caring for people, and not financial gain.

Third, the respect given to physicians comes in part because they are viewed as nonjudgmental. Health professionals learn a great deal of intimate information about patients. Patients often disclose their thoughts and feelings more readily to physicians and nurses than to their closest friends or spouses. The physician's role involves simply learning as much as he or she can about the patient, avoiding negative judgments about the patient as a person, and helping the patient to engage in healthful behaviors. When doctors fulfill these expectations, they are accorded a tremendous amount of respect and credibility by their patients. Anything that makes it clear that the physician really does have special knowledge and really does have the patient's interests at heart will serve to increase the doctor's influence. On the other hand, if a person believes that his or her physician is incompetent or after money, the advice will not be followed.

A related source of influence is the power of the physician to certify illness. People need a doctor's approval to enter the sick role and receive all sorts of social benefits such as sick leave, sympathy, and special treatment. To maintain this status, many must often attempt to follow the doctor's advice.

It is important to note that these sources of influence derive from the physi-cian's traditional position of power and authority. But as that position changes, what other types of influence will be effective?

Cognitive Consistency

Years of research on social influence shows us that people will bring their attitudes into line with their behaviors. This is especially true if the behaviors are seen as free choices and if some commitment is involved. Taking small steps, making public commitments, and investing resources in new ways may all be effective. So, for example, patients who can be encouraged to join a health club, buy an attractive jogging suit, visit a nonsmoking restaurant, or announce to the whole office that they have given up smoking will be more likely to change their behavior. The physician is not convincing the patient to start exercising, lose weight, or stop smoking. Such "New Year's resolutions" are generally not kept. Rather the physician is gently inducing the patient to voluntarily make a public commitment to a new behavior. The behavior change will then often follow.

Changes in Self-Concept: The Social Self

Probably the best source of influence involves the patient's social identity. This identity—which arises from interactions with other people—is called the *social self*. If we can induce people to think of themselves as health-seeking, as nonsmokers, as cooperative eaters, and so on, they are likely to engage in healthy behaviors. This approach is even more effective if the person has support, advice, and encouragement from other people—termed *social support*. It is one reason groups like Alcoholics Anonymous are so effective.

Besides referral to such identity-forming support groups, what can physicians do? For the most part, the greatest influence that the physician can have on the patient's health behavior is through the use of referent power, the process of forming a social unit with the patient. If patients come to trust the health care professional and to *model themselves* after the health care professional as someone who values healthy, responsible behavior, they are likely to cooperate with healthy behaviors. We have all heard about the fat, harried physician who sits at his desk smoking a cigarette and telling his patient that the patient is at high risk for another heart attack. This doctor might be seen as kind of low on proper referent power. Enough said on that. Here again, the quality of the doctor–patient relationship is critically important for the care of patients and for building patient motivation.

THE PHYSICIAN'S LIMITS

Now that I have described some ways that physicians can be effective, it is necessary to point out some serious limits.

Consider the following scenario: A married man, father of three and prominent in his church, comes into the doctor's office complaining that he has had a number of infections and illnesses during the past year. The physician decides to do a complete physical exam. One of the questions asked is, "Have you been having anal intercourse with promiscuous males?"

In these days of AIDS, this is a question that the physician should ask. However, how many doctors will actually be able to ask such questions? For a variety of reasons, many of which are obvious, this and other relevant questions are not likely to be asked (Lewis, Freeman, & Corey, 1987). In short, physicians do not do everything that seems theoretically reasonable to help their patients adopt healthy life-styles. Physicians in our society usually are really only expected to intervene to treat a specific illness. Of course, we might want to change the structure of medicine, but that is a big issue and should not be undertaken lightly (Friedman & DiMatteo, 1989; Shorter, 1985).

A second important limit on what physicians can do comes from a lack of training. Not long ago, at a meeting of the California Medical Association in Anaheim, Dr. Donald Francis, the California advisor from the Centers for Disease Control, urged the several hundred physicians at the meeting to assume the classical role of counselor and community leader to teach people how to stop the spread of AIDS. I am not sure whether physicians ever had such a classic role, but they surely do not have it now. Although there are some exceptions, physicians are not trained as counselors and they are not trained to be community leaders. Most physicians, through no fault of their own, are simply not able to assume such responsibilities.

Could they get the necessary training? I recently received the following interdepartmental memo: "Students in the UCR—UCLA joint medical school program [a program at the University of California which leads to a bachelors degree and M.D. in 7 years] will no longer be required to take Psychology 178, Psychology and Medicine. The committee thought that other courses such as history and philosophy would also provide a rounded education in the humanities." This course, Psychology 178, is one that Robin DiMatteo and I codeveloped 10 years ago to be a model for the training of future physicians in the social and behavioral aspects of medicine (DiMatteo & Friedman, 1982). But it is very difficult to keep such courses in a medical curriculum that is still dominated by the traditional medical model of illness. Social science has not yet assumed its rightful role in health care.

Interestingly, the same day that I got the memo, I also received a letter from a former undergraduate who had done some work with me on nonverbal communication to cancer patients. She is a resident in surgery, about to enter surgical oncology, and she wrote that she appreciates the tremendous importance of what she does with her patients *outside* the operating room. If we want physicians to promote health we have to teach them how (Bok, 1984), but such educational reform may not be imminent.

The final important point concerns the limits of the physician in promoting patient cooperation with health recommendations. Although one goal of this chapter is to show what a good physician can do, in reality the evidence suggests that physicians by themselves often cannot do that much in the grand scheme of things.

Consider the case of diet and nutrition. People eat and drink what they do because of (1) what is *available* at the supermarket, at restaurants, and at McDonald's; (2) *family expectations*: they eat omelettes every Sunday morning and ham every Christmas because that's what they grew up eating; (3) *cultural norms*: they drink diet Pepsi rather than Bosco chocolate milk because that's what everyone else (including Michael Jackson) is drinking; (4) *peer pressure*, such as to drink beer in college; (5) *addiction*, such as to caffeine and alcohol; (6) *affordability and convenience*—for example, frozen pizza (much of which is quite healthy) is a big seller these days; and (7) *habit*: often people eat what they eat because that is what they have always eaten.

Similarly, although physician-delivered interventions can have an impact on smoking cessation (Ockene, 1987), they cannot work in isolation. The far greater influences on smoking are the social expectations reflected in our laws, customs, social models, and philosophies. Physicians have been warning against smoking for years, but simply berating patients will not work; it is the enlisting of the patient's cooperation and shared responsibility and supportive changes in society as a whole that produce dramatic reductions in smoking.

In short, individuals often do not make conscious decisions about their health behaviors. Therefore, for much ongoing health behavior, physicians are not the only relevant influence. The greatest influences on people's health behaviors are the societal structures over which physicians may have little direct control. However, physicians can expand their roles and help to change these structures by being advocates if this fits their interests. A physician's therapeutic partnership with a patient can act synergistically with policies such as seat belt laws and American Heart Association-approved meals in restaurants to promote healthy behavior. Individual education works best in the presence of supportive social and societal influences on self-concept. The physician and the health care system represent one of the channels that provide this influence and support.

CONCLUSION

Boxing is not going to be eliminated because a physician says it is not healthy to get punched in the head. A large number of patients fail to follow medical advice. Although many physicians believe that patients' failures to cooperate are the fault of the patients, research indicates this is not the case. Patient cooperation is dependent upon a number of social–psychological variables.

As other chapters in this book describe, cooperation with treatment regimens is more likely when patients believe they are susceptible to serious disease, trust in the efficacy of the treatment, and believe treatment benefits outweigh the costs. Thus education plays a role, but it is not the most important factor. Rather, cooperation is most likely when patients have clear, open communication with physicians who provide understandable, sensible explanations to them, when physicians enlist patients' motivation to heal themselves, and when physicians prescribe regimens compatible with the patients' social and cultural norms.

Recent research strongly supports the notions of the turn-of-the-century physicians like Shattuck, Peabody, and Osler, who wrote of the importance of the interpersonal quality of the doctor–patient relationship. However, such matters should not be considered medical "art." A social scientific approach to assessment, communication, and influence is possible. Maybe, given our knowledge of effective doctor–patient relations, we can eliminate the boxing between doctors and patients.

REFERENCES

Becker, M. H., & Maiman, L. A. (1980). Strategies for enhancing patient compliance. *Journal of Community Health, 6*, 113–135.

Ben-Sira, Z. (1976). The function of the professional's affective behavior in client satisfaction: A revised approach to social interaction theory. *Journal of Health and Social Behavior, 17*, 3–11.

Blau, P. (1968). Social exchange. In D. Sills (Ed.), *International encyclopedia of the social sciences* (pp. 452–457). New York: Macmillan.

Bloom, S. W. (1963). *The doctor and his patient: A sociological interpretation.* New York: Russell Sage Foundation.

Blum, R. H. (1960). *The management of the doctor–patient relationship.* New York: McGraw-Hill.

Bok, D. (1984). *The president's report, 1982–83.* Cambridge, MA: Harvard University Press.

Booth-Kewley, S., & Friedman, H. S. (1987). Psychological predictors of heart disease: A quantitative review. *Psychological Bulletin, 101*, 343–362.

Boyd, J. R., Covington, T. R., Stanaszek, W. F., & Coussons, R. T. (1974). Drug-defaulting. II. Analysis of noncompliance patterns. *American Journal of Hospital Pharmacy, 31*, 485–491.

Chafetz, M. E. (1970). No patient deserves to be patronized. *Medical Insight, 2*, 68–75.

Charney, E. (1972). Patient–doctor communication: Implications for the clinician. *Pediatric Clinics of North America, 19*, 263–279.

Cobb, B. (1954). Why do people detour to quacks? *The Psychiatric Bulletin, 3*, 66–69.

Davis, M. S. (1966). Variations in patients' compliance with doctors' orders: Analysis of congruence between survey responses and results of empirical investigations. *Journal of Medical Education, 41*, 1037–1048.

DiMatteo, M. R. (1979). A social-psychological analysis of physician–patient rapport: Toward a science of the art of medicine. *Journal of Social Issues, 35*(1), 12–33.

DiMatteo, M. R., & DiNicola, D. D. (1982). *Achieving patient compliance*. New York: Pergamon Press.

DiMatteo, M. R., & Friedman, H. S. (1982). A model course in social psychology and health. *Health Psychology, 1*, 181–193.

DiMatteo, M. R., Friedman, H. S., & Taranta, A. (1979). Sensitivity to bodily nonverbal communication as a factor in practitioner–patient rapport. *Journal of Nonverbal Behavior, 4*, 18–26.

Engel, G. L. (1977a). The care of the patient: Art of science? *The Johns Hopkins Medical Journal, 140*, 222–232.

Engel, G. L. (1977b). The need for a new medical model: A challenge for biomedicine. *Science, 196*, 129–136.

Eraker, S. A., Kirscht, J. P., & Becker, M. H. (1984). Understanding and improving patient compliance. *Annals of Internal Medicine, 100*, 258–268.

Francis, V., Korsch, B. M., & Morris, M. J. (1969). Gaps in doctor–patient communications: Patients' response to medical advice. *New England Journal of Medicine, 280*, 535–540.

Friedman, H. S. (1982). Nonverbal communication in medical interaction. In H. S. Friedman & M. R. DiMatteo (Eds.), *Interpersonal issues in health care* (pp. 51–66). New York: Academic Press.

Friedman, H. S., & Booth-Kewley, S. (1987). The "disease-prone personality": A meta-analytic view of the construct. *American Psychologist, 42*, 539–555.

Friedman, H. S., & DiMatteo, M. R. (1979). Health care as an interpersonal process. *Journal of Social Issues, 35*, 1–11.

Friedman, H. S., & DiMatteo, M. R. (1989). *Health psychology*. Englewood Cliffs, NJ: Prentice-Hall.

Friedman, H. S., Hall, J., & Harris, M. J. (1985). Type A behavior, nonverbal expressive style, and health. *Journal of Personality and Social Psychology, 48*, 1299–1315.

Friedman, H. S., Prince, L. M., Riggio, R. E., & DiMatteo, M. R. (1980). Understanding and assessing nonverbal expressiveness: The affective communication test. *Journal of Personality and Social Psychology, 39*, 333–351.

Gillum, R. F., & Barsky, A. J. (1974). Diagnosis and management of patient noncompliance. *Journal of the American Medical Association, 228*, 1563–1567.

Haynes, R. B., (1979). Introduction. In R. B. Haynes, D. W. Taylor, & D. L. Sackett (Eds.), *Compliance in health care* (pp. 1–7). Baltimore: Johns Hopkins University Press.

Haynes, R. B., Taylor, D. W., & Sackett, D. L. (Eds.). (1979). *Compliance in health care*. Baltimore: Johns Hopkins University Press.

Headlee, R. (1973). The tacit contract between doctor and patient. *Medical Insight, 5*, 30–37.

Hippocrates. (1923). *On decorum and the physician* (Vol. II) (W. H. S. Jones, Trans.). London: William Heinemann.

Hulka, B. S. (1979). Patient-clinician interactions and compliance. In R. B. Haynes, D. W. Taylor, & D. L. Sackett (Eds.), *Compliance in health care* (pp. 63–77). Baltimore: Johns Hopkins University Press.

Illich, I. (1976). *Medical nemesis: The expropriation of health*. New York: Random House.

Janis, I. L. (1984). Improving adherence to medical recommendations. In A. Bau, S. E. Taylor, & J. Singer (Eds.), *Handbook of psychology and health, Vol. 4: Social psychological aspects of health* (pp. 113–148). Hillsdale, NJ: Erlbaum.

Janz, N. K., & Becker, M. H. (1984). The health belief model: A decade later. *Health Education Quarterly, 11,* 1–47.

Kasl, S. V. (1975). Issues in patient adherence to health care regimens. *Journal of Human Stress, 1,* 5–17.

Korsch, B. M., Gozzi, E. G., & Francis, V. (1968). Gaps in doctor–patient communication. I. Doctor–patient interaction and patient satisfaction. *Pediatrics, 42,* 855–871.

Lander, L. (1978). *Defective medicine: Risk, anger, and the malpractice crisis.* New York: Farrar, Straus, & Giroux.

Lewis, C. E., Freeman, H. E., & Corey, C. R. (1987). AIDS-related competence of California's primary care physicians. *American Journal of Public Health, 77,* 795–799.

Moos, R. (Ed.). (1977). *Coping with physical illness.* New York: Plenum.

Ockene, J. K. (1987). Physician-delivered interventions for smoking cessation. *Preventive Medicine, 16,* 723–737.

Osler, W. (1904). The master-word in medicine. *Aequanimitas with other addresses to medical students, nurses, and practitioners of medicine* (pp. 369–371). London: H. K. Lewis.

Peabody, F. W. (1927). The care of the patient. *Journal of the American Medical Association, 88,* 877–882.

Rodin, J., & Janis, I. L. (1982). The social influence of physicians and other health care practitioners as agents of change. In H. S. Friedman & M. R. DiMatteo (Eds.), *Interpersonal issues in health care* (pp. 33–49). New York: Academic Press.

Roter, D. L. (1984). Patient question asking in physician–patient interaction. *Health Psychology, 3,* 395–409.

Sackett, D. L., & Snow, J. C. (1979). The magnitude of compliance and noncompliance. In R. B. Haynes, D. W. Taylor, & D. L. Sackett (Eds.), *Compliance in health care* (pp. 11–22). Baltimore: Johns Hopkins University Press.

Salzman, C., Shader, R., Scott, D. A., & Binstock, W. (1970). Interviewer anger and patient dropout in a walk-in clinic. *Comprehensive Psychiatry, 11,* 267–273.

Shapiro, A. K. (1960). A contribution to a history of the placebo effect. *Behavioral Science, 5,* 109–135.

Shapiro, A. K. (1971). Placebo effects in medicine, psychotherapy, and psychoanalysis. In A. E. Bergin & S. L. Garfield (Eds.), *Handbook of psychotherapy and behavior change: An empirical analysis* (2nd ed.) (pp. 439–473). New York: John Wiley.

Shattuck, F. C. (1907). The science and art of medicine in some of their aspects. *Boston Medical and Surgical Journal, 157,* 63–67.

Shorter, E. (1985). *Bedside manners: The troubled history of doctors and patients.* New York: Simon and Schuster.

Stiles, W. B., Putnam, S. M., Wolf, M. H., & James, S. A. (1979). Interaction exchange structure and patient satisfaction with medical interviews. *Medical Care, 17,* 667–679.

Stone, G. C. (1979). Patient compliance and the role of the expert. *Journal of Social Issues, 35,* 34–59.

Svarstad, B. (1976). Physician–patient communication and patient conformity with medical advice. In D. Mechanic (Ed.), *The growth of bureaucratic medicine: An inquiry into the dynamics of patient behavior and the organization of medical care* (pp. 220–238). New York: John Wiley.

Szasz, T. S., & Hollender, M. H. (1956). A contribution to the philosophy of medicine: The basic models of the doctor-patient relationship. *Archives of Internal Medicine, 97,* 585–592.

Tumulty, P. A. (1970). What is a clinician and what does he do? *New England Journal of Medicine, 283,* 20–24.

Vaccarino, J. M. (1977). Malpractice: The problem in perspective. *Journal of the American Medical Association, 238,* 861–863.

5

Issues in the Measurement of Adherence

Cynthia S. Rand

The frequent failure of patients to adequately adhere to prescribed medication and behavioral regimens has been a continual source of frustration to clinicians and a frequent topic of empirical investigation by health researchers (Masur, 1981; Sackett & Haynes, 1976).

Adherence is generally defined as the degree to which patient behaviors coincide with the clinical recommendations of health care providers. While this standard definition of adherence has some conceptual utility, it is far too broad to be of much value in specific clinical or research settings. Instead, adherence must be situationally defined, with the parameters of good adherence explicitly delineated and appropriate for the health behavior under study. Clearly, the way in which we define and measure our variable of interest will fundamentally influence the nature of our findings. There is no gold standard for what defines "good" or "acceptable" adherence across all health behaviors. Factors such as necessary therapeutic levels, research versus clinical setting, the risks of nonadherence, and the complexity of the regimen will all influence the criteria for good adherence. Regardless of the specific standard chosen to categorize or quantify levels of patient adherence, in a research setting the selected adherence criteria should be carefully evaluated, clearly defined, and precisely documented. Clinicians may need less precision than researchers in their adherence criteria; however, they also could benefit from a more thoughtful evaluation of what constitutes "good" patient adherence to commonly recommended medical regimens.

How one chooses to define good adherence is integrally related to the way in which adherence will be best measured. A broadly defined, gross criteria of adherence may not need precise measurement methodology. For example, a physician treating hypertension may recommend a modest salt-restricting diet to a patient. If that physician defines adequate adherence to this prescription as having "eliminated or limited the use of table salt," then patient self-report may be both an appropriate and adequate means of assessing adherence. In contrast, when detailed and exact adherence data are necessary, then the measurement instruments should be comparably precise. Assessment of adherence in a clinical trial, for example, must be as rigorous as possible in order to ensure the fundamental integrity of the study's conclusions.

METHODS FOR MEASURING ADHERENCE

Several investigators have published excellent reviews of adherence measurement research, and the reader is referred to them for greater detail (Dunbar, 1980; Gordis, 1979; Masur, 1981). As these reviewers have noted, all of the most commonly used methods for assessing adherence have both strengths and weaknesses that must be considered in their use. Certainly the poorest (and undoubtedly most widespread) measure of patient adherence is physician's judgment.

Clinician Judgment

Several studies have shown that physicians generally greatly overestimate the degree to which their patients comply with their directives (Davis, 1966; Kasl, 1975; Paulson, Krause, & Iber, 1977). A study by Mushlin and Appel (1977) found that when medical interns and residents attempted to make assessments of individual patients' medication adherence they were accurate only 25% of the time. Physicians not only overestimate patient adherence, they are also poor predictors of which specific patients will be good or poor adherers (Davis, 1966). Whether clinicians are unredeemably poor judges of adherence, or simply unskilled and inconsistent in their methods of assessment, is unclear.

Self-Report

Self-report of medication adherence (an inexpensive and quick measure) has been compared to an objective measure (i.e., pill counts) and found to have a highly variable degree of accuracy (Francis, Korsch, & Morris, 1969; Sheiner, Rosenberg, Marathe, & Peck, 1974). A study by Spector et al. (1986) compared asthmatic patients' self-reports of inhaler usage with the objective adherence data collected by a medication monitoring device called a nebulizer chronolog (discussed below). They found that while all subjects self-reported using the inhaler on more than half of the study days, the measured medication usage indicated that only 52.6% of the subjects actually did so. Self-reports of adherence are influenced by both patient and provider characteristics. Elderly patients with memory impairment (often taking multiple medications) may not be able to accurately self-report their usage pattern of any one medication. Patients on long-term medication regimens may be able to correctly recall recent usage patterns, but may fail to report their adherence patterns 4 months prior to their physician visits. Physicians' sensitivity and skill in eliciting patients' self-reports will certainly influence the reliability and usefulness of the information they receive. While self-report may not be a sufficient measure of adherence in many settings (particularly in research), it is probably a necessary measure in all settings, for, when carefully collected, this information can provide invaluable insight into the nature of patients' problems with adherence. In addition, because there is no evidence to suggest that adhering patients will misrepresent themselves as nonadherers (Gordis, 1976), this measurement technique will allow the simple identification of many candid nonadherers.

Medication Measurement

Medication measurement has frequently been used as a relatively simple yet objective measure of adherence (Gordis, 1976; Roth & Berger, 1960). Counting pills, checking prescription refills, and weighing inhaler canisters or liquid medication are examples of measures that allow researchers to infer the degree of medication adherence. This method requires that the clinician or investigator know exactly how much medication the patient began the measurement period with and how much medication should have been used during this period. While these adherence data are both objective and reasonably simple to collect, they are limited by several factors. Medication measures can easily be influenced by a patient's efforts to deceive the investigator, for example, the guilty patient who discards pills on the morning of his or her appointment. Medications are often shared within households, particularly when family members are on the same medication (i.e., common antihypertensives) and for particular types of medications (i.e., tranquilizers, antibiotics, and sleeping pills). In addition, medication measures give no indication of the accuracy of dosages or the timing of medication (Christensen, 1978). However, in situations where patients are unthreatened by the consequences of reporting nonadherence, the pattern of medication use is not critical, and where the likelihood of medication sharing is low, then medication measurement is a useful, objective, and valid means of assessing adherence.

Biochemical Analysis

Clinical analysis of blood, urine, or other bodily excretions has frequently been used to objectively measure medication or byproduct levels, as well as to detect tracer or marker substances (such as riboflavin) that have been deliberately added to medications to track adherence (Bergman & Werner, 1963; Colcher & Bass, 1972; Markowitz & Gordis, 1968). This is the only method of adherence measurement that confirms that medications have actually been taken by a patient, and for this reason biochemical analysis is one of the most valuable techniques available for assessing adherence. Biochemical analysis is also popular in studies of smoking cessation adherence, where rather than looking for byproducts of medication use, analysis is done for the presence of smoking byproducts, such as carbon monoxide or cotinine (Pechacek, Fox, Murray, & Luepker, 1984). While biochemical analysis allows a very direct assessment of drug use, it also has some limitations. In order for the excretion pattern of the drug, tracer, or byproduct to be clearly understood, drug adherence is best assessed by repeated measures and analyses (Marston, 1970). This type of repeated assessment is probably clinically practical only when the monitoring is also necessary for determining appropriate therapeutic levels of medication (i.e., theophylline levels). Particularly when biochemical analysis requires the use of an invasive procedure to collect a sample, repeated measures solely for confirming adherence are usually impractical. Even when biochemical monitoring is feasible, not all medications can be easily detected or tagged with tracer substances. Biochemical analysis can provide a measure of adherence for a single test, or for multiple tests, but it cannot realistically be used to measure day-to-day adherence with long-term medication. And finally, even this technique can be compromised if a patient deliberately or inadvertently begins taking the medication just prior to the clinical analysis.

Medication Monitors

A fifth strategy for determining adherence has been the development of a variety of medication monitors. These devices are designed to tally medication use, generally by means of specialized medication packaging. Perhaps the most familiar form of medication monitor is those commonly used to package contraceptive pills. This type of special packaging provides a more precise record of medication use than does the usual form of medication measurement. Often medication monitors are employed to promote patient adherence because their design facilitates the patient's ability to self-monitor. Wong and Norman (1987) found that the use of a calendar blister-pak to package medications did reduce nonadherence in a sample of geriatric patients. Becker et al. (1986), however, failed to find a significant adherence-promoting effect when they examined the use of special blister packaging of antihypertensive medication in a randomized trial. Patients in this study reported that they found the blister packaging somewhat inconvenient and more difficult to use than conventional packaging. In both of these studies, the medication monitors were both an independent variable and a dependent variable, because pill counts of the medication remaining in the blister-paks were used (along with other techniques) to assess adherence. Tallying the pills remaining in a blister-pak, like other forms of medication measurement, still does not provide information about a patient's pattern of medication use over time, nor does it eliminate the possibility of patient deceit. A study by Moulding (1979) addressed these problems by using a unique pill dispenser that produced a record of exposure dots on a film strip for each pill taken. Not only did this record document the number of pills taken, it also reflected in the shading of the exposure dots the regularity with which the pills were taken. While such devices provide no guarantee that the medication was actually taken, they do provide strong inferential evidence of daily use.

The Johns Hopkins Lung Health Study (a National Heart, Lung, and Blood Institute-sponsored clinical trial center) will be utilizing a unique medication monitor in a large-scale assessment of subject adherence. A major component of the Lung Health Study is the evaluation of the prophylactic use of an inhaled bronchodilator in the treatment of subjects with early obstructive lung disease. These asymptomatic participants will be asked to use their assigned inhaler (bronchodilator or placebo) three times a day, with each dose consisting of two puffs spaced 2 to 5 minutes apart. Because participant adherence was believed to be both critical and problematic, participant adherence will be measured not only by self-report and canister weighing, but also with a device called the nebulizer chronolog (NB), a microprocessor-based medication monitor. This instrument can be attached to a handheld inhaler, where it will record the day and time of each inhaler usage for up to 4 months. When a subject returns for a follow-up visit the nebulizer chronolog is read by an interpreting device coupled with an IBM PC. The computer will provide the investigators with adherence data, ranging from the exact time and day of each inhaler use to summary reports of average morning usage during January. After being read, each chronolog is re-initialized and can then record another 4 months of adherence data. The use of this innovative adherence measurement technology in the Lung Health Study will not only provide an unparalleled data set on long-term adherence with daily medication in an asymptomatic study population, it may also enhance overall subject adherence. The nebulizer chronolog can potentially improve participants' adherence in several ways. First, the participants' awareness that adherence feedback to the clinical trial staff will be precise and detailed may encourage increased vigilance with the prescribed regimen. Second, the complete adherence record provided by the chronolog will allow the study's behavioral staff to accurately identify subjects with adherence problems early in the study. And third, when a subject is identified as a poor user the detailed record of time and day usage provided by the chronolog will supply the data base necessary to design a tailored adherence promotion program for that subject. For example, if a review of the usage data indicates that inhaler use is worst on weekend mornings, then specific behavioral strategies can be suggested that focus on this problem time period. The chronolog will then be able to provide both the investigators and the participant with rapid feedback on the implemented behavioral intervention's effectiveness.

ISSUES IN ADHERENCE MEASUREMENT
Reactivity

When adherence behavior is monitored by methods that are known by both the clinician and the patient to be both accurate and revealing, there is a strong possibility that patients' adherence behavior will be altered to meet the demand characteristics of the monitoring situation. In fact, there may well be a direct relationship between the detail and precision of any measurement strategy and its impact on adherence. How troublesome this reactivity will be will depend upon the goals of the study or clinical interaction. When the focus of a study is on the generalizability of the study's conclusions (i.e., will most patients use enough bronchodilator to achieve therapeutic goals?), then the use of a specialized, highly reactive measurement methodology would be inappropriate (Dunbar, 1980). If, however, the goal is improved adherence for either research purposes (i.e., is this bronchodilator efficacious?) or clinical purposes, then the use of reactive measurement techniques may be desirable. It therefore is important to clarify the goals of adherence assessment in each research or clinical application and to then select the most appropriate measurement strategies.

Multiple Measures

Because of the relative strengths and weaknesses of each of the adherence measures discussed, the optimal strategy for assessing adherence will usually involve the use of multiple measures. Patient contacts in both clinical and research settings should almost certainly include the eliciting of self-report information. Skillfully collected, these data will not only identify adherence difficulties, but will also provide the investigator with information about the circumstances of nonadherence. The correction of adherence difficulties may well depend upon the investigator understanding the whys of nonadherence and working with the patient toward a solution.

The inclusion of one or more objective measures when assessing adherence will confirm patients' self-report, but their potential reactive effect should be weighed. Self-report combined with an unannounced biochemical analysis of a urine sample is unlikely to have any impact on patients' adherence behavior, while self-report combined with blister-pak medication monitoring and repeated drug-screening urinalysis probably will alter either the patient's adherence behavior, self-report, or both.

The Use of Adherence Data

Clinicians interested in assessing patient adherence should clarify to themselves and then in turn to their patients why this information is being collected and what exactly the information is to be used for. In a research context, where the value of a drug or therapeutic regimen is being evaluated, the purpose of adherence assessment may be well defined for the investigator, but unclear to the participant. In clinical care, adherence assessment can easily be interpreted by patients as paternalistic intrusion, the doctor checking for who's been "naughty" or "nice." Unfortunately, for some clinicians that is exactly the intent and tone of their adherence assessment, with patients being categorized as "good" (adherers) or "bad" (nonadherers). If the goal of adherence determination is the evaluation of a treatment's efficacy, rather than a judgment of the patient's reliability or trustworthiness, then this goal should be both explicit and implicit in the patient–physician interaction.

FUTURE DIRECTIONS FOR ADHERENCE RESEARCH

The better a behavior can be observed, the more complete will be our understanding of that behavior. The recent explosion in microcomputer technology has opened up remarkable new opportunities in adherence monitoring technology. The possibility now exists for the investigator to examine real-life adherence behavior with close to the control and observation allowed by a laboratory setting. While specialized adherence monitors such as the nebulizer chronolog are hardly a panacea for patient adherence difficulties, incorporating their use in both clinical and research settings would not only improve measurement precision, but would also offer increased opportunities for adherence-promoting interventions.

Whether sophisticated new technology or a simple clinical interview is utilized to measure and promote adherence, the patient or subject should be recognized as an active partner in the patient–provider exchange. No technology now or in the future will replace the good listening and sincere concern of a first-rate therapeutic relationship.

REFERENCES

Becker, L. A., Glanz, K., Sobel, E., Mossey, J., Zinn, S. L., & Knott, K. A. (1986). A randomized trial of special packaging of antihypertensive medication. *The Journal of Family Practice, 22,* 357–361.

Bergman, A. B., & Werner, R. J. (1963). Failure of children to receive penicillin by mouth. *New England Journal of Medicine, 268,* 1334–1338.

Christensen, D. B. (1978). Drug-taking compliance: A review and synthesis. *Health Services Research, 13,* 171–187.

Colcher, I. S., & Bass, J. W. (1972). Penicillin treatment of streptococcal pharyngitis: A comparison of schedules and the role of specific counseling. *Journal of the American Medical Association, 222,* 657–659.

Davis, M. S. (1966). Variations in patients' compliance with doctors' orders: Analysis of congruence between survey responses and results of empirical investigations. *Journal of Medical Education, 41,* 1037–1048.

Dunbar, J. M. (1980). Assessment of medication compliance: A review. In R. B. Haynes, M. E. Mattson, & T. O. Engelbretson (Eds.), *Patient compliance to prescribed antitensive regimens: A report to the National Heart, Lung, and Blood Institute* (pp. 63–82) (N.I.H. Publication No. 81-2102). U.S. Department of Health & Human Services, Public Health Service, Bethesda, MD.

Francis, V., Korsch, B. M., & Morris, M. J. (1969). Gaps in doctor–patient communications. *New England Journal of Medicine, 280,* 535–540.

Gordis, L. (1979). Methodologic issues in the measurement of patient compliance. In D. L. Sackett & R. B. Haynes (Eds.), *Compliance with therapeutic regimens.* Baltimore: Johns Hopkins University Press.

Kasl, S. V. (1975). Issues in patient adherence to health care regimens. *Journal of Human Stress, 1,* 5–17.

Markowitz, M., & Gordis, L. (1968). A mail-in technique for detecting penicillin in urine: Application to the study of maintenance of prophylaxis in rheumatic fever patients. *Pediatrics, 41,* 151–153.

Marston, W. V. (1970). Compliance with medical regimens: A review of the literature. *Nursing Research, 19,* 312–323.

Masur, F. T. (1981). Adherence to health care regimens. In C. K. Prolop & L. A. Bradley (Eds.), *Medical psychology.* New York: Academic Press.

Moulding, T. (1979). The unrealized potential of the medication monitor. *Clinical Pharmacology and Therapeutics, 25,* 131–136.

Mushlin, A. I., & Appel, F. A. (1977). *Archives of Internal Medicine, 137*(3), 318–321.

Paulson, S. M., Krause, S., & Iber, R. (1977). Development and evaluation of a compliance test for patients taking disulfiram. *Johns Hopkins Medical Journal, 141,* 119–125.

Pechacek, T. F., Fox, F. H., Murray, D. M., & Luepker, R. V. (1984). Review of techniques for measurement of smoking behavior. In J. D. Matarazzo, J. D. Weiss, A. J. Herd, N. E. Miller, & S. M. Weiss (Eds.), *Behavioral health: A Handbook of health enhancement and disease prevention*. New York: John Wiley & Sons.

Roth, H. P., & Berger, D. G. (1960). Studies on patient cooperation in ulcer treatment. I. Observation of actual as compared to prescribed antacid intake on a hospital ward. *Gastroenterology, 38*, 630-633.

Sackett, D. L., & Haynes, R. B. (1976). *Compliance with therapeutic regimens.* Baltimore: Johns Hopkins University Press.

Sheiner, L. B., Rosenberg, B., Marathe, V. V., & Peck, C. (1974). Differences in serum digoxin concentrations between outpatients and inpatients: An effect of compliance? *Clinical Pharmacology and Therapeutics, 15*, 239-246.

Soutter, B. R., & Kennedy, M. B. (1974). Patient compliance assessment in drug trials: Usage and methods. *Australian and New Zealand Journal of Medicine (Sydney), 4*, 360-364.

Spector, S. L., Kinsman, R., Mawhinney, H., Siegel, S. C., Rachelefsky, G. S., Katz, R. M., & Rohr, A. S. (1986). Compliance of patients with asthma with an experimental aerosolized medication: Implications for controlled clinical trials. *Journal of Allergy and Clinical Immunology, 77*, 65-70.

Wong, B. S. M., & Norman, D. C. (1987). Evaluation of a novel medication aid, the calendar blister-pak and its effect on drug compliance in a geriatric outpatient clinic. *Journal of the American Geriatrics Society, 35*, 21-26.

Commentary: Theory and Measurement in Adherence Research

Andrew Baum

As has been amply discussed and documented in this section of the book, adherence is a vitally important aspect of curative and preventive medical regimens. This is so for several reasons. First, assuring that patients do as they have been advised is necessary to maximize treatment and to optimize the relationship between patient and health care specialists. In addition, the basis upon which health care delivery, diagnostic procedures, and so on depends on one's willingness to maintain adherence to one or another regimen or prescription. Perhaps the most compelling reason to study adherence, though, lies in the fact that many people do not correctly follow medical advice, hobbling the physician and medical staff charged with patient care. Whether deliberate, caused by poor doctoring skills, or simply a matter of poor communication, lack of adherence is a major problem in health care and requires clever and imaginative research.

Studying adherence, however, is not an easy thing to do. Understanding why people do or do not comply with prescriptions for medicines, habitual behavior change, preventive screening, and so on is not well served by laboratory investigation, and reporting rates on adherence may not accurately reflect whether patients are in fact doing as they were advised. As Rand notes in her chapter, self-report of medication adherence is often in error, subject to recall problems, the desire to please the physician, and other patient and care provider characteristics. Judgments by the provider are not very good indices of adherence, and measurement of medication to determine whether proper doses have been taken is also limited. We can assay patients' blood or urine and determine whether appropriate levels of a medication are present or whether tracer substances are detectable, but this is expensive and is not entirely without problems: it is best done several times, may vary with metabolism changes and stress, and is invasive. Rand goes on to discuss medication monitors, designed to count medication use through packaging of the medicine. Research suggests that this measurement strategy yields more accurate and useful data, though simultaneous use of multiple measures probably offers the most effective assessment of adherence.

It should be clear that measures of adherence will be imperfect, as the refinements and measures discussed above pertain only to compliance with medication regimens. Preventive advice to change one's life-style or diet or otherwise alter longstanding behavior can only be inferred from ultimate change in behavior, weight, or other outcomes and cannot be measured objectively if one leaves the environment intact. Regardless, research has progressed and a number of theoretical perspectives derived. Becker reviews 10 of these models. Some are heavily determined by antecedent conditions such as predispositions, beliefs, and knowledge, others are characterized by emphasis on one's ability to secure services or gain access to health resources, and most consider patient needs and/or physician behavior. Many are descriptive: use of health care depends on whether one is predisposed to use it, whether it is accessible, whether the consequences of not doing so are serious, whether we are reminded to use these services. Other models are derived from the attitude change literature in social psychology, focusing on intentions and other mental constructs to predict behavior. Though they capture the basis on which many decisions are based, all of these models presuppose that the patient will be scientific or at least rational in his or her decision making. Clearly, some adherence problems are neither intentional nor rational.

The most important direction for research on adherence to take is in deriving programs and strategies for improving compliance. Much of the other work we do in this area ultimately translates into improvements in our ability to measure or predict adherence, but the bottom line is that adherence should be increased. Whether we will accomplish "better" behavior or not or whether we are struggling against a ceiling imposed by organismic limits depends in part on how one views the problem. Are we attempting to increase the frequency of good behavior (i.e., following regimens), or are we trying to extinguish behaviors that interfere with adherence (e.g., forgetting, naive theories)? The assumptions underlying these orientations are different and would likely lead us to different approaches to the problem.

Much of the research that has been done appears to be based on the notion that the obstacles to adherence must be eliminated. Friedman's chapter, for example, considers the interaction between patient and physician to be a crucial source of these "bad" behaviors. Improving the interpersonal quality of these interactions and reducing barriers to adherence is the goal of this work, and there is clear evidence of the problems that characterize the doctor–patient relationship. The extent to which the systematic elimination of these problems will yield increments in adherence is not yet clear.

The questionnaire discussed by Goodwin and his colleagues begins to combine a focus of adherence as a skill or quality with the notion that better adherence will follow elimination of factors that interfere with it. Assessing a patient's skills and reinforcing those that are less well-developed, measuring those characteristics of one's environment that might interfere and minimizing them, and assessing social support and other situational variables that may help to reduce the effects of interfering factors is a broad strategy combining several perspectives.

One final issue is related to the belief that characteristics of the situation are of primary importance in determining adherence. The stage of treatment or type of behavior that is of interest is key in understanding or attempting to modify one's compliance with the regimen. Long-term behavior change that is often directed toward elimination of habitual or addictive behavior or treatment/prevention of asymptomatic conditions offers perhaps the greatest challenge. Marlatt and George discuss one important aspect of adherence with long-term changes, focusing on the postintervention maintenance of healthy behavior. Relapse prevention is not just a matter of stamping out the behavior being modified. The meaning of relapse and how a patient is oriented toward one or more failures appear to be important determinants of successful maintenance. Interpretation of their causes and significance in the long run contribute to the effects of relapses in the ultimate success of attempts to modify life-style, drug use, and other problem behaviors.

Whether dramatic improvements in adherence can be achieved remains largely unanswered. Interventions designed to do so must address basic skills and motivation as well as situational factors and aspects of the nature of the target of adherence in different regimens. The continued development of theories that specify the dynamics of medication taking, life-style modification, and so on is necessary for this effort to achieve success. At the same time, better understanding of the methodological problems in evaluating these factors is needed.

SECTION II

Life-Style Interventions and Maintenance of Behaviors

Joan M. Wolle, Editor

The theoretical bases for affecting health behavior change were presented in the first section of this book. This section focuses on the implementation of life-style interventions and maintenance of behaviors for several chronic health conditions. The targeted populations include HIV-positive hemophiliacs, older adults with progressive chronic obstructive pulmonary disease (COPD), youngsters with asthma, middle-aged people with high cholesterol levels, and those recovering from myocardial infarction.

In Chapter 6, Agle discusses the psychological and social factors that may influence compliance with safer sex behaviors. In counseling HIV-positive hemophiliacs, Agle advises using a biopsychological rather than a biomedical approach. He further advises that all patients and couples may not be responsive to counseling and may require instructions delivered in a benevolent, authoritative manner.

In Chapter 7, Kaplan et al. present evidence indicating that exercise and rehabilitation interventions result in an enhanced health status and improved quality of life without necessarily directly affecting pulmonary functioning. The COPD patients are an example of a type of patient for whom it may not be possible to devise interventions that will change the course of the disease but it may be possible to devise interventions that may help them live fuller lives.

In Chapter 8, Evans et al. describe a school-based program for young children with asthma. As a result of the educational interventions, the children increased their asthma self-management skills and peer social support, reduced the frequency and duration of episodes of asthma, and improved their academic performance.

In Chapter 9, Ewart develops a performance model to explain change, incorporating the diverse social pressures and personal problems encountered when people try to maintain health behaviors over the long term. The proposed Social Problem-Solving Model integrates critical behavioral processes that are necessary for long-term maintainance. A potential application of the model is indicated for tertiary prevention after uncomplicated myocardial infarction.

In Chapter 10, McCann et al. present an overview of current knowledge about adherence to cholesterol-lowering diets and a broad-based model for organizing a review of efforts to identify gaps in knowledge about implementing dietary recommendations. The authors draw upon their experiences in a study of dietary alternatives for lipid lowering in Seattle, Washington.

In his discussion of the chapters in this section, Secker-Walker has emphasized that despite the diversity of behaviors addressed, interventions used, and target populations, common themes emerge that are significant in enhancing adherence. He also points to the need to include a broader environmental context to describe behavior changes and recommends the use of the Social Problem-Solving Model, described in Chapter 9, to test the hypotheses implicit in the model.

The authors of the chapters in this section have discussed the implementation and evaluation of several programs to influence human behavior among populations with chronic health conditions and have indicated research needs. The theoretical model that has been proposed can be used as a framework to guide efforts to encourage adherence. Both researchers and practitioners should find the concepts in these chapters useful and the suggestions for future studies challenging.

6

Life-Style Interventions For HIV-Antibody-Positive Hemophiliacs

David Agle

AIDS and its causative agent—the human immunodeficiency virus, HIV—present major challenges for health education today. Massive educational programs are generated to promote the critical health behavior—the practice of safer sex. There is, however, little compelling evidence that patient education consistently influences health behavior. This suggests that efforts to encourage compliance with safer sex recommendations must include more than just the provision of information. One critical intervention is the recognition and management of psychological and social factors that impact on health behavior. There is no quick and easy way to do this. The promotion of safer sex must be an ongoing process and not a single educational encounter.

This chapter describes certain psychological and social factors that appear to influence compliance with safer sex recommendations and a program approach to deal with them. These ideas come from clinical experience with the hemophilic population.

Hemophilia is a genetically inherited bleeding disorder generally passed from carrier mother to recipient son. People with hemophilia have been infected with HIV through contaminated blood products. It is estimated that 85% of all hemophiliacs who regularly used clotting factor concentrates prior to 1985 are seropositive for HIV antibodies, and many show immunologic dysfunction (Agle, Gluck, & Pierce, 1987). Their sexual partners are also in jeopardy. A 1985 study found that 9.5% of wives of seropositive hemophiliac husbands were themselves seropositive, and this rate is increasing (Kriess, Kitchen, Prince, Kasper, & Essex, 1985).

Essentially, then, the majority of adolescents and adults with hemophilia are capable of transmitting this deadly virus through sexual behaviors. In the face of this impending catastrophe, the sexually active hemophiliac has three disagreeable choices: sexual abstinence, risking behaviors that may be lethal to others, or using safer sex and avoiding pregnancies. The choice may seem easy, but human behavior does not always follow apparent logic.

COMPLIANCE IN GENERAL

Illness Factors

What do compliance studies tell us that is relevant to safer sex behaviors? First, compliance with doctor's orders is greater when the patient feels the most discomfort (Blackwell, 1973). Conversely, compliance is least in disorders such as silent hypertension where no symptoms are present (Kirscht, Kirscht, & Rosenstock, 1981). The incentive of personal discomfort is lacking to support safer sex behaviors.

Patient Knowledge

While it is reasonable to assume that patients who are more knowledgeable about their disease and its treatment would be more compliant, study results are not convincing. For example, Sackett found only spotty response to massive education regarding the life-saving properties of antihypertensives (Sackett, Haynes, & Gibson, 1975).

Fear Techniques

Fear is a double-edged sword. While some patient apprehension facilitates compliance, actual threats of dire consequences for noncompliance are more apt to damage the doctor–patient relationship and increase patient denial (Higbee, 1969). It would seem naive, then, to assume that massive education concerning the real horrors of AIDS would be sufficient to ensure safer sex behaviors.

Patient Attitude Toward Health and Disease

Becker and others have defined the health belief model emphasizing patient attitude about health as the critical determinant of compliance (Becker et al., 1977). Their work suggests that compliance is better when the patient (1) feels susceptible to the illness, (2) believes that the illness can have severe consequences, (3) believes that the treatment can be effective, and (4) sees no major obstacles to using the recommended behavior.

This model is based on cognition—a framework for what the patient says he or she knows or believes. This seems to ignore the enormous complexities and multideterminants of behavior—character, affect and behavior control, defensive and coping patterns, socioeconomic state, and social support. Yet, when viewed as the final common pathway of these multideterminants, the health belief model can have considerable utility in organizing counseling approaches. Hemophiliacs themselves will suffer no direct physical consequences from practicing unsafe sex. Here the model is applicable to their desire to protect others from these consequences.

SAFER SEX AND THE CONDOM

Simple and ritualistic behaviors are more apt to be adopted than complex ones (Stoudemire & Thompson, 1983). The recommended health behavior to prevent the spread of HIV is simply to prevent the transmission of body fluids from a seropositive donor to a noninfected partner. The best available method is the careful use of condoms to prevent the passage of semen and other body fluids during sexual activity. Unfortunately, this is not a simple, easily adapted behavior. At the least, condoms are considered a nuisance. They are intrusive, and many feel that they significantly reduce pleasurable sexual sensations. Condom use requires considerable self-control, somewhat of a contradiction to the compelling nature of sexual excitement and the common mix of sex and alcohol. In fact, condoms do not have a wonderful track record. A 10 to 20% failure rate in contraception over a 12-month period of usage has been reported (Johns Hopkins University, 1982).

HEMOPHILIC PATIENT COMPLIANCE
WITH SAFER SEX BEHAVIORS

What are patient responses so far to safer sex education, and what can we anticipate? The results of an anonymous questionnaire survey of a portion of the clinical population of the Mt. Sinai Hemophilic Treatment Center in New York City demonstrated that 98% of respondents were highly knowledgeable about HIV infection and how to prevent its spread. Yet the same knowledgeable patients use condoms less than 50% of the time. Even this figure may be an overestimate of condom usage because of nonresponse bias (Aledort, 1987).

This is an alarming, but not surprising, finding. As in most behaviors, patient response to initial educational efforts will include a group who will readily comply, a group who will never comply, and a large group who will need much attention in order to achieve consistent safer sex behavior. This response variation cannot be understood without attention to psychological factors.

Ready Compliers

Part of the group who readily comply are those who become sexually abstinent. Many of these are young men already uncomfortable about sexual behaviors and other forms of intimacy. Under the impact of AIDS education, they choose abstinence with little discomfort or even some relief. Others who are readily compliant are those patients who possess character traits allowing them to consider and trust the opinion of experts, to work for future goals, to consider the welfare of others, and to exercise reasonable self-control.

FACTORS IN NONCOMPLIANCE OF HEMOPHILIC PATIENTS

Anxiety

The state of anxiety is both a friend and a foe of the health educator. As any teacher knows, some anxiety helps by increasing attention and alertness, but excessive anxiety leads to panic and a variety of mental responses that defeat the educational goal. Best known of these is the defensive maneuver of denial (Stoudemire & Thompson, 1983). Denial is an effort to ward off anxiety by avoiding or not recognizing frightening information, by forgetting it, or by minimizing its significance. The use of denial is clearly an obstacle to safer sex compliance.

Hargraves and others at the Centers for Disease Control recently found that a group of hemophilic respondents showed greater knowledge about AIDS risk factors for the gay population than for themselves (Hargraves, 1987). The obvious conclusion is that the hemophilic population needs more education. But denial would also explain this finding—a blindness to an unacceptable problem in the self that is seen more clearly in others. More education generally does not reduce denial. Efforts to reduce anxiety levels are required.

Excessive anxiety may lead to daredevil or counterphobic behaviors. The daredevil repeats dangerous behaviors in an attempt to prove invulnerability. Such behaviors are often seen in hemophilic boys and adolescents who seem unusually attracted to such activities as motorcycle racing (Agle, 1964). The counterphobic response could lead to dangerous avoidance of condoms—an exciting version of Russian roulette played by both sexual partners. Patient anger is another important factor. A potential interference with a trusting counselor-patient relationship is the hidden anger of some patients that their dangerous situation has been caused by blood products prescribed by the treatment center itself.

The Condom as a Symbol

What does the condom symbolize? Some patients report that the condom is the horrible reminder of AIDS and their own potential destructiveness to their loved ones. Rather than a reassurance of safety, it brings to mind a partially denied worry and can lead to sexual dysfunction.

Others describe the condom as a blow to self-esteem. These men have struggled all their lives to prove that they are as good or better than others in spite of having a chronic disease. The condom destroys this barely won victory. Once more they are made to feel not only different and defective, but, in fact, unclean and harmful to others. The condom then destroys self-esteem, a so-called narcissistic blow. Small wonder that denial and avoidance of safer sex instruction occur.

Psychopathology

Included in the noncompliant group are patients with sociopathic tendencies, that is, people whose character structure features little or no conscience or regard for the rights of others. They are controlled only by the fear of being caught.

Central Nervous System Damage

Others will not be able to comply because they cannot attend to and use information. Since HIV tends to attack the central nervous system, early deliriums and dementias may be a significant threat to safer sex practices.

Mood Disorders

Significant mood disorders may impair adaptation to safer sex. Patients with major depression feature apathy, impaired concentration, low energy levels, and overt and covert self-destructive tendencies. The significantly depressed person has little interest in health practices (Stoudemire & Thompson, 1983). Depression is seen in the HIV-positive individual and, even more commonly, in patients with AIDS-related complex and AIDS itself. In contrast, the manic phase of bipolar illness features grandiosity and lack of interest in controlled behavior.

THE COUPLE RELATIONSHIP

The couple relationship is, of course, critical. The sexual partner's logical fear and temporary loss of sexual interest may mean a variety of things to the hemophiliac mate. For some, it confirms their own sense of being defective and unworthy of being loved. One response is to demand reassurance through sex without condoms.

Dangerous behaviors can be initiated by the hemophiliac's partner. One young woman said that she proved her love for her hemophiliac fiancé by not insisting that he use a condom. Another said that since she worked in a hospital, she was just as much at risk for AIDS as her hemophiliac lover, so no condoms were necessary. This is a form of rationalization that borders on the delusional.

The examination of the couple relationship clarifies the issue of incentive for safer sex compliance. The hemophiliac's incentive is basically altruistic—the desire to protect others or at least to avoid their anger. The incentive for his sexual partner, on the other hand, is to avoid HIV infection. It seems logical that the drive for self-preservation is a more powerful force than altruism. This suggests that the sexual partner should be a key target of education and counseling. This, in turn, raises ethical and legal problems. Each treatment center must develop guidelines regarding patient confidentiality versus aggressive outreach to sexual partners.

PRINCIPLES OF MANAGEMENT

This brief review of some of the obvious and the more hidden obstacles to safer sex compliance helps define some principles of management. First, one must avoid the naive view that compliance is merely a matter of enough information; rather, it must be a multistaged process. Second, this process will require skilled people; for example, counselors with sufficient training and experience to recognize and deal with complex psychological issues. Finally, the approach to compliance should follow a biopsychosocial rather than biomedical model.

The Biomedical Model

The narrow biomedical approach assumes that the patient will do as he or she is told. Noncompliant responses trigger more education, persuasion, and even threats. Patients are told that recommended behaviors are good for them, they are warned that noncompliance is silly and bad, and they are threatened with dire consequences if they do not behave.

The Biopsychosocial Model

In contrast, the biopsychosocial approach is nonjudgmental. Rather, the noncompliant patient is viewed as a person dealing with feelings and ideas that produce resistance. Empathy is used to understand the patient's feelings, and dialogue replaces lecture. The ingredients of noncompliance are identified as ideas and feelings that eventually can be mastered. The patient's own self-control and self-efficacy are emphasized. In order to achieve these results, the care provider/

patient relationship should be carefully scrutinized. The patient becomes a colleague in the effort, not a passive recipient of information (Brody, 1980).

This attitudinal difference in the counseling relationship is important. The traditional concept of the doctor–patient relationship views the patient as a passive, dependent person whose role is to seek competent help and cooperate with the doctor who is granted dominance. This traditional relationship is ineffective with many patients, particularly those with chronic disorders; self-care and self-determination are becoming increasingly emphasized in patient management. Unless the patient sees him or herself as an active colleague in counseling, the more hidden ideas and feelings that interfere with safer sex behaviors can never be addressed.

The process of safer sex instruction involves several steps. First is getting the patient's attention and extending the concept of patient to include the sexual mate. Dialogue is emphasized rather than lecture as the counselor carefully monitors the patient's anxiety and ability to comprehend the information. Safer sexual pleasures receive considerable emphasis, not just attention to restrictions. Common problems in using condoms, both mechanical and emotional, are anticipated, along with the clear message that these can be overcome through further work and understanding. The patient must feel comfortable about returning and talking about failure if failure is to be overcome.

Follow-up is critical. Follow-up does not mean an interrogation to determine if the patient is behaving, but rather a dialogue examining any problems in accepting the health behavior. There are no shortcuts in this work; counselors must be prepared for repeated sessions for some patients and referral of others with identified psychiatric disorders.

Counseling methods will vary depending upon specific patient's or couple's needs as well as the training and the skills of the counselor. Insight psychotherapy will be valuable for some, helping the patient to understand and master the hidden ideas and feelings that lead to noncompliance. For others, a cognitive behavioral approach will be more useful. The health belief model provides one framework for a cognitive approach (Becker et al., 1977).

This biopsychosocial approach to safer sex instruction will not be applicable to all patients or couples. It is a guideline that will require modification according to the needs of individual patients and couples. For example, not all patients can take part in counseling as a colleague. Rather, they require instructions (both oral and written) provided in a benevolent, authoritative manner.

IMPLEMENTATION

How can such a program be implemented? For the hemophilic population, the burden of this counseling falls largely to the staff of comprehensive hemophilic treatment centers. Fortunately, many of these centers now have effective psychosocial programs. As the AIDS epidemic has intensified the needs of the population, more sophisticated and larger mental health programs have developed. The National Hemophilia Foundation in partnership with the Bureau of Maternal and Child Health and the Centers for Disease Control has assisted these programs through staff education. These efforts have included medical bulletins, guidelines for AIDS counseling, and a series of regional workshops devoted to psychosocial issues. Workshop curricula include ethical and legal issues, problems of compliance, the methodology of safer sex instruction, and dealing with staff burnout.

RESEARCH DIRECTIONS

There are a number of potentially valuable studies for this at-risk and stressed population. These include observations of stress response and coping, the impact of stress on the immune system, and efficacy studies of safer sex counseling approaches. One testable hypothesis is that a comprehensive program, including psychosocial case finding and counseling, will more effectively control seroconversion in sex partners than education alone. The methods of safer sex counseling with the sexual partner and the adolescent require special attention.

CONCLUSION

The most compelling issue facing the medical care system today is the control of HIV infection. Clinical experience with the hemophilic population suggests certain critical psychosocial factors that impact on the practice of safer sex. Safer sex counseling must include careful attention to these relevant psychosocial issues.

REFERENCES

Agle, D. P. (1964). Psychiatric studies of patients with hemophilia and related states. *Archives of Internal Medicine, 114*, 76–82.
Agle, D. P., Gluck, H., & Pierce, G. F. (1987). The risk of AIDS: Psychologic impact on the hemophilic population. *General Hospital Psychiatry, 9*, 11–17.
Aledort, L. (1987). Personal communication.
Becker, M. H., Haefner, D. P., Kasl, S. V., Kirscht, J. P., Maiman, L. A., & Rosenstock, I. M. (1977). Selected psychosocial models and correlates of individual health related behaviors. *Medical Care, 15*, 27–46.

Blackwell, B. (1973). Drug therapy: Patient compliance. *New England Journal of Medicine, 289*, 249–252.

Brody, D. S. (1980). The patient's role in clinical decision making. *Annals of Internal Medicine, 93*, 718–722.

Hargraves, M. (1987). Hemophilic patient's knowledge and educational needs concerning AIDS. *American Journal of Hematology.*

Higbee, K. L. (1969). Fifteen years of fear arousal: Research on threat appeals. *Psychological Bulletin, 17*, 426–444.

The Johns Hopkins University. (1982). Update on condoms—Products, protection, promotion. *Population Reports, 10*(5), 121–156.

Kirscht, J. P., Kirscht, J. L., & Rosenstock, I. M. (1981). A test of interventions to increase adherence to hypertension medical regimens. *Health Education Quarterly, 8*, 261–272.

Kriess, J. M., Kitchen, L. W., Prince, H. E., Kasper, C. K., & Essex, M. (1985). Antibody to human T-lymphotrophic virus type III in wives of hemophiliacs—Evidence for heterosexual transmission. *Annals of Internal Medicine, 102*, 623–626.

Sackett, D. L., Haynes, R. B., & Gibson, E. S. (1975). Randomized clinical trial of strategies for improving medical compliance in primary hypertension. *Lancet, 1*, 1205–1207.

Stoudemire, A., & Thompson, T. L. (1983). Medication noncompliance: Systematic approaches to evaluation and interventions. *General Hospital Psychiatry, 5*, 233–239.

7

Adherence to Prescribed Regimens for Patients with Chronic Obstructive Pulmonary Disease

Robert M. Kaplan, Michelle Toshima,
Catherine J. Atkins, Andrew L. Ries

Chronic obstructive pulmonary disease (COPD) is a major cause of disability in most Western countries. Behavior and COPD are inseparably intertwined. Extensive evidence over the past 30 years suggest that smoking behavior is the major risk factor for the development of emphysema and chronic bronchitis (Higgins, 1958; National Institutes of Health, 1983). In addition, several epidemiologic studies have shown that the rate of decline in pulmonary function for afflicted patients decreases with cessation of smoking behavior (Astin, 1976). Thus, individual behavior is a major risk factor for the development and maintenance of COPD. Once diagnosed, COPD patients are asked to comply with a complex regimen that may incude multiple medications, chest physiotherapy, and exercise. Thus, behavioral management strategies are also important in the care of

COPD patients. In this chapter we focus on behavioral programs for COPD patients. As the review will suggest, the contemporary literature contains few descriptions of systematically evaluated programs. Before considering the behavioral interventions, it will be worthwhile to review the definition of COPD and its etiology, prevalence, and medical management.

THE THREE CHRONIC OBSTRUCTIVE PULMONARY DISEASES

The American College of Chest Physicians and the American Thoracic Society define COPD as a "disease of uncertain etiology characterized by persistent slowing of airflow during forced expiration" (ACCP-ATS Joint Committee, 1976). Chronic bronchitis, emphysema, and asthma are the three diseases most commonly associated with COPD. The common denominator of these disorders is expiratory flow obstruction due to airway narrowing, although the cause of airflow obstruction is different in each. Also, in many patients airflow obstruction may be attributed to more than one specific condition.

Emphysema

Emphysema is characterized by abnormal enlargement of the air spaces resulting from destruction of the walls of the alveoli. Alveoli are clusters of air spaces at the ends of the airways in the lung. As the alveolar walls break down, individual alveoli coalesce, and the lung gradually loses its elasticity. This loss of lung elasticity means that the airways are not held open during expiration and tend to collapse. Air gets trapped in these damaged areas, and the lungs become inflated and enlarged (Tisi, 1980; West, 1977).

Chronic Bronchitis

Chronic bronchitis is the result of chronic inflammation of the cells lining the breathing passages (bronchi). The inflammation causes the cells to swell and produce excess quantities of mucus. The swelling and excess mucus result in a narrowing of the bronchi, which, in turn, obstructs the airflow. The irritation of excess mucus also produces a chronic cough (Tisi, 1980; West, 1977).

Asthma

Asthma is a disease in which the muscles of the bronchial tubes experience spasm in response to some irritant such as an infection, allergy, cold air, or cigarette smoking. The spasm produces airway narrowing, which may reverse spontaneously or after treatment. In addition, the irritant causes an oversecretion of mucus, which further narrows the airways.

The common feature shared in emphysema, chronic bronchitis, and asthma is difficulty in expelling air from the lungs during expiration. In practice, the clinical signs and symptoms of these three diseases are often very similar. In fact, many patients with COPD have varying combinations of emphysema, chronic bronchitis, and asthma (West, 1977). However, asthma differs from chronic bronchitis and emphysema in that a component of the obstruction can be reversed by the administration of a brochodilator medication.

ETIOLOGY

The specific etiologies of emphysema, asthma, and chronic bronchitis have not been definitely determined (Tisi, 1980). While the exact cause of each of the three diseases may be somewhat different, it appears that some etiologic features are common to each. Smoking is clearly the major risk factor for the development of emphysema and chronic bronchitis and is an irritant that may exacerbate chronic asthma. Genetic factors contribute to the development of COPD in some cases (Petty, 1978a; U.S. Government Task Force, 1979). For these individuals, a deficiency in alpha-1 antitrypsin enzyme leads to the development of the disease. In addition, allergy may play a major role in the development of asthma (Tisi, 1980).

The roles of air pollution, occupational fumes, and repeated lung infections in producing COPD are all subjects of considerable study (Brashear, 1980; Petty, 1978a; U.S. Government Task Force, 1979). It appears that all of these factors make COPD worse (Petty, 1978a; Tisi, 1980). In addition, a number of occupational exposures are believed to be causally related to asthma and chronic bronchitis, leading to pulmonary damage in susceptible patients (West, 1977).

PREVALENCE

COPD has become an important public health problem for at least four reasons: (1) it is a major cause of death, (2) it affects a large number of persons, (3) incidence is increasing, and (4) it has a major impact upon activities of daily living (Crystal, 1987). Deaths due to COPD are rising at a rate of 1.4% per year (U.S. Government Task Force, 1979). From 1970 to 1975, the mortality rate from chronic obstructive pulmonary diseases increased from 16 per 100,000 of the population to 19 per 100,000 of the population (Brashear, 1980). COPD now ranks fifth as a cause of death in the U.S. and accounted for nearly 70,000 deaths in 1985. In addition, COPD was a contributing cause of death for nearly 80,000 individuals (Crystal 1987). Another indicator of the severity of COPD can be measured in years of potential life lost before age 55 as a result of the disease. Although COPD ranks 12th in this category, it has rapidly increased in recent years. A 1987 report suggests that COPD ranks third for increases in years of potential life lost between 1984 and 1985. The change in rate was 4.5%. Only diabetes mellitus (6.4%) and AIDS (82.4%) had more rapid rates of increase.

Respiratory diseases are generally considered to be of greater importance as causes of disability and ill health than as causes of death. Studies that deal with long-term course and prognosis of COPD indicate that the process covers a time span of at least several decades (Petty, 1987b). Moribidy from COPD results in approximately 34 days of restricted activity per 100 persons per year (Brashear, 1980). Respiratory diseases account for approximately 14% of all office visits for any condition and COPD accounts for approximately one-fifth of these visits (Brashear, 1980; U.S. Government Task Force, 1979). Although direct estimates of the number of physician visits for COPD vary, these have been estimated recently to be 2,220,000 per year (Centers for Disease Control, 1986).

Total costs for COPD have been estimated to be $27 billion per year (Lenfant, 1982). Recent reports suggest that 1,140,000 years of potential life are lost to COPD each year (Centers for Disease Control, 1986).

COMPLIANCE WITH PHARMACOLOGICAL INTERVENTIONS

Despite major advances in diagnosis and medical therapeutics, many patients do not receive optimal benefit from medical care. While some aspects of COPD are treatable, the medical regimen is extremely complex. Traditional medical management of COPD consists primarily of aggressive pharmacologic intervention. However, treatment may also include chest physiotherapy, exercise, and suggestions to quit smoking. Most patients are confronted with complex combinations of antibiotics, bronchodilators, anti-inflammitory drugs, and, in some cases, supplemental oxygen.

Two comprehensive reviews of the literature prior to 1980 (Atkins, 1981; Haynes, Taylor, & Sackett, 1979) did not identify studies on compliance to medical regimens for COPD patients. For example, the exhaustive Haynes et al. annotated bibliography does not include a single reference to a study limited to COPD patients. Because earlier comprehensive reviews had been conducted, the computer searches date back only to 1980. The results of the search, summarized in Table 7.1, revealed few studies that have directly addressed the issue of compliance with traditional medical regimens for COPD patients. The studies considered different treatments in diverse samples and employed various definitions of, and measurements for, compliance. Unfortunately, few conclusions, if any, can be drawn from the current literature.

TABLE 7.1 Summary of Studies on Compliance in COPD

Citation	Regimen	Sample	Measure	Definition	Compliance
Taylor et al. (1984)	Theophylline	63 patients in General Practice clinics (Northern Ireland)	Plasma theophylline levels before and after treatment	Δ Plasma levels <5.8 µg/ml at 350 mg dose/day and <9.6 µg/ml at 700 mg/day	
			Tablet counting	Taking >80% of prescribed medications	60% of patients
Chryssidis et al. (1981)	Aerosol therapy (Salbutamol and Beclomethasone diproprionate)	84 outpatients and 30 recently discharged inpatients (South Australia)	Estimation of compliance by weight of canisters at 1 and 2 months	Compliance score = #doses used #doses prescribed	Mean compliance scores at 1 month = 98.5%, at 3 months = 110.8%

Study	Therapy	Sample	Measure	Definition	Result
James et al. (1985)	Prescribed drug therapy	185 patients in chest/asthma/allergy clinics (London)	Self-report of drug taking patterns by questionnaire	Maintenance therapy—patients who took prescribed medication regularly	49% of patients
				Full compliance—patients who took prescribed medication regularly + adjusted therapy according to symptom exacerbation	31% of patients
IPPB Clinical Trial (1983)	Intermittent Positive Pressure Breathing therapy	500 patients in multicenter trial	Number of minutes on therapy as measured by recording devices attached to the machines	Did assigned therapy >25 minutes/day	50% of patients
	Compressor Nebulizer therapy	485 patients in multicenter trial			
Kaplan et al. (1984b)	Exercise prescription	76 patients randomized into 1 of 5 experimental groups	Self-report of time spent walking (walking logs)	Mean cumulative time spent walking in minutes	Cognitive/Behavioral modification group had greatest compliance

Estimated or measured compliance values do not appear to converge on a specific rate or even a specific pattern. James et al. (1985) reported that only half of their London patients took their medicine regularly. The Intermittent Positive Pressure Breathing (IPPB) clinical trial, which used objective assessments of actual time on oxygen therapy, found only half of the patients using oxygen at least 25 minutes per day, the minimal level for clinical efficacy. However, a noteworthy similarity among studies investigating pharmacological therapy was the mention of "overcompliant" patients, referring to those individuals who regularly took more than their prescribed amount of medication. In the Chryssidis, Frewin, Frith, and Dawes (1981) study, for example, the use of high doses of aerosol therapy often exceeded prescription rates. The mean percentage of prescribed dose actually used was 98.5% at 1-month follow-up and 110.8% at 2-month follow-up. Since there was variability for each of these estimates, it appears that some portion of the patients took considerably more medication than was prescribed. It is not surprising that patients suffering from COPD, a highly symptomatic disorder, would overuse a medication that provides rapid symptomatic relief.

The traditional view of compliance/noncompliance in the literature, in which the patient either strictly follows or fails to follow a treatment recommendation, may no longer be the optimal direction of compliance research in the future. The degree of compliance required for the desired outcome, be it adherence to a prescribed regimen or maximizing quality of life, varies from treatment to treatment and should be considered. To date, few studies have systematically evaluated compliance with medical treatments for the COPD patient, and in these few cases the focus has been on drug and oxygen therapy. Further, no studies evaluating interventions to improve compliance for COPD patients have been reported. Several commentaries have offered strategies for enhancing compliance; however, none have been systematically studied. At present, the measures of compliance used in the studies, such as the mean number of pills consumed, self-report of regimen adherence, or percentages of patients who complied with "all recommendations," no longer provide sufficient information.

MEDICAL MANAGEMENT

Since COPD is generally recognized at an advanced stage, medical management requires close supervision and attention from physicians and other allied health professionals. Treatment may include a variety of modalities (Ingram, 1983; Petty, 1978b). It is most important to encourage patients to stop smoking to retard further progression of disease. Because the diseases may be largely irreversible when recognized, however, smoking cessation may not result in significant return of lost lung function. Chest physiotherapy techniques may be very helpful in controlling chronic cough and sputum. General health measures including regular exercise may promote improved health and fitness.

A variety of medications may also be used. Antibiotics are used to control infections and acute exacerbations of bronchitis. Bronchodilator medications are used to treat any reversible component of the airway obstruction and should generally be tried in all patients. Theophylline and sympathomimetic drugs are the mainstays of bronchodilator therapy. Both types of medicines result in relaxation of bronchial smooth muscle, but because they act by different mechanisms, their effects are additive. Newer theophylline medications are slow-release, longer-acting medicines that give stable blood levels. These levels can be measured and titrated to an optimal level for each individual patient. Sympathomimetic drugs may be given either orally or by inhalation. Newer medications are selective beta-2 agonists that act more selectively on bronchial smooth muscle and have a lower incidence of side effects from action at other sites. Inhaled sympathomimetics generally have the advantage of fewer systemic side effects than oral preparations. In addition, many patients may be tried and managed on corticosteroids, both oral and inhaled, to control imflammation and to treat reversible airway obstruction. Other types of medications may also be indicated for individual patients.

COPD patients with significant hypoxemia (low blood oxygen levels) may be treated with oxygen. Two important clinical trials demonstrated the benefits of oxygen therapy. In the NIH-sponsored multicenter Nocturnal Oxygen Therapy Trial (NOTT), hypoxemic COPD patients were randomly assigned to receive oxygen therapy for either 12 or 24 hours (Nocturnal Oxygen Therapy Trial Group, 1980). In the British Medical Research Council study, hypoxemic COPD patients received either no oxygen or 15 hours of therapy (Medical Research Council Working Party, 1981). Both studies demonstrated a significant reduction in mortality associated with the use of oxygen. Patients receiving continuous oxygen therapy had significantly reduced mortality compared with patients receiving intermittent oxygen (12 or 15 hours). The highest mortality rate was seen in patients who received no oxygen. In addition, the 24-hour oxygen group experienced higher scores on general quality of life measures (McSweeney, Grant, Heaton, Adams, & Timms, 1982) and, after 1 year, on selected tests of cognitive function (Heaton, Grant, McSweeny, Adams, & Petty, 1983). Although oxygen is expensive and inconvenient for patients to use, there are now several types of oxygen therapy systems available, including portable units for ambulation, that allow for continuous therapy. Therefore, with the use of oxygen, hypoxemic COPD patients can remain active and engage in a variety of physical activities and beneficial exercises. At present, no eminent medical or surgical cure awaits most COPD patients. Yet behavioral programs may offer some benefits.

BEHAVIORAL AND REHABILITATION PROGRAMS IN COPD

In addition to drug interventions, behavioral changes, especially in the areas of smoking and physical activity, are usually recommended for COPD patients. Because of the well-documented association between smoking and COPD, successful smoking prevention programs are expected to reduce the incidence of these diseases. Smoking cessation programs are also valuable. However, by the time patients become function-limited, substantial proportions have stopped smoking on their own. There is considerable interest in the effects of smoking cessation for smokers with mild airway obstruction who may be at risk for COPD. The NIH is currently conducting an experimental trial to evaluate the benefits of smoking cessation for these high-risk individuals.

Although COPD patients can benefit greatly from exercise (Bell & Jensen, 1977), adherence to a physical regimen is often poor because activity can cause shortness of breath and fatigue. The more severely disabled patients often complain that their situation is hopeless and one over which they have little control (Fix, Daughton, & Kass, 1981). Long-term maintenance of physical exercise is difficult even when patients are initially motivated, and it may be an even more serious problem for the chronically ill (National Institutes of Health, 1981).

There is no medical cure for COPD. Because of the insidious origin of the disease and the large pulmonary reserve, COPD is generally not recognized until late in its course. Although standard medical treatment provides some relief for patients with COPD, the disease is largely irreversible and patients are left disabled with symptoms (e.g., breathlessness) that limit their daily activities significantly.

Comprehensive pulmonary rehabilitation programs have been developed to provide a multidisciplinary therapeutic program tailored to the needs of the individual patient (Lertzman & Cherniack, 1976). Such programs may include several components, including individual assessment, education, instruction in respiratory and chest physiotherapy techniques, psychosocial support, and supervised exercise training. The primary goal of pulmonary rehabilitation is to restore the patient to the highest possible level of independent function. Successful programs can help patients to become better educated and more involved in their own care. In addition, patients will have reduced symptoms, improved exercise tolerance, fewer hospitalizations and physician visits, and more gainful employment (American Thoracic Society, 1981; Lertzman & Cherniack, 1976; Moser, Bokinsky, Savage, Archibald, & Hansen, 1980). Pulmonary rehabilitation programs have expanded substantially in the last decade and are now an accepted form of comprehensive therapy for many COPD patients. In 1981, the American Thoracic Society recommended standards for pulmonary rehabilitation programs (1981).

An important component of most pulmonary rehabilitation programs has been the establishment of a regular exercise regimen. Specific physical conditioning exercises, such as walking, can be undertaken by the patient to help maintain lung function and improve the remainder of the oxygen delivery system (Bell & Jensen, 1977). In several published studies, the improvements in COPD patients following rehabilitation training have been striking (Bass, Whitcomb, & Forman, 1970; Fishmen & Petty, 1971; Moser et al., 1980; Pierce, Paez, & Miller, 1965; Unger, Moser, & Hansen, 1980). Specifically, appropriate physical conditioning exercises can improve maximum oxygen consumption and endurance, reduce heart rate, improve ventilatory efficiency, and increase tolerance for exercise.

There have been few controlled studies evaluating COPD rehabilitation programs or their components. Reports from nonrandomized studies typically suggest that the objectives can be achieved (Bass, Whitcomb, & Forman, 1970; Moser et al., 1980; Unger, Moser, & Hansen, 1980). Recently, a few controlled trials documented the benefits of exercise programs for COPD patients. Cockcroft, Saunders, and Berry (1981) randomly assigned 39 patients to a 6-week exercise program or to a no-treatment control group. In comparison to the control group, patients in the exercise group experienced subjective benefits and increased the amount of distance they could walk in 12 minutes. However, the length of follow-up was only 2 months. McGavin and co-workers (1977) randomly allocated 24 COPD patients to a 3-month unsupervised stair-climbing home exercise program or to a nonexercise control group. The 12 patients in the exercise group noted subjective improvements and an increased sense of well-being and decreased breathlessness. They also reported an objective increase in the 12-minute walk distance and maximal level of exercise on a cycle ergometer. These changes did not occur in the control group. However, the length of follow-up was liited to 3 months. Ambrosino and coworkers (1981) randomly assigned 23 patients to a 1-month medical and rehabilitative therapy group and 28 patients to medical therapy alone (without exercise training). The experimental group improved in exercise tolerance and respiratory pattern (as evidenced by decrease in respiratory rate and increase in tidal volume). Again, these changes were not present in the control group. To date, none of these studies has evaluated comprehensive pulmonary rehabilitation programs. Further, it was not possible to link the results of published studies to important outcomes such as those suggested by Petty and Cherniak (1981).

Although the data on exercise and rehabilitation programs for COPD patients appear promising, there still is no evidence from randomized, controlled studies on their efficacy. The results of an experimental trial designed to evaluate behavioral and cognitive–behavioral programs for increasing exercise among COPD patients were recently reported. (Atkins, Kaplan, Timms, Reinsch, & Lofback, 1984b). COPD patients underwent exercise testing on a treadmill and were given an exercise prescription. Then they were randomly assigned to one of five experimental or control groups. The experimental groups were designed to improve compliance with the exercise prescription. They included Behavior Modification, Cognitive–Behavior Modification, and a Cognitive Modification Condition.

The behavior modification treatment included goal-setting, functional analysis of reinforcers, mediating walking, a behavioral contract, contingency management, and two sessions of relaxation training. In the cognitive treatment, subjects experienced didactic interactions in which they learned to identify negative self-statements and to replace them with positive thoughts, to identify specific cues for promoting positive self-talk, and other similar strategies. The experimenter attempted to challenge irrational beliefs about walking whenever possible. The cognitive–behavioral group experienced many of the same positive self-talk exercises. However, they also received training in contingency management and two relaxation sessions. The attention control group received attention but did not have training specifically directed toward increasing compliance. During six sessions, they completed a variety of questionnaires including the MMPI, a life stress questionnaire, and the Trailmaker test from the Halstead-Reitan Battery (Reitan, 1971). The results of these tests and their relationship to lung disease were discussed during the sessions. A more detailed description of the treatments is given in Atkins et al. (1984b). The first four sessions were held weekly during the month following the initial interview. Sessions were held biweekly the second month. Three months following the initial assessment, patients were reevaluated on all measures in the clinic. Outcome measures included a general Quality of Life Index, Pulmonary Function tasks, Exercise Tolerance tasks, and measures of Self-Efficacy.

Analysis of the data suggested that those in the Cognitive–Behavior Modification Group complied more with the advice to walk than those in the other experimental or control groups. All three treatment groups complied more than those in the two control groups (Atkins et al., 1984b). These changes were reflected in changes in exercise tolerance measured 1 month after the treatment. However, there were no significant changes in spirometric parameters. Several analyses were performed using a General Health Index (Kaplan, 1985) and a General Health Policy Model. Over the course of 18 months, the experimental and control groups showed significant differences on a quality of life index. These differences were used to calculate quality-adjusted life years and perform cost–effectiveness studies. There is considerable debate about the value of insurance reimbursement for behavioral and rehabilitation programs. The cost-effectiveness analyses suggested that behavioral and rehabilitation programs for COPD patients produce an equivalent of a well-year for approximately $23,000. This is comparable to other widely advocated health care programs (Toevs, Kaplan, & Atkins, 1984).

These same patients were studied again 3 years after the beginning of the program. At this time, observed differences between the experimental and control groups remained for the Quality of Well-being measure (Atkins, Hayes, & Kaplan, 1984a); yet substantial increases in variability precluded statistically significant effects. Analysis of the data using concepts derived from social learning theory (Bandura, 1977) suggested that perceived self-efficacy mediated changes in behavior and function (Kaplan, Atkins, & Reinsch, 1984).

FOR OPTIMAL HEALTH
Measurement of Outcomes

Both behavioral and biomedical interventions should be evaluated in terms of their potential to improve health status and the quality of life. No behavioral or medical intervention can repair damaged lung tissue and restore pulmonary function (Unger, Moser, & Hansen, 1980). The objective of the interventions is to improve function and the quality of life. Several studies have demonstrated that function can improve in the absence of changes in measures of pulmonary function (Atkins et al., 1984b; Petty & Cherniak, 1981). Capturing these benefits requires a technology for measuring functioning and the quality of life.

It has been suggested that diseases and disabilities may have at least three important effects on health status: They may affect current functioning (quality of life), they may affect future functioning, or they may affect life expectancy (Kaplan, 1985; Kaplan, Atkins, & Timms, 1984). A variety of measures reviewed by Kaplan (1984) are designed to measure these effects. At least three different approaches have been used to evaluate COPD patients. The Sickness Impact Profile (SIP) has been employed in a variety of major clinical trials. The SIP includes 136 items, which are divided into 12 categories. These categories are further clustered into three groups: Independent Categories, Physical, and Psychosocial (Bergner, Bobbitt, Carter, & Gilson, 1981). In the Nocturnal Oxygen Therapy Trial, the SIP was used to demonstrate that COPD patients experienced severely curtailed quality of life in comparison to age-matched controls (McSweeney et al., 1982). The second approach is a questionnaire developed for the RAND Health Insurance Study. The RAND instruments include specific measures for Physiologic Health, Physical Health, Mental Health, and Social Health. In one study, it was demonstrated that the Physical Health measures correlate substantially with forced expiratory volume in 1 second ($FEV_{1.0}$) (Allen, 1985). In addition, a recent study by Guyatt and colleagues (1985) demonstrated that the RAND instrument was highly correlated with performance on a walking test. A laboratory bicycle ergometer test was not as strongly correlated with other indices of disease severity.

In a previous paper, it was proposed that a General Health Policy and in particular a subcomponent known as the Quality of Well-being Scale had validity as an outcome measure for evaluating interventions for COPD patients (Kaplan et al., 1984b). In medical research, program or treatment effectiveness is often measured using single indicators. In chronic lung disease, those indicators may be physiologic parameters such as pulmonary function, exercise preference, pulmonary hemodynamics, and so forth. These measures are essential for monitoring the course of a specific disease. Yet disease-specific indicators often fail to capture the total impact of a treatment because they may allow side effects of treatment to be overlooked (Jette, 1980). Steroid drugs can modify many symptoms for COPD patients, but they may also be associated with decreased immunity and increased susceptibility to many problems in the long run. A measure focusing only on pulmonary function may miss the overall impact of the treatment upon function and symptoms.

This approach expresses the benefits of medical care, behavioral intervention, or preventive programs in terms of well-years. These well-years integrate mortality and morbidity to express health status in terms of equivalence of well-years of life. Mortality effects can be assessed through years of life lost. For example, a COPD patient with a life expectancy of 73 years would have lost 13 years if he died at age 60. If 100 COPD patients died at age 60 (and had a 73-year life expectancy), they collectively would have lost $100 \times 13 = 1,300$ life-years.

Although COPD may result in early death, it is also a major cause of disability. Patients with decreased lung function experience reduced quality of life over an extended period of time. Our system allows the integration of quality-of-life information with mortality. For example, if the quality of life for the COPD patient is reduced by one half, we say that the disease takes away 0.5 well-years over the course of 1 year. If it effects two people, it will take away 1.0 well-years ($= 2 \times 0.5$) over a 1-year period. Our previous work has suggested that behavioral programs can improve the quality of life by as much as .073 units of well-being for 1 year. Thus, for each 100 patients receiving this benefit, 7.33 well-years would be produced (Toevs et al., 1984).

FUTURE DIRECTIONS

Given the importance of COPD in terms of death, disability, and medical expense, it is surprising that so little attention has been devoted to systematic behavioral studies in this area. In contrast to nearly every other major medical condition, there are few published intervention studies evaluating the benefits of behavioral interventions to improve compliance. In addition, there are no population-based studies on compliance, and the extent to which compliance is a problem is not known. Also the extent to which problems such as overcompliance affect detrimental outcomes for COPD patients is unknown. At present, the measures of compliance used, such as the mean number of pills consumed, self-report of regimen adherence, or percentages of patients who complied with "all recommendations," no longer provide sufficient information.

Recently, the Task Force on Lung Diseases for the NHLBI workshop "Adoption and Maintenance of Behaviors for Optimal Health" suggested five directions for future research. These will be discussed briefly.

The regimen for patients with COPD requires many different behaviors. These might include the use of several different medications, exercise, respiratory therapy, and other aspects of self-care. It is not known whether or not these different behaviors are intercorrelated. In other chronic illnesses, for example, hypertension, adherence with one aspect of the regimen is often not correlated with adherence to other components. More research is necessary to define the interrelationships between behaviors relevant to the management of COPD.

A second issue identified in this literature review is that overcompliance with the regimen for COPD patients may be a problem. This is a particular concern for inhaled medications that provide symptomatic relief. More research is necessary in order to document overcompliance and evaluate effects upon health outcome.

These studies have attempted to link adherence with measureable health outcomes. More research is necessary to establish the links between adherence and obtainment of health benefits. At present, little is known about how to improve adherence for COPD patients. There are no published studies on increasing adherence to prescribed medications. Only a few studies consider improving adherence to behavioral regimens. The problem of smoking cessation among the elderly has also received insufficient study. These problems require further systematic investigation.

Finally, there is very little research on rehabilitation programs for COPD patients. Although these programs are common, little is known about their effectiveness. We are currently conducting an experimental evaluation of rehabilitation programs for COPD patients. The program is a traditional rehabilitation program. The control group for the experiment is education and patient support. In the trial, a wide variety of outcome measures are being used, including physiologic measures and measures of pulmonary function, blood gases, and exercise tolerance. In addition, psychosocial measures are being used; these include general quality-of-life measures, measures of depression, and measures of self-efficacy. Early data suggest there are systematic associations between exercise and quality of life and inverse relationships between compliance and depression. Detailed reports of the study should be available within the next few years.

Rehabilitation programs for COPD patients include many different components. For example, comprehensive programs often include exercise, education, chest physiotherapy, and psychosocial support. If the programs are shown to be effective, it is not clear what aspects of the program caused the benefits. Further studies are needed to identify the essential components of a successful program. Research on mechanisms of delivery and reimbursement for rehabilitation programs is also required.

In summary, COPD is an important health problem that requires further systematic investigation. There has been very little behavioral research relevant to COPD. Yet behavior change, in the form of adherence to various recommendations, may be essential for obtaining optimal patient outcomes. Further research relevant to the clinical management of COPD should be encouraged.

REFERENCES

ACCP–ATS Joint Committee. (1976). Pulmonary terms and symbols: A report of the ACCP–ATS joint committee on pulmonary nomenclature. *Chest, 67,* 583–593.

Allen, H. (1985, August). *Validity of measures in the RAND health insurance study.* Paper presented at the meeting of the American Psychological Association, Los Angeles, CA.

Ambrosino, N., Paggiaro, P. L., Macchi, M., Felieri, M., Toma, G., Lombard, F. A., DeiCesta, F., Parlanti, A., Loi, A., & Baschieri, L. (1981). A short-term effect of rehabilitative therapy in chronic obstructive pulmonary disease. *Respiration, 41,* 40–44.

American Thoracic Society. (1981). Pulmonary rehabilitation. *American Review of Respiratory Diseases, 124,* 683–686.

Astin, T. W. (1976). Cigarette smoking and chronic bronchitis. *British Medical Journal, 2,* 1261.

Atkins, C. J. (1981). *A randomized clinical trial comparing cognitive and behavioral strategies for exercise compliance among chronic obstructive pulmonary disease patients.* Unpublished doctoral dissertation, University of California, Riverside.

Atkins, C. J., Hayes, J., & Kaplan, R. M. (1984a, June). *Four year follow-up of behavioral programs in COPD.* Paper presented at the University of California Health Psychology Conference, Lake Arrowhead, CA.

Atkins, C. J., Kaplan, R. M., Timms, R. M., Reinsch, S., & Lofback, K. (1984b). Behavioral programs for exercise compliance in COPD. *Journal of Consulting and Clinical Psychology, 52,* 591–603.

Bandura, A. (1977). Self-efficacy: Toward a unifying theory of behavior change. *Psychological Review, 84,* 191–215.

Bass, H., Whitcomb, J. F., & Forman, R. (1970). Exercise training: Therapy for patients with chronic obstructive pulmonary disease. *Chest, 57,* 116–120.

Bell, C. W., & Jensen, R. H. (1977). Exercise and stress testing in physical conditioning. In R. H. Jensen & I. Kass (Eds.), *Pulmonary rehabilitation medical manual.* Omaha: University of Nebraska Medical Center, 50–91.

Bergner, M., Bobbitt, R. A., Carter, W. B., & Gilson, B. S. (1981). The sickness impact profile: Development and final revision of a health status measure. *Medical Care, 19,* 787–806.

Brashear, R. E. (1980). Chronic obstructive pulmonary disease. In D. H. Simmons (Ed.), *Current Pulmonology* (Vol. 2). Boston: Houghton-Mifflin.

Centers for Disease Control. (1986). Premature mortality in the United States: Public health issues in the use of years in potential life lost. *Morbidity & Mortality Weekly Report*, 35 (supp. 2).

Chryssidis, E., Frewin, D. B., Frith, P. A., & Dawes, E. R. (1981). Compliance with aerosol therapy in chronic obstructive lung disease. *New Zealand Medical Journal*, 94, 375-377.

Cockroft, A. E. (1981). Randomize controls trial of rehabilitation in chronic respiratory disease. *Thorax*, 36, 200.

Crystal, R. G. (1987). Chronic obstructive pulmonary disease. In *Forty years of achievement in heart, lung, and blood research: A collection of essays in selected papers of biomedical research accomplishment.* Bethesda, MD: National Institutes of Health, National Heart, Lung, and Blood Institute.

Fishmen, D. B., & Petty, T. L. (1971). Physical, symptomatic and psychological improvement in patients receiving comprehensive care for chronic airway obstruction. *Journal of Chronic Diseases*, 24, 775-785.

Fix, A. J., Daughton, D., & Kass, I. (1981). Behavioral sciences in pulmonary rehabilitation. *Applied Techniques in Behavioral Medicine*, I, 263-294.

Guyatt, G. H., Thompson, P. J., Berman, L. B., Sullivan, M. J., Townsend, M., Jones, N. L., & Pugsley, S. O. (1985). How should we measure function in patients with chronic heart and lung disease? *Journal of Chronic Diseases*, 38, 517-524.

Haynes, R. B., Taylor, D. W., & Sackett, D. L. (1979). *Compliance in health care.* Baltimore: Johns Hopkins University Press.

Heaton, R. K., Grant, I., McSweeny, A. J., Adams, K. M., & Petty, T. L. (1983). Psychological effects of continuous and nocturnal oxygen therapy in hypoxemic chronic obstructive pulmonary disease. *Archives of Internal Medicine*, 143, 1941-1947.

Higgins, I. T. T. (1958). Tobacco smoking, respiratory symptoms, and ventilatory capacity: Studies in random samples of the population. *British Medical Journal*, 2, 325-329.

Ingram, R. H., Jr. (1983). Chronic bronchitis, emphysema, and airways obstruction. In R. G. Petersdorf, R. D. Adams, E. Braunwald, K. J. Isselbacher, J. B. Martin, & J. D. Wilson (Eds.), *Harrison's principles of internal medicine* (10th ed) (pp. 1545-1553). New York: McGraw-Hill.

Intermittent Positive Pressure Breathing Trial Group. (1983). Intermittent positive pressure breathing therapy of chronic obstructive pulmonary disease. *Annals of Internal Medicine*, 99, 612-620.

James, P. N. E., Anderson, J. B., Priar, J. G., White, J. P., Henry, J. A., & Cochrane, G. M. (1985). Patterns of drug taking in patients with chronic airflow obstruction. *Postgraduate Medical Journal*, 61, 7-10.

Jette, A. M. (1980). Health status indicators: Their utility in chronic disease evaluation research. *Journal of Chronic Diseases*, 33, 567-579.

Kaplan, R. M. (1984). Quality-of-life measurement. In P. Karoly (Ed.), *Measurement strategies in health psychology* (pp. 115-146). New York: Wiley-Interscience.

Kaplan, R. M. (1985). Quantification of health outcomes for policy studies in behavioral epidemiology. In R. M. Kaplan & M. H. Criqui (Eds.), *Behavioral epidemiology and disease prevention* (pp. 31-54). New York: Plenum.

Kaplan, R. M., Atkins, C. J., & Reinsch, S. (1984a). Specific efficacy expectations mediate exercise compliance in patients with COPD. *Health Psychology*, 3, 223-242.

Kaplan, R. M., Atkins, C. J., & Timms, R. M. (1984b). Validity of a quality of well being scale as an outcome measure in chronic obstructive pulmonary disease. *Journal of Chronic Diseases, 37*, 85-95.

Lenfant, C. (1982). Lung research: Government and community. *American Review of Respiratory Diseases, 126*, 753-757.

Lertzman, M. M., & Cherniack, R. M. (1976). Rehabilitation of patients with chronic obstructive pulmonary disease. *American Review of Respiratory Diseases, 114*, 1145-1165.

McGavin, C. R., Gupta, S. P., Lloyd, E. L., & McHardy, J. R. (1977). Physical rehabilitation of chronic bronchitis: Results of a controlled trial of exercises in the home. *Thorax, 32*, 307-311.

McSweeny, A. J., Grant, I., Heaton, R. K., Adams, K. M., & Timms, R. M. (1982). Life quality of patients with chronic obstructive pulmonary disease. *Archives of Internal Medicine, 142*, 473-478.

Medical Research Council Working Party. (1981). Long term domiciliary oxygen therapy in chronic hypoxic cor pulmonale complicating chronic bronchitis and emphysema. *Lancet, 1*, 681-686.

Moser, K., Bokinsky, G., Savage, R., Archibald, C., & Hansen, P. (1980). Results of a comprehensive rehabilitation program: Physiologic and functional effects on patients with chronic obstructive pulmonary disease. *Archives of Internal Medicine, 140*, 1596-1601.

National Institutes of Health. (1981). *Chronic obstructive pulmonary disease* (NIH Publication No. 81-2020). Bethesda, MD: U.S. Department of Health and Human Services.

National Institutes of Health. (1983, February). *Report on workshop on lung disease and behavior.* Bethesda, MD: U.S. Department of Health and Human Services.

Nocturnal Oxygen Therapy Trial Group. (1980). Continuous or nocturnal oxygen therapy in hypoxemic chronic obstructive lung disease: A clinical trial. *Annals of Internal Medicine, 93*, 391-398.

Petty, T. L. (1978a). *Chronic lung disease: A practical office approach to early diagnosis* (2nd ed.). New York: Beon Laboratories.

Petty, T. L. (Ed.). (1978b). *Chronic obstructive pulmonary disease.* New York: Marcel Dekker.

Petty, T. L., & Cherniak, R. M. (1981). Comprehensive care of COPD. *Clinical Notes on Respiratory Diseases, Winter*, 3-12.

Pierce, A. K., Paez, P. N., & Miller, W. F. (1965). Exercise training with the aid of a portable oxygen supply in patients with emphysema. *American Review of Respiratory Diseases, 91*, 653-659.

Reitan, R. M. (1971). Trial making test results for normal and brain damaged children. *Perceptual and Motor Skills, 33*, 575-581.

Taylor, D. R., Kinney, C. D., & McDevitt, D. G. (1984). Patient compliance with oral theophylline therapy. *British Journal of Clinical Pharmacology, 17*, 15-20.

Tisi, G. M. (1980). *Pulmonary physiology in clinical medicine.* Baltimore: Williams and Wilkins.

Toevs, C. T., Kaplan, R. M., & Atkins, C. J. (1984). The costs and effects of behavioral programs in chronic obstructive pulmonary disease. *Medical Care, 22*(12), 1088-1100.

Unger, K., Moser, K., & Hansen, P. (1980). Selection of an exercise program for patients with chronic obstructive pulmonary disease. *Heart and Lungs, 9,* 68–76.

U.S. Government Task Force. (1979). *Epidemiology of respiratory diseases: Task force report on state of knowledge, problems, and needs* (NIH Publication No. 81-2019). Washington, D.C.: National Institutes of Health.

West, J. B. (1977). *Pulmonary pathophysiology: The essentials.* Baltimore: Williams and Wilkins.

8

School-Based Health Education for Children with Asthma: Some Issues for Adherence Research

David Evans, Noreen M. Clark, Charles H. Feldman,
Yvonne Wasilewski, Moshe J. Levison,
Barry J. Zimmerman, Bruce Levin, Robert B. Mellins

Approximately 5% of the children in the United States suffer from asthma (National Institute of Allergy and Infectious Diseases [NIAID], 1979). Despite advances in pharmacologic therapy, childhood asthma continues to take a tremendous toll on families and communities each year, causing increased school absences, frequent use of emergency health care services, and disruption

The work described in this paper was supported in part by grant No. 1-R18-HL-28907 from the Division of Lung Diseases, the National Heart, Lung, and Blood Institute, and by a gift from the Spunk Fund.

of the daily life of family and child (NIAID, 1979). Recent studies have shown that health education programs for childhood asthma delivered in ambulatory care settings can improve self-management skills, improve school attendance and performance, and reduce use of emergency health care services (Clark et al., 1986a, b; Creer et al. 1988; Hini-Alexander & Cropp, 1984; Lewis, Rachelevsky, Lewis, de la Sota, & Kaplan, 1984; McNabb, Wilson-Pessano, Hughes, & Scamagas, 1985; Parcel, Nader & Tiernan, 1980). Studies conducted by the authors in the Department of Pediatrics at Columbia University developed and evaluated an asthma self-management program called *Open Airways* for families of children being treated in an outpatient clinic setting (Clark et al., 1986a, b, National Heart, Lung, and Blood Institute, 1984).

There are limits to making health education accessible in ambulatory health care settings. First, health education programs are difficult to offer in solo or small-group practices, especially outside urban areas. It is not easy to locate or pay for the services of a health educator or to train an already employed nurse to assume the responsibility of organizing and conducting health education programs. Second, some children do not have a health care provider who cares for their asthma on a regular basis and thus have no access to asthma health education through the health care system. Third, because most ambulatory health care facilities are administratively independent of one another, it is not easy for them to minimize costs by sharing the services of a health educator.

The school system provides an alternative setting for asthma health education that does not have these limitations. All children are required to attend school, and schools usually have the physical and human resources (classroom space, teaching equipment, and health teachers) to offer health education programs. Because public school systems are centrally organized, it is possible for schools in a district to share a health educator with special training in asthma or other chronic diseases. Because of this potential for providing children with asthma the broadest possible access to health education, a study was conducted to develop and evaluate an asthma self-management program for use in elementary schools (Evans et al., 1987).

The research had four specific objectives. The first was to demonstrate the feasibility of offering asthma health education in the schools. Would the schools cooperate? Could accurate identification of children with asthma be accomplished in the schools? The second objective was to overcome the problem of low parental attendance encountered in the ambulatory health care study and in a pilot test of asthma health education conducted in the schools (Kaplan et al., 1986). In both cases, parents attended approximately half the sessions. The initial health education program centered on the role of the parent and the interaction of parent and child in self-management. Participation by parents was essential. Children were embarrassed and learned less when their parents were absent. To overcome this barrier to teaching children self-management skills, the program was redesigned to emphasize the child's role and capacity to independently initiate asthma management steps. The children were educated in groups at school. Parents were educated at home through written materials and joint homework assignments to be completed with their children. The third objective was to explore children's capacity to initiate appropriate health behavior and exert influence on their parents' management decisions. Developmental theory suggests that 8- to 11-year-olds can make independent decisions (Piaget, 1967), and one study has shown that children can decide independently when to use school health services (Lewis, Lewis, & Lorimer, 1977). No work, however, had yet explored the extent to which children can take independent management steps, can provide relevant health information to parents, and can be acknowledged as participants in decision making about health by their parents. The fourth objective was to explore the concept of self-efficacy. Self-efficacy has been strongly associated with change in health behavior (O'Leary, 1985; Strecher, DeVellis, Becker, & Rosenstock, 1986). Because parents' and children's levels of confidence in their asthma self-management skills were shown to be low in previous studies (Clark et al., 1980), the authors decided to explore the role of self-efficacy plays in learning new self-management skills for childhood asthma.

The hypotheses for this study were that school-based asthma health education for children aged 8 to 11 years would improve asthma management skills, increase children's influence on parents' management decisions, increase children's self-efficacy, reduce school absences, and improve academic grades in school.

STUDY METHODS

The methods have previously been described in detail (Evans et al., 1987). In brief, the study population consisted of 239 children in the third, fourth, and fifth grades of 12 public elementary schools in Manhattan and the south Bronx in New York City. The schools were cooperative because schools officials recognized that asthma created problems for both the family and the school, including poorer academic performance, increased absences, and the occurrence of asthma attacks at school. All children in grades three, four, and five in the 12 schools were given a letter to take home to their parents that described the symptoms of asthma and the program to be offered. Parents who responded by returning a tearoff sheet (9%) were interviewed by telephone to confirm that the child had asthma. Children were eligible to participate if their parents reported that the child had experienced symptoms of asthma at least three times during the preceding year. Using this criterion, 5% of the children in the three grades had asthma. Ninety-three percent of the parents of the children who enrolled in the study reported that a physician had diagnosed asthma in their child.

An experimental research design was used to evaluate the effectiveness of the health education program. After the enrollment procedure was completed, the 12 schools were paired according to ethnic composition and size. One school in each pair was randomly selected to receive the health education program, while the other school served as a control. A total of 134 children received the program, while 105 children served as controls. All control group children received the program after the follow-up data were collected.

A sociodemographic profile of the study population showed that 71% received Medicaid. Seventy percent were Hispanic, 28% were non-Hispanic blacks, and 2% were from other groups. Fifty-nine percent of the children were male, and the mean age was 9.1, with a range from 7 to 12 years. Nineteen percent of the children had no source of health care other than the emergency room (Kaplan et al., 1986). This confirmed our conjecture that there were children who were not receiving continuing primary health care for asthma and thus had no access to health education through the health care system. The average number of annual emergency room visits was 0.56 per child, and only 4% of the children had been hospitalized in the year preceding the study, indicating that this population was characterized by mild asthma (Evans et al., 1987).

The asthma self-management program consisted of six hour-long group sessions for children that were held during the school day. Makeup sessions were provided, and all children completed the program, with the exception of one child who missed a single session. Written materials given to the children were also sent home to the parents to familiarize them with what their child was learning and to build parental support for the child's new skills. Children were given homework assignments to complete with their parents to increase family communication about asthma and to encourage children to rehearse their new skills at home.

The learning objectives of the program were to teach children to recognize asthma symptoms when they first occur, to initiate management steps immediately, to communicate with parents and teachers, and to recognize when medical care is needed. The session topics included (1) information and feelings about asthma, (2) recognizing and managing asthma symptoms (3) using prescribed medicines appropriately and deciding when to seek help, (4) keeping physically active, (5) identifying and controlling asthma triggers, and (6) handling asthma problems at school.

The learning activities were all led by health educators using group process methods to get children to share problems and develop solutions. The learning activities were desinged to enable children to acquire and practice skills needed to manage asthma at home and at school. All the activities were very concrete in their treatment of asthma problems and focused on mastery of skills. Both these attributes were considered essential to learning by children aged 8 to 11 years, who are considered to be in the concrete operational stage of development

(Piaget, 1967). Activities included modeling of new behaviors by the health educator, use of stories to stimulate problem solving, use of games to practice decision making, role play to rehearse new skills in lifelike situations, and making clay figures to express and share feelings. Children were also taught relaxation exercises to help them stay calm and control feelings. Strong reinforcement was given when they made good suggestions or described use of management strategies in the home or school environment.

The curriculum for each of the six sessions was designed to enhance self-efficacy. The learning activities intended to increase self-efficacy drew on the four sources of efficacy information described by Bandura (1977): enactive mastery of skills through practice and feedback, vicarious learning from models or from other children's experience, verbal persuasion by the health educator, and reduction of anxiety through learning how to relax. For example, in the session on recognizing and managing asthma symptoms, children were taught to perform a breathing exercise to help them relax while experiencing symptoms. The health educator first modeled this skill and then had children practice it in easy steps until they had mastered it. She taught the children how to observe themselves so that they could see if they were doing the exercise correctly and gave direct feedback about their progress. Children were encouraged to teach the breathing exercise to another member of the family and to use it the next time they had symptoms of asthma.

In developing and evaluating the health education program, two issues were encountered that are important for programs designed to increase adherence to therapeutic regimens.

1. *Removing barriers to the adoption of new health behaviors.* In addition to activities designed to teach skills and increase self-efficacy, a problem-solving approach was used to help children anticipate and prepare to overcome some of the barriers to self-management activities that can erode adherence. For example, one problem was children's embarrassment about performing productive cough in school, that is, purposefully and effectively coughing up mucus and spitting it into a tissue to relieve asthma symptoms. The solutions developed included teaching children how to perform productive cough in relative privacy (by going to the hall or a corner) and how to deflect criticism from other children ("I know it sounds gross, but it helps me breathe better"). We found that both parents and children experienced a variety of barriers to adherence and that the only reliable way to identify them was to ask the family members about their problems or concerns with the treatment plan during the educational intervention. We think that educational interventions to promote adherence can be strengthened by specifically including procedures for identifying such frequently overlooked barriers and helping the family to overcome them.

2. *Measuring adherence when treatment plans include self-management.* The self-management intervention was designed to promote adherence to the specific regimen that the child's physician had prescribed. In addition, it was designed to teach children and their families to adopt and adhere to general guidlines for self-management of asthma. Examples of guidelines include such recommendations as increasing the child's physical activity levels within tolerable limits, improving communication with school teachers and physicians about asthma, and increasing the child's responsibility for managing asthma. To follow guidelines such as these, the family must embellish them with specific behaviors that they choose and evaluate primarily by themselves. Adherence to guidelines for self-management is harder to define and measure than adherence to the specifics of a medical regimen because the specific behaviors chosen by the family can be idiosyncratic, are not set in advance, and may vary in how well they fit the guidelines. Measuring family adherence to guidelines may be further complicated because self-management may require many complex behaviors that are difficult for parents or children to recall or describe to researchers.

The approach used to measure adherence to the health messages and skills taught in the intervention was to count all the behaviors that children reported using to manage asthma that fit within the guidelines taught in the self-management program. Children were asked during the baseline and follow-up interviews to describe what they did to manage symptoms of asthma at home and at school. Open-ended questions were used to avoid response bias. An index of self-management behavior by children was developed that consists of responses to questions about preventive measures, steps to control symptoms at home, steps to control symptoms at school, and efforts to communicate information about asthma to parents and teachers (Evans et al., 1987).

RESULTS

The results of this study are reported in detail elsewhere (Evans et al., 1987). The principal findings are summarized below.

Self-Management, Self-Efficacy, and Influence

Compared with the control group, children from schools that participated in the program had statistically significant increases in use of self-management steps, level of self-efficacy in managing asthma, and influence on parents' management decisions (as reported by parents). A regression analysis was conducted to explore further the role of self-efficacy in acquiring self-management skills. Children's self-efficacy level at baseline was associated with the use of increased self-management steps at follow-up, controlling for baseline self-management scores and the effect of the program (beta $= 0.19$; $p < 0.05$).

School Absences and Performance

Both program and control group children had reduced school absences in the follow-up year, but the difference between groups was not statistically significant. Program children showed a statistically significant improvement on an index of academic grades, however, while the grades of control children remained the same. No difference between groups was observed in the teachers' ratings of the children's classroom behavior.

Quality of Life and Social Support

Children were asked to rate their feelings about asthma and about school; in both cases, program children reported statistically significant increases in positive feelings compared with control children at follow-up. In addition, there was a marked increase in the percentage of children in the program group who reported receiving help from other children during their last asthma episode at school ($+62\%$ vs $+9\%$; $p < 0.05$).

Episodes of Asthma

The annual frequency of episodes of asthma and the average duration of an episode reported by the children's parents decreased in the program group and increased in the control group; both differences between groups were statistically significant. By multiplying these two numbers, estimates were made of the annual frequency of days with symptoms of asthma. Program children averaged 14 fewer days with symptoms per year, compared with an increase of 2 days for control children.

DISCUSSION

These data indicate that school-based health education for children with asthma aged 8 to 11 years can (1) increase the child's use of self-management steps, self-efficacy, and influence on parents' management decisions; (2) improve the quality of the child's life and social support received from peers; (3) improve academic performance; and (4) reduce the frequency and duration of episodes of asthma. Health education for children with asthma can be efficiently delivered to children in the public schools, can reach children who do not have access to health education through the health care system, and can improve children's ability to manage asthma and live normally.

Considered in light of other recent studies, these findings also have important implications for future directions in research on adherence. The data suggest that self-efficacy is an important motivational factor in adherence. In addition to this study, there is already a small but growing body of research, reviewed recently by Strecher et al. (1986) and O'Leary (1985), that demonstrates that self-efficacy plays an important role in promoting the adoption and maintenance of new health behaviors. Developing feelings of self-efficacy, however, is only part of the larger process of self-regulation of behavior (Bandura, 1986). The first component of self-regulation is self-observation, also referred to as self-monitoring. Recording self-observations in a diary has been shown to be an important tool by itself for controlling health behavior problems, including smoking (Blittner, Goldberg, & Merbaum, 1978), overeating (Romanczyk, 1974), and alcohol abuse (Marlatt, 1979). The second component of self-regulation is self-evaluation, which involves making judgments about success from self-observations. The third component is the process of self-reaction, which includes both developing feelings of self-efficacy and providing self-rewards for success.

There is evidence that these processes interact with and reinforce each other and that interventions that combine training in self-observation, self-evaluation, and the development of self-efficacy are more effective than interventions that focus on monitoring or self-efficacy alone (Bandura & Cervone, 1986; Bellack, 1976; Ewart, 1978). These findings suggest that additional studies are needed to (1) explore the interrelationships between these three components of self-regulation and (2) examine the potential for training in self-regulation to increase adherence to medical regimens and healthy behaviors.

REFERENCES

Bandura, A. (1977). *Social learning theory.* Englewood Cliffs, NJ: Prentice-Hall.

Bandura, A. (1986). *Social foundations of thought and action: A social cognitive theory* (pp. 335–453). Englewood Cliffs, NJ: Prentice-Hall.

Bandura, A., & Cervone, D. (1986). Differential engagement of self-reactive influences in cognitive motivation. *Organizational Behaviors and Human Decision Processes, 38,* 92–113.

Bellack, A. S. (1976). A comparison of self-reinforcement and self-monitoring in a weight reduction program. *Behavior Therapy, 7,* 68–75.

Blittner, M., Goldberg, J., & Merbaum, M. (1978). Cognitive self-control factors in the reduction of smoking behavior. *Behavior Therapy, 6,* 553–561.

Clark, N. M., Feldman, C. H., Evans, D., Dttzey, O., Levinson, M. J., Wasilewski, Y., Kaplan, D. L., Rios, J. L., & Mellins, R. B. (1986a). Managing better: Children, parents, and asthma. *Patient Education and Counseling, 8,* 27–38.

Clark, N. M., Feldman, C. H., Evans, D., Levinson, M. J., Wasilewski, Y., & Mellins, R. B. (1986b). The impact of health education on the frequency and cost of health care use by low income children with asthma. *Journal of Allergy and Clinical Immunology*, 78, 108–115.

Clark, N. M., Feldman, C. H., Freudenberg, N., Millman, E. J., Wasilewski, Y., & Valle, I. M. (1980). Developing education for children with asthma through study of self-management behavior. *Health Education Quarterly*, 7, 278–297.

Creer, T. L., Baikiel, M., Burns, K. L., Leung, P., Marion, R. J., Miklich, D. R., Morrill, C., Tapiln, P. S., & Ullman, S. (1988). Living with asthma: I Genesis and development of a self-management program for childhood asthma. *Journal of Asthma*, 25(6), 15–42.

Evans, D., Clark, N. M., Feldman, C. H., Rips, J. L., Kaplan, D. L., Levinson, M. J., Wasilewski, Y., Levin, B., & Mellins, R. B. (1987). A school health program for children with asthma aged 8 to 11 years. *Health Education Quarterly*, 14, 267–279.

Ewart, C. K. (1978). Self-observation in natural settings: Reactive effects of behavior desirability and goal-setting. *Cognitive Therapy and Research*, 2, 39–56.

Hindi-Alexander, M. C., & Cropp, G. J. A. (1984). Evaluation of a family asthma program. *Journal of Allergy and Clinical Immunology*, 74, 505–510.

Kaplan, D. L., Rips, J. L., Clark, N. M., Evans, D., Wasilewski, Y., & Feldman, C. H. (1986). Transfer of a clinic-based health education program for children with asthma to a school setting. *Journal of School Health*, 56, 267–271.

Lewis, C. E., Lewis, M. A., & Lorimer, A. (1977). Child-initiated care: The use of school nursing services by children in an adult-free system. *Pediatrics*, 60, 449–456.

Lewis, C. E., Rachelevsky, G., Lewis, M. A., de la Sota, A., & Kaplan, M. (1984). A randomized trial of A.C.T. (asthma care training) for kids. *Pediatrics*, 74, 478–486.

Marlatt, G. A. (1979). Alcohol use and problem drinking: A cognitive behavioral analysis. In P. C. Kendall, & S. D. Hollen (Eds.), *Cognitive behavioral interventions: Theory, research, and procedures*. New York: Academic Press.

McNabb, W. L., Wilson-Pessano, S. R., Hughes, G. W., & Scamagas, P. (1985). Self-management education of children with asthma: AIR WISE. *American Journal of Public Health*, 75, 1219–1220.

National Heart, Lung, and Blood Institute. (1984). *Open Airways/Respiro Abierto: Asthma self-management program* (NIH Publication No. 84-2365). Washington, D.C.: U.S. Government Printing Office.

National Institute of Allergy and Infectious Diseases. (1979). *Asthma and other allergic diseases: NIAID task force report.* (NIH Publication No. 79-397). Bethesda, MD: National Institute of Allergy and Infectious Diseases.

O'Leary, A. (1985). Self-efficacy and health. *Behavioral Research and Therapy*, 23, 437–451.

Parcel, G. S., Nader, P. R., & Tiernan, K. (1980). A health education program for children with asthma. *Developmental and Behavioral Pediatrics*, 1, 128–132.

Piaget, J. (1967). *Six psychological studies* (pp. 38–60). New York: Random House.

Romanczyk, R. G. (1974). Self-monitoring in the treatment of obesity: Parameters of reactivity. *Behavior Therapy*, 5, 531–540.

Strecher, V. J., DeVillis, B. M., Becker, M. H., & Rosenstock, I. M. (1986). The role of self-efficacy in achieving health behavior change. *Health Education Quarterly*, 13, 73–91.

9

A Social Problem-Solving Approach to Behavior Change in Coronary Heart Disease

Craig K. Ewart

Patients with coronary heart disease are told to stop smoking, start exercising, eat fewer foods they enjoy, and do so for the rest of their lives. Although a surprising number manage to follow this advice, it is unclear why some succeed where many fail. Factors critical to prolonged adherence are poorly represented in popular health decision models. Until recently, behavioral scientists have been more interested in explaining why individuals make particular health choices than in understanding how people develop the ability to adhere to choices they have made. The better-known health decision models resemble *competence* models in learning theory: They identify personal attributes or qualities (knowl-

Preparation of this chapter was supported in part by grants R01-HL29431 and R01-HL36298 from the National Heart, Lung, and Blood Institute of the National Institutes of Health, Bethesda, Maryland. I wish to thank Marilyn Bergner, Jeffrey Johnson, Margaret Ensminger, and Barbara Curbow for their helpful comments on an earlier draft. Thanks are also due to Dorothy Pumphrey for her assistance in typing and editing the manuscript.

edge, beliefs, attitudes) individuals must possess in order to arrive at a given health choice. But to explain long-term change, a *performance* model is needed, one encompassing the diverse social pressures and personal dilemmas people encounter when trying to maintain healthy behavior patterns "forever."

The present chapter develops such a model. It underscores the role of social interactions in moderating the impact of behavioral interventions on long-term change. Moreover, the ever-shifting demands of daily living place a premium on personal problem-solving activities, phenomena insufficiently explored in previous adherence research. The "social problem-solving" model here proposed integrates core *behavioral processes* that are critical for long-term maintenance. Persistence in life-style change is a direct function of continued problem-solving activity that is motivated by social reinforcement and self-efficacy enhancement processes. As time passes, interactions with family, co-workers, and significant others play in increasingly important role in strengthening or weakening problem-solving efforts. By focusing attention on *processes*, here defined as observable and potentially modifiable behavioral event sequences, the model provides a practical map to guide adherence promotion efforts.

This approach originated in the author's research on behavioral factors affecting patients' return to work soon after uncomplicated acute myocardial infarction (MI). In its current form, the model provides a flexible framework for explaining and treating a wide variety of behavioral adherence problems in adults and children. This chapter illustrates potential applications by emphasizing the model's contributions to tertiary prevention after uncomplicated MI.

RECOVERY FROM ACUTE MYOCARDIAL INFARCTION

Acute MI is a frightening experience that disrupts patients' lives in many ways. Intense anxiety and depression are common soon after the acute event, and later patients often experience unexpected difficulties when trying to resume normal physical activities, perform family roles, or return to their jobs (Garrity et al., 1981). By the late 1970s, it had become apparent that psychological or behavioral reactions to MI often were greater barriers to recovery than was the myocardial damage resulting from infarction. Cardiologist Robert DeBusk and his colleagues at Stanford (1983) had conducted an important series of studies to determine the diagnostic value of early (3 weeks post-MI) treadmill exercise testing as an alternative to more expensive and invasive medical tests. Uncomplicated male patients who had been carefully prescreened were turning out to be more fit than anyone had expected. Only 3 weeks after MI, most patients were able to perform a maximal (symptom limited) exercise stress test that showed them to be capable of slow jogging. Of the more than 700 patients evaluated, none suffered harm attributable to the test, and most were found to be physically capable of returning to their usual employment far sooner than had been anticipated (Davidson & DeBusk, 1980).

Maximal treadmill exercise (TME) showed them to have a relatively well-preserved functional capacity 3 weeks after MI and disclosed that by 11 weeks post-MI their performance was nearly normal. Moreover, these gains were achieved even without special exercise training programs: Men who engaged in routine low-intensity exertion at home improved as rapidly as men who participated in supervised group training in a gymnasium (Miller, Haskell, Berra, & DeBusk, 1984).

DeBusk's data (DeBusk et al., 1983) indicated that in nearly half of the men between the ages of 30 and 70 years who survive 21 days following acute MI, the proportion who will suffer a fatal cardiac event in the next 12 months is only 1.5%. Patients at lower risk can be identified on the basis of their medical history (no prior angina pectoris, infarction, or recurrent chest pain), absence of clinical indications (unstable angina pectoris or heart failure), or by graded treadmill exercise test. Unfortunately, most of these patients worry excessively and may even curtail their activities to a degree that causes financial hardship (from prolonged unemployment) or seriously disrupts family ties (Croog & Levine, 1977). Such individuals have trouble developing the program of frequent, safe physical exercise needed to reduce unnecessary fears, build self-confidence, and improve physical functioning.

Exercise is a central focus of rehabilitation because it benefits the cardiac patient in a number of important ways. In the first few months after MI, appropriate physical exertion reassures patients that they are recovering and can safely resume normal activities. Later, an exercise program improves cardiovascular functioning and may help reduce risk. Regular exercise can reduce the burden on the damaged heart by increasing the efficiency of oxygen use in the skeletal muscle while facilitating weight control and helping to modify lipid profiles (Clausen, 1976; Shephard, 1981). In the early stages of recovery, the chief barrier to initial life-style change is the patient's fear of exertion, while later on major barriers are behavior patterns and preferences that interfere with patient involvement in continuing exercise and diet programs (Oldridge, 1982). The challenge to behavioral scientists is to discover ways to identify patients who will have trouble making life-style changes and to develop methods to modify inappropriate fears and preferences so as to promote sustained change.

ORIGIN AND CORE COMPONENTS OF A SOCIAL PROBLEM-SOLVING MODEL

The first part of this challenge, prediction, requires determination of which measurable characteristics of individuals reliably indicate their future actions.

Prevention, the second task, might then become feasible if powerful causal mechanisms that are amenable to change can be determined. For years the favored method in health research was to characterize patients in terms of broad, stable, personality dispositions or traits, presumably reflected in their responses to items on paper and pencil tests. But in the late 1960s this approach came under attack. In an influential monograph, Walter Mischell (1968) demonstrated that there was surprisingly little correlation between people's trait scores on conventional personality tests and their trait-relevant behaviors in specific situations. The lively debate that followed led many to question the meaning of popular personality measures and the trait theories on which they were based (Pervin, 1985). Was the consistancy seen in an individual's day-to-day actions attributable to "inner" dispositions, traits, or drives? Or did this apparent stability merely reflect enduring consistencies in the person's social environment? If individual consistency was attributable to the *interaction* of personal and environmental factors, how should this interplay be modeled and measured?

In the face of these questions, traditional trait theories appeared conceptually sterile. Even if the predictive power of trait measures could be improved (for example, by repeated testing over many occasions), a high trait score would imply only that, *on average*, an individual will tend to exhibit characteristics of a given type (e.g., friendliness, hostility, shyness) over a wide range of situations. While often useful, this information alone does not reveal the personal or environmental *causes* of the person's actions. Nothing in trait theory suggested how to modify a trait or develop an appropriate intervention plan.

The attack on conventional personality testing stimulated attempts to ground personality assessment in current theory about causal mechanisms. For example, research on cognitive processes was suggesting that people could be described in terms of their characteristic ways of thinking, of processing information about themselves and their world, or the cognitive skills they employed to manage their lives and solve challenging problems (Epstein & O'Brien, 1985; Mischel,, 1973). This was exciting because it connected personality theory with advances in cognitive science. Cognitive processes were measurable and modifiable behavioral phenomena acquired through learning according to empirically testable principles. The cognitive approach held promise both for predicting behavior and for suggesting specific interventions to alter maladaptive patterns.

These developments in psychology, together with advances in social interaction research, have important implications for efforts to predict and enhance long-term maintenance of health-promoting behavior. Unfortunately, they have not been assimilated adequately into the mainstream of research on behavioral compliance with medical advice. The present Social Problem-Solving Model is designed to facilitate this assimilation. By constructing a causal framework integrating major theoretical advances in cognitive-behavioral research, the Model suggests how more powerful approaches to health behavior change could be achieved. Three important theoretical developments comprise the "core" of the Social Problem-Solving Model.

Self-Efficacy

The first development is an improved understanding of how health and coping are influenced by patients' perceptions of their ability to predict and control the flow of events that shape their lives. Experimental work by Julian Rotter, Martin Seligman, Ellen Langer, and many other investigators amply demonstrates the role of perceived lack of control or helplessness in stimulating fear, depression, and diminished coping (Langer & Rodin, 1976; Rotter, 1966; Seligman, 1975). While earlier health belief models had emphasized the importance of patients' expectations concerning the efficacy and value of medical treatments, research on perceived control suggests that perceptions of personal efficacy or ability to change may be equally important. Albert Bandura's (1977) Self-Efficacy Theory provides a novel way to synthesize a wide variety of data on human coping and offers highly specific guidelines for modifying patient expectations to promote behavior change. This theory was an early focus of the present Social Problem-Solving Model and plays a central role in its current formulation. When patients are told they should change their behavior, they must first appraise the difficulty of the task and gauge the resources available to meet this challenge. These appraisal processes strongly influence initial motivation to comply with medical advice.

Problem-Solving

The second major development reflected in the Social Problem-Solving Model is the discovery that patients' success at implementing demanding behavior changes is greatly affected by their ability to exercise critical problem-solving skills. Growing recognition that problem-solving competence is central to personal adjustment and change reflects a convergence of findings from research in clinical psychology (D'Zurilla & Goldfried, 1971), decision counseling (Janis & Mann, 1977; Krumboltz & Thoresen, 1976), and studies of cognitive processes in depression (Beck, 1967). This work has succeeded in identifying cognitive and social skills that are critical to solving personal problems, including the ability to recognize and define problems, envisage multiple coping alternatives, evaluate potential solutions, and develop realistic plans of action. Unlike previous health decision models, the Social Problem-Solving Model accords problem-solving competencies central importance, holding that they mediate the relationship between motivational influences and behavioral outcomes and, therefore, constitute proximal determinants of personal change. This helps explain why patients who want to change their behavior frequently fail to do so: In many cases, they lack the problem-solving skills needed to envisage potential challenges and develop effective behavioral coping strategies.

Social Interaction Processes

The third core component of the Model derives from advances in social interaction research. Recall that a challenge to traditional personality trait theory arises from the need to account for the interaction of environmental influences and personal dispositions. By the early 1960s, work by social learning theorists had begun to yield important insights into how environmental and personal factors might interact to establish significant, enduring behavior patterns (Eron, 1987). In a famous series of experiments, Bandura had demonstrated the effects of social modeling and reinforcement in stimulating aggression in normal children (Bandura, 1973). Further advances were being made by Gerald Patterson, John Gottman, and Ewart Thomas (Patterson, 1982), who were studying disturbed children and families in a novel way. Using field observation methods borrowed from ethology, these investigators found they could examine the flow of parent–child interaction much as the ethologist might analyze the complicated bonding rituals of nesting storks. Their work was full of suprises, of which the most striking was the discovery that the chaotic behavior of troubled families was not really as chaotic as it appeared. Family interactions were, in fact, highly structured. The structure became visible only when one examined moment-to-moment interaction sequences: In this perspective, aberrant behavior of one family member was often highly predictable from behaviors of other family members earlier in the interaction sequence. Moreover, certain repetitive, stereotyped interactions occurring frequently in famlilies of aggressive children provided a potent mechanism (coercion) by which violent behavior could be developed and consistently maintained (Patterson, 1982).

To many, this suggested that social interaction analysis might yield insights into behavioral consistency and causation that would not be achieved by measuring personality characteristics of isolated individuals. This is not to say that individual attributes were deemed unimportant, but that their "expression" was now seen to be regulated extensively by interpersonal transactions within one's social milieu. The social interactionist approach could explain why children who were equally skilled in aggressive behavior could differ greatly in their rates of aggressive acts, or why children who were highly aggressive in one setting (e.g., school) might be quite nonaggressive in another (e.g., the family). Apart from improving our ability to understand and predict problem behavior, social interaction analysis also was appealing because it identified specific event sequences that might be modified in order to test a hypothesis or promote change. In the context of MI, this approach seemed especially relevant to a problem encountered regularly in the clinic but that was not addressed by attitudinal models prevalent at the time: What to do about the patient who responds readily to behavioral intervention early in recovery but later succumbs to subtle or overt counterpressures exerted by family or friends?

OVERVIEW OF THE MODEL

The remainder of this chapter describes the Social Problem-Solving Model and illustrates its application to coronary heart disease. Following a brief overview of the model, component processes are presented in detail. Within each component, specific implications for clinical intervention and research are developed. The final section of the chapter presents a developmental perspective on adherence, showing how the various components can assume greater or lesser importance as a patient progresses from deciding whether or not to comply with medical advice, through early efforts to change, to routine maintenance of recommended health behaviors.

Figure 9.1 outlines the Social Problem-Solving Model. Note that unlike many health decision models, the present model was not designed to predict a specific health choice, such as to undergo cancer screening, or a discrete behavioral event, such as relapsing after having abstained from alcohol. Instead, it is a performance model designed to: (1) specify behavioral activities or processes critical to sustaining performance of desired health behaviors; (2) show how these activities or processes are related to one another; and (3) generate practical guidelines and research hypotheses for improving long-term maintenance of health behavior.

The model can be viewed as a causal model indicating how component processes interact to influence long-term adherence. On the other hand, the causal directions indicated by the arrows in Figure 8.1 are not meant to be unidirectional, implying that causation operates only in the direction specified. In fact, they are bidirectional. For example, motivation to change may lead to effective problem-solving for adherence as shown in Figure 9.1, but success at problem-solving also can lead to increased motivation to solve future problems. The causal directions specified in the figure are meant to highlight relationships I believe to be especially important for understanding and enhancing peoples' ability to sustain long-term change. Thus the model contains motivational processes critical to the initial decision to attempt change and to early adoption, but "nests" these influences within a larger conceptual framework that includes behavioral processes necessary to prolonged maintenance.

The resulting conceptual structure addresses a need not currently met by research on health behavior change processes or by health education approaches, such as the popular PRECEDE diagnostic framework developed by Green and his associates (Green, Kreuter, Deeds, & Partridge, 1980). The former

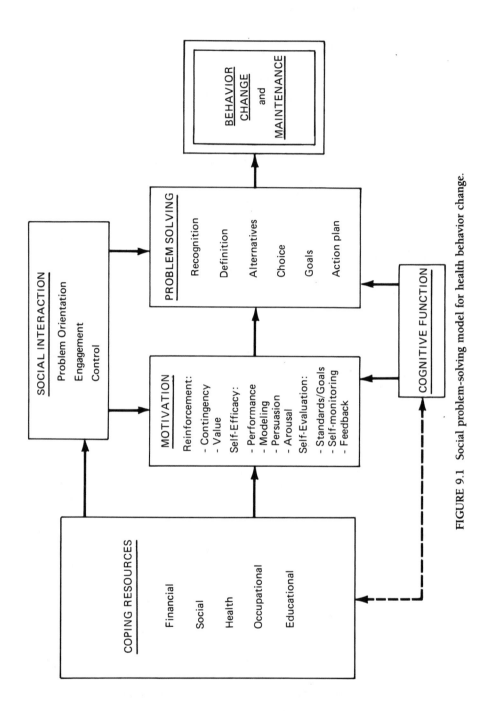

FIGURE 9.1 Social problem-solving model for health behavior change.

activities tend to focus on more narrowly defined influence processes and their application. At the other pole, the PRECEDE framework catalogues a broad range of behavioral factors to consider when planning for an educational program, but does not link these to causal mechanisms that have been the object of rigorous empirical investigation and theory building. PRECEDE notes that influences such as attitudes or social reinforcement are important, but offers little explicit guidance on how best to define, quantify, and activate these influences. Although PRECEDE represents an important step toward a more comprehensive, social-environmental approach to intervention and assessment, it does not specify how the behavioral influences it enumerates might interact as parts of an integrated system. Thus, it is often difficult to decide which of multiple influences might be most critical or should be targeted first by a given health promotion effort. The importance of increased specificity regarding causal processes and their possible interactions should become evident below as the components of the Social Problem-Solving Model are examined.

PROBLEM-SOLVING PROCESSES

In a problem-solving model, emotional reactions and life disturbances occasioned by MI are construed as problems the patient must learn to solve. Following D'Zurilla and Goldfried (1971), a *problem* is here defined as a life situation that demands a response for effective functioning but for which no effective response is immediately apparent or available to the individual confronted with the situation. For many patients, sexual intimacy poses a problem due to fears that sexual arousal could cause another heart attack. Such fears often pose serious barriers to resuming rewarding personal relationships or to engaging in activities that would promote health and speed recovery. A *solution* to this problem could be defined as a coping response that alters the situation or one's reactions to it so that it is no longer perceived as a problem. For example, a patient might be encouraged to seek advice from a physician and to experiment by monitoring heart rate while engaging in less feared activities, such as walking or climbing stairs. *Problem solving* refers to the process by which the patient discovers a solution to a problem. Techniques for solving threatening life problems have been reviewed by D'Zurilla (1986), who presents a highly developed prescriptive problem-solving model applicable to a wide range of challenges and situations.

Figure 9.1 emphasizes that problem-solving activities and competencies function as critical proximal determinants of long-term behavior change. The Model highlights specific cognitive–behavioral activities patients must perform regularly if they are to develop the ability to maintain a diet, exercise, or other behavior routines. Making a new behavior pattern part of one's normal routine entails repeated cycles of adjustment, disruption, and readjustment; to borrow a phrase from evolutionary biology, maintenance might be viewed as the achievement of a "punctuated equilibrium." To accomplish this, the individual must learn to: (1) recognize when threats to "equilibrium" exist or might arise; (2) envision a variety of alternative ways to cope with threats; (3) use appropriate criteria to evaluate these alternatives; (4) select a coping strategy that is likely to work; and (5) decide upon a specific course of action, including ways to overcome obstacles to implementing the solution (D'Zurilla, 1986). Together, these performance skills define patient *competence* to engineer and maintain behavioral life-style changes. The lack of these critical abilities can doom to failure even strongly motivated patients who sincerely want to change their harmful habits.

Although problem-solving processes have long been a focus of research on health decision making (Janis & Mann, 1977), their vital role in long-term behavior change became more evident when researchers began to attack the problem of preventing relapse after successful behavioral treatment for smoking, alcohol and drug use, or obesity. G. Allan Marlatt, Judith Gordon, and their associates developed behavioral interventions specifically designed to help patients anticipate lapses and prevent their leading to treatment failure. The relapse-prevention training is designed to develop a problem-solving orientation to these episodes and build coping skills: Patients are taught to anticipate occasions in which slips could occur, define the slip as a problem that must be solved (instead of a "failure"), and generate realistic goals and plans of action to prevent recurrences (Marlatt & Gordon, 1984). This problem-solving approach has also been shown to increase long-term adherence to aerobic exercise programs in healthy adults (Belisle, Roskies, & Levesque, 1987) and to enhance maintenance of weight loss in a behavioral weight reduction program (Black & Scherba, 1983). In the latter study, patients who wrote behavioral contracts to problem solve when tempted to overeat achieved significantly greater weight reduction than did a comparison group that contracted to practice only self-monitoring and reinforcement techniques.

Intervention Guidelines

This analysis suggests that behavior change programs should provide extensive modeling of adherence problem-solving skills, encourage patients to practice solving a range of hypothetical maintenance problems, and provide prompt feedback to support these efforts. Such practice receives too little attention in many cardiac rehabilitation programs, which typically emphasize nutrition knowledge and safe exercise skills. While this information is essential, more time should be devoted to increasing patients' ability to apply their knowledge by showing them how to anticipate adherence threats, define them as behavior problems, generate coping alternatives, and implement solutions. To keep patients from becoming discouraged, inevitable failures to adhere perfectly to exercise, diet, or other plans should be attributed to the patient's inexperience in solving that type of behavior problem, instead of to a "character defect" or to lack of "will power" (cf., Marlatt & Gordon, 1984).

Research Issues

Problem-solving skills can be assessed by observing patients' responses when they are asked to explain how they might solve various real-life problems. Measures of competence include the amount of time the individual spends deliberating about the problem, the degree to which potential threats are specified, number and type of coping alternatives considered, use of explicit criteria to evaluate the alternatives, ability to anticipate barriers to implementing solutions, and specification of a plan of action (Blechman & McEnroe, 1985; Kendall & Fischler, 1984; Shure & Spivack, 1972). Individuals and families at risk for emotional or behavioral disorder can be identified by their performance on these tasks (Leff & Vaughn, 1985; Urbain & Kendall, 1980). In the MI patient, denial or excessive fear may impair ability to envision coping alternatives, think flexibly, and evaluate potential solutions against appropriate criteria.

The Social Problem-Solving Model holds that: (1) intervention to reduce fear will improve behavioral problem-solving performance; and (2) measures of problem-solving ability like those above will predict patient success at implementing health behavior changes. Research to test these hypotheses could yield valuable data on how behavioral adherence to rehabilitation guidelines might be predicted and enhanced.

MOTIVATION

Patients and their families do not solve adherence problems unless they want to solve them. What factors strengthen or weaken one's desire to engage repeatedly in problem-solving activities? Social psychologists have made significant strides in identifying influences that shape health choices (Becker, 1989; Maiman & Becker, 1974). Their work has been strongly influenced by "expectancy-value" theories of motivation. This general approach holds that health choices are determined by one's beliefs that (1) the recommended action will significantly affect one's health (expectancy) and (2) the health impact is desirable (value). Expectancy-value analyses have improved our ability to anticipate public response to public health programs and forecast population trends.

The approach to motivation advocated in the present Model is compatible with expectancy-value notions, but differs from previous health belief formulations in at least two important respects. First, the Social Problem-Solving Model incorporates motivational processes governing the maintenance of complicated and demanding behaviors like diet and exercise as well as comparatively simple and time-limited actions (such as attending a clinic for health screening) that were often the focus of earlier models. Second, motivational influences specified in the present Model are behavioral processes for which there exists a well-developed set of empirically tested principles telling how to manipulate these influences to promote change. Earlier health belief models often measured factors (e.g., "norm awareness") that, while useful for prediction, offer scant procedural guidance when one is trying to establish lasting behavior change.

From a behavior-change perspective, motivation is best analyzed in terms of reinforcement, self-efficacy, and self-evaluation processes, which in the Social Problem-Solving Model are conceived as hierarchically integrated behavioral systems. This analytic framework has a number of important implications that shall now be considered.

Reinforcement Processes

The Social Problem-Solving approach holds that behavior is a function of its anticipated and experienced consequences: Behavior patterns are strengthened or weakened by the reinforcing or punishing effects they generate. This view is quite compatible with expectancy-value formulations. As used here, "expectancy" is the perception of *contingency*, or the expectation that a given health behavior will produce a given consequence. The "value" component refers to the combined *desirability* of a consequence. Contingency and desirability perceptions combine to generate *outcome expectancies* (Bandura, 1977a), or the perception that the positive benefits of a given behavior do or do not outweigh the behavior's undesired effects of costs.

Outcome expectancies include the immediate as well as the delayed effects of engaging in a behavior; for example, outcome expectancies for jogging might include the physical sensations, thoughts, emotions, or social companionship experienced during running as well as more delayed outcomes such as weight loss, approving comments from friends, and reduced cardiovascular risk. Outcome expectancies are specific events, behaviors, or sensations people expect to experience in consequence of making recommended changes. They include experiences intrinsic to the activity itself as well as more extrinsic outcomes (Lepper & Greene, 1978).

The motivational importance of behavioral consequences is demonstrated by research on factors affecting patient compliance with exercise programs in cardiac rehabilitation. Data from major long-term programs in Canada, the United States, New Zealand, and Sweden reveal that patients who drop out of exercise programs are usually individuals who encountered important aversive consequences when they tried to exercise regularly (Oldridge, 1982). These punishing outcomes included physical injury or discomfort, excessive fatigue, inconveniences involved in getting to the program site or incorporating exercise into a demanding work schedule, and problems with a nonsupportive spouse or family. Especially likely to drop out were persons with more severe disease, smokers, the obese, and individuals who had rarely exercised before. People with these problems are unusually vulnerable to unpleasant sensations or symptoms during vigorous physical exertion.

Analyzing motivation in terms of specific reinforcing and punishing consequences has several advantages. First, measuring specific expectations instead of more general motives focuses attention on precisely those events and experiences one must change in order to increase adherence to the recommended behavior. Second, it becomes possible to identify areas of misinformation or ignorance that may contribute to nonadherence. Above all, the focus on expected consequences of behavior gives health promotion efforts a sounder empirical base. Principles for altering behavior by restructuring its consequences are well developed in operant behavior analysis (Kazdin, 1984) and Social Learning Theory (Bandura, 1986). Extensive experimental work has elucidated fundamental principles that determine the degree to which a behavior's consequences influence the future occurrence of similar behaviors. For example, health-promoting behaviors are influenced most by consequences that are immediate rather than delayed, frequent rather than rare, strongly desired or feared rather than of neutral valence, and of larger rather than smaller magnitude (Baldwin & Baldwin, 1986; Kazdin, 1984).

When planning an intervention, it is extremely useful to construct "contingency grids" to examine the consequences of adopting a recommended diet or exercise change (Marlatt & Gordon, 1984). Perceived consequences of the behavior change are enumerated and then sorted into four cells created by crossing the time (immediate vs. delayed) dimension with the valence (desired vs. undesired) dimension. This process quickly discloses potential motivational problems due to a lack of immediate positive outcomes or a surfeit of immediate aversive consequences that might discourage change attempts. Intervention then can focus on finding ways to increase immediate positives and decrease immediate negatives. Contingency (outcome) analysis can reveal which benefits to emphasize when trying to persuade patients to change. For example, it is often more effective to emphasize immediate positive effects of a desired behavior (e.g., money saved by not drinking or smoking) than emphasizing more delayed health outcomes such as avoiding cancer or heart disease.

Self-Efficacy Enhancement

Until fairly recently, perceptions of contingency and value were thought to be the prime movers determining whether people adopted or shunned health behavior changes. This view has changed with the advent of Self-Efficacy Theory (Bandura, 1986), which asserts that motivation is driven not only by desiring a given outcome but also by believing that one is capable of performing the actions necessary to produce the desired result. Whereas Outcome Expectancies describe perceived consequences of behavior, Self-Efficacy (SE) refers to the person's *confidence* that he or she can actually carry out the behavioral tasks necessary to produce the outcome. As developed by Bandura, the SE concept is of theoretical importance because it identifies a significant, conceptually distinct judgmental process and specifies causal factors that can be manipulated to support behavior change. Moreover, it turns out that SE theory is especially helpful for predicting and enhancing recovery following acute MI, when fear causes many patients to become excessively cautious and leads others to deny or minimize the health threat.

According to SE theory, confidence in one's abilities (SE) is not static but changes continually in response to new experiences. These experiences can enhance or diminish one's sense of personal efficacy. One of SE theory's most salient contributions is its analysis of the origins of SE perceptions (Bandura, 1977b, 1982, 1986). By showing how specific modifiable behavioral processes enhance or undermine SE, the theory provides practical guidelines for building personal confidence. The theory asserts that SE perceptions are derived from four major sources of information. Listed in order of their power of influence behavior, these sources are the following: (1) prior experiences performing similar behaviors; (2) opportunities to observe others similar to oneself performing the behavior; (3) persuasion by a respected authority; and (4) one's self-perceived level of physiological arousal. Stated simply, the most effective way to increase SE is to have the person perform a feared activity in gradually increasing doses while providing reassuring feedback and counseling. These assertions led to research testing the value of the theory for understanding and treating psychological problems of patients with coronary heart disease. Studies conducted with colleagues at Stanford and Johns Hopkins have demonstrated that brief cost-effective interventions derived from SE theory can modify inaccurate self-perceptions that constitute barriers to recovery (Ewart, 1989).

Not only did DeBusk's exercise studies show that early treadmill testing was informative and safe, they suggested that TME could have dramatic psychological effects. Patients who were excessively anxious prior to testing became more confident after performing the test and showed a new eagerness to resume their normal routines. It seemed that SE theory might suggest powerful new ways to measure, monitor, and modify patient fears. The result could be a less costly and more effective alternative to conventional personality testing and psychotherapy.

The first challenge was to develop reliable and valid SE measures. The theory asserts that "self-confidence" is not a broad and stable trait but is comprised of many highly specific judgments of personal abilities that change with experience or with fluctuations in one's mood (Bandura, 1977b). To assess SE in our patients, we developed scales measuring self-perceived ability to walk various distances, jog, climb stairs, perform sexual intercourse, and lift objects of varying weights (see Figure 9.2). Patients are asked to indicate their level of confidence in their ability to perform each task, using a scale ranging from 0 (not at all confident) to 100 (completely confident). A series of studies has shown that these scales yield very reliable (reproducible) measures of patients' self-perceived abilities and that they permit highly sensitive and specific measures of intervention effects. As predicted by SE theory, SE perceptions change after exposure to safe graded exercise and counseling (Ewart, Taylor, Reese, & DeBusk, 1983). Perceptual changes are largest for activities resembling the walking, jogging, or lifting task performed during the test (Ewart, Stewart, Gillilan, & Kelemen, 1986).

Most important, the SE scales appear to tap important motivational processes: Changes in SE after testing have predicted changes in patients' home activity levels (assessed by portable monitor) more accurately than did the treadmill test performance measures. In a study of patients who participated regularly in a supervised group jogging program, Jog SE ratings obtained prior to the program predicted later noncompliance with exertional guidelines when patients were monitored during the jogging exercises. Again, the SE perceptions were better predictors than was a TME test administered prior to the jogging program (Ewart et al., 1986b). Finally, another study assessed SE, arm strength, leg strength, and aerobic fitness in patients participating in an evaluation of a circuit weight training program (Ewart et al., 1986a). Multiple regression analyses revealed that Strength SE judgments obtained prior to the 10-week weight training program predicted posttest strength gains, even after controlling for baseline strength and frequency of participation. These findings suggest that SE judgments reflect important motivational processes and are not simply reflections of measured physical abilities.

Self-Evaluation Processes

Health care providers who work with MI patients find that many patients react to their sudden illness with feelings of diminished self-esteem or self-worth. Along with biochemical changes occurring during MI, the realization that one is no longer free to conduct one's usual affairs (decreased self-efficacy) or do things one enjoys (diminished reinforcement) can trigger depressive reactions, including excessive self-depreciation. Patients also become more vulnerable to inappropriate self-disparagement when they find they can no longer meet important self-standards.

Notions of "self-concept" or "self-esteem" long played a leading role in phenomenological theories whose proponents made little effort to validate their central constructs through rigorous empirical observation and experiment. In

SELF-EFFICACY SCALES

NAME_____   DATE_____

This form asks you how much physical activity you think you can handle right now. It gives the medical team a better picture of how you are feeling.

Activities are listed on the page that follows . You show how <u>confident</u> you are that you could do each activity <u>now</u> by writing a number in the blank to the right of the activity. Use one of the following numbers to show how confident you are.

Definitely <u>Cannot</u> Do It		Probably Cannot		Maybe (50/50)		Probably Can		Definitely <u>Can</u> Do It

0%	10%	20%	30%	40%	50%	60%	70%	80%	90%	100%

<u>Example:</u> Jim is asked how far he thinks he can throw a football. Can he throw it 10 yards? 15 yards? 30 yards? 40 yards? 60 yards? Jim decides that he can <u>definitely</u> throw the football 10 yards—he is 100% confident about that. He is pretty sure he can throw the football 15 yards—he feels 80% certain. He feels there is about a 50/50 chance he could throw the ball 30 yards, but thinks his chances of hitting the 40-yard marker are slim. He is <u>definitely</u> sure he cannot throw the ball 60 yards.

Jim should write his answers to the question like this:

<u>Throw a football</u>	<u>Confidence</u>
10 yards	<u>100%</u>
15 yards	<u>80%</u>
30 yards	<u>50%</u>
40 yards	<u>20%</u>
60 yards	<u>0</u>

If Jim was definitely sure he could throw the ball 60 yards he would have put 100% in every blank. If he was definitely sure he could not throw the ball even as far as 10 yards, he would have put a 0 in every blank.

Now look at each activity and show how confident you are that you could do it NOW.

FIGURE 9.2 An example of a self-efficacy scale.

Lifting objects:	Confidence
Lift a 10 pound object	_____
Lift a 20 pound object	_____
Lift a 30 pound object	_____
Lift a 40 pound object	_____
Lift a 50 pound object	_____
Lift a 60 pound object	_____
Lift a 70 pound object	_____
Lift an 80 pound object	_____
Lift a 90 pound object	_____
Lift a 100 pound object	_____
Lift a 110 pound object	_____
Lift a 120 pound object	_____

Jogging at a steady pace (5 miles per hour) without stopping:	Confidence
Jog 1 block (1 minute)	_____
Jog 2 blocks (2 minutes)	_____
Jog 3 blocks (3 minutes)	_____
Jog 4 blocks (4 minutes)	_____
Jog 1/2 mile (6 minutes)	_____
Jog 3/4 mile (8 minutes)	_____
Jog 1 mile (12 minutes)	_____
Jog 1 1/2 miles (18 minutes)	_____
Jog 2 miles (24 minutes)	_____
Jog 2 1/2 miles (30 minutes)	_____
Jog 3 miles (36 minutes)	_____
Jog 3 1/2 miles (42 minutes)	_____
Jog 4 miles (48 minutes)	_____
Jog 4 1/2 miles (54 minutes)	_____
Jog 5 miles (60 minutes)	_____

Walking at a steady pace (3 miles per hour) without stopping:

	Confidence
Walk 1 block (2 minutes)	_____
Walk 2 blocks (4 minutes)	_____
Walk 3 blocks (6 minutes)	_____
Walk 4 blocks (8 minutes)	_____
Walk 1/2 mile (10 minutes)	_____
Walk 3/4 mile (15 minutes)	_____
Walk 1 mile (20 minutes)	_____
Walk 1 1/2 miles (30 minutes)	_____
Walk 2 miles (40 minutes)	_____
Walk 2 1/2 miles (50 minutes)	_____
Walk 3 miles (60 minutes)	_____
Walk 3 1/2 miles (1 hour, 10 minutes)	_____
Walk 4 miles (1 hour, 20 minutes)	_____
Walk 4 1/2 miles (1 hour, 30 minutes)	_____
Walk 5 miles (1 hour, 40 minutes)	_____

Climbing stairs at a steady pace without pausing:

	Confidence
Walk up several steps	_____
Walk up 1 flight of stairs	_____
Walk up 2 flights of stairs	_____
Walk up 3 flights of stairs	_____
Walk up 4 flights of stairs	_____
Walk up 5 flights of stairs	_____
Walk up 6 flights of stairs	_____
Walk up 7 flights of stairs	_____
Walk up 8 flights of stairs	_____

Push-ups at a steady pace without stopping:

	Confidence
Do 1 push-up	_____
Do 3 push-ups	_____
Do 6 push-ups	_____
Do 10 push-ups	_____
Do 15 push-ups	_____
Do 20 push-ups	_____
Do 25 push-ups	_____
Do 30 push-ups	_____
Do 35 push-ups	_____
Do 40 push-ups	_____

Sex (engage in intercourse, not including foreplay):

1–5 minutes	_____
6–10 minutes	_____
11–15 minutes	_____
16–20 minutes	_____
More than 20 minutes	_____

From Ewart, C. K., & Taylor, C. B. (1985). The effects of early postmyocardial infarction exercise testing on quality of life. *Quality of Life in Cardiovascular Care, 1,* 162–175.

recent years, however, a growing interest in cognitive processes has stimulated critical scrutiny of the ways self-perceptions are created and, in turn, influence behavior. The older idea of a single global self-concept has been replaced by the view that behavior is guided by multiple, more specific "self-concepts" in the form of "self-schemas," "scripts," or rules (Markus & Wurf, 1987). In the present model, self-concepts assume motivational importance when defined as specific self-evaluative behaviors that lead to self-reinforcement or self-punishment (Bandura, 1977a). Levels of self-satisfaction and self-dissatisfaction (high or low self-esteem) are determined by one's behavioral accomplishments and by the standards one uses to evaluate them.

Social learning research has shown how self-standards are acquired and maintained through observational learning and reinforcement. People are more likely to emulate self-standards that are modeled by persons they judge to be similar to themselves (Bandura & Whalen, 1966), who consistently apply to their own behavior the standards they use to evaluate others, and who apply the same standard across a variety of tasks (Bandura & Mahoney, 1974). As people develop through adulthood, they learn to evaluate their functioning in various domains according to standards modeled by influential reference groups. Attaining an emulated standard occasions self-reinforcement in the form of self-approval and tangible reward (e.g., taking a break from one's work, indulging in a hobby, relaxing with friends, enjoying a favorite meal). These reinforcing activities can generate further good feelings. On the other hand, prolonged striving to attain excessively high goals or repeated failure to meet important personal standards leads to self-criticism, lack of reinforcement, or even to various forms of self-punishment (Stone & Hokanson, 1969). These restrictions may contribute to depression (Beck, Rush, Shaw, & Emery, 1979).

As different activities require different competencies and performance standards, people learn to evaluate themselves against a variety of criteria, generating multiple self-evaluations or "self-concepts." A person's self-conception will vary according to the performance domain (e.g., professional attainments, personal attractiveness, popularity, athletic ability) and the respective standard used for self-evaluation. Depressive reactions are presumed to occur when individuals perceive themselves to perform "inadequately" in a variety of domains or in certain highly valued performance areas.

Recent research on Type A behavior, a risk factor for MI, suggests that the intense competitive striving and hostility associated with the Type A pattern may be caused by a dysfunctional self-evaluation system (Grimm & Yarnold, 1984; Friedman & Ulmer, 1984; Ward & Eisler, 1987). Research has shown that in achievement situations, Type A individuals tend to set more difficult performance goals than do Type B persons (Grimm & Yarnold, 1984; Snow, 1978), more often fail to achieve these goals, and express greater dissatisfaction with their actual levels of performance (Ward & Eisler, 1987). Presumably, the tendency to focus on an overly narrow range of goals and to set excessively high and inflexible achievement standards leaves these individuals vulnerable to the frequent anxiety, depression, and anger associated with increased cardiovascular risk (Friedman & Booth-Kewley, 1987).

After MI, patients are often unable to perform tasks they value at levels sufficient to meet long-held self-evaluative standards. Familiar clinical examples include the male patient who has always taken pride in his physical strength, emotional aggressiveness, or ability to work long hours on the job (e.g., Type A pattern). To such persons, advice to cut back or take it easy can be extremely threatening. Resulting self-disparagement, nonreward, and despondency can become barriers to recovery, either by causing the individual to withdraw from involvement in rehabilitation or by stimulating excessive and dangerous striving to regain lost competence (Garrity, 1981). These patients require intervention to help reduce the perceived discrepancy between their performance ideals and their actual capabilities.

Social learning research suggests that an effective approach would involve exposing patients to respected peer models who could demonstrate self-approval and reinforcement for other kinds of success. A male factory worker was seen who, proud of his physical strength, became depressed and angry after MI when he was forced to hire a neighbor's son to finish a building project he had started in his backyard. Months later the clinic staff were nonplussed when this patient proudly showed them a sweater he was learning to knit! He had asked his wife to teach him after seeing a television show about a popular professional football player who had learned to do needlepoint to pass the time while recuperating from an injury. Noting everyone's surprise, the patient explained: "If it's macho enough for the NFL, it's macho enough for me!" Assessment should determine if recommended changes conflict with important self-standards and arrange corrective counseling and modeling experiences accordingly.

Hierarchical Integration of Reinforcement, Self-Efficacy, and Self-Evaluative Processes

It is useful to think of the above processes as hierarchically linked systems, such that changes in one system can affect the functioning of the others (Hyland, 1987). Self-efficacy would be above reinforcement processes in the hierarchy because self-efficacy perceptions are usually created by the degree of success a person experiences in obtaining specific valued reinforcers. Self-evaluative processes probably occupy the highest level because self-evaluations are created both by the amount and type of reinforcement one experiences and by self-perceived ability to control reinforcers (self-efficacy). Processes higher in the hierarchy can also influence lower-level processes. Self-efficacy perceptions determine how hard and how long people will strive to obtain specific reinforcers (Bandura, 1977b; Ewart et al., 1986a), and self-evaluative processes influence the kind of performances people undertake as well as the type and amount of a particular reinforcer they seek (Hyland, 1987).

This hierarchical structure has important implications for interventions with patients. Depressed individuals who manifest excessive anxiety should be exposed gradually to a variety of self-efficacy-enhancing performances that build confidence in one's ability to resume desired activities safely. On the other hand, depressed persons who engage in excessive self-disparagement should be exposed to respected models who demonstrate self-approval and reinforcement for skills and pursuits more in keeping with their postinfarction capabilities. These patients should simultaneously be introduced to self-efficacy-enhancing experiences that create confidence in one's ability to perform the new activities.

Intervention Guidelines

The outcome expectancy model developed above suggests that attempts to promote behavior changes should begin with a careful analysis of the short- and long-term consequences to the patient. If the contingency grid reveals no important long-term benefits, the behavior change probably should not be recommended in the first place. If the behavior has long-term benefits but fails to generate immediately experienced positive effects, intervention should focus on producing desirable short-term benefits and removing or reducing immediately felt negative effects.

Once benefits are evident to the patient, SE perceptions should be assessed using highly specific SE scales like the ones developed by Ewart and Taylor (1985). If SE deficits are detected, those attributable to deficient knowledge or skill (e.g., calorie counting, pulse monitoring) can be remedied via appropriate education, while low SE due to excessive fear can be treated by exposing the patient to feared tasks or situations at gradually increasing intensities (Bandura, 1986). Care should be taken to expose the patient to a range of behaviors or situations to promote SE generalization (Ewart et al., 1986a).

Self-evaluative reactions should be assessed to identify persons in whom MI occasions excessive self-disparagement in one or more valued performance domains. Corrective social modeling and self-efficacy-enhancing interventions can be implemented as mentioned above. Self-evaluative processes are also important to consider when recommending specific changes in life-style patterns, as some changes (e.g., becoming a jogger or a nonsmoker) may conflict with a patient's self-evaluative standards. These standards may be modified via social modeling, or needed behavior changes may be introduced in ways that are more consistent with a valued self-standard.

Research Issues

Future research should test the assertion that people who perceive many immediate positive benefits of diet or exercise relative to short-term costs (favorable
Outcome Expectancies), are confident they can perform the component behaviors (high Self-Efficacy), and view recommended changes as goals whose attain-
ment will occasion positive self-appraisal and self-reward (Self-Esteem enhancing) will be better adherence problem solvers than will people who see few
advantages in changing, lack confidence, or feel that life-style modification
violates their self-image. Compared to the latter, the former patients will be more
likely to anticipate barriers to adherence, generate practical ways to overcome
them, and propose realistic action plans. Patients who fail to perceive potential
reinforcers, who evidence low self-efficacy or low self-esteem, will either fail to
acknowledge obstacles or will mention them without being able to identify
possible solutions. Remember, however, that desire to change one's habits does
not automatically lead to adherence. Only those patients who express a desire to
change *and* are able to state a specific and appropriate plan of action (effective
problem solvers) are likely to achieve success.

SOCIAL INTERACTION

Especially frustrating in post-MI care are the success stories that turn sour: the
many patients who make important changes in the early months after MI but
lapse later when faced with social pressures and conflicts at home and at work.
The Social Problem Solving Model suggests new ways to understand and prevent
these failures. In Figure 9.1, interpersonal processes are accorded a critical role
as "moderator" variables, meaning that they limit (moderate) the degree to which
motivational influences (Reinforcement, Self-Efficacy enhancement, Self-Evaluation) stimulate the persistent problem solving needed to establish frequent
exercise (Baron & Kenny, 1986). The Model identifies three mechanisms
through which social processes may affect patient motivation and problem
solving.

Intimate social relationships entail mutual interdependence: They can be
described in terms of the amount of emotional, informational, or practical
assistance partners in the relationship typically provide each other (Thoits,
1986). This analytic approach has been developed extensively in *behavior exchange* theories of marital or family functioning. In these theories, relationship
quality is determined by partners' satisfaction with prevailing rates of "behavioral
exchange," that is, with the number and type of supportive acts contributed by
each partner (Homans, 1961; Thibaut & Kelley, 1959). Circumstances that create
unacceptable "imbalances" in these (often implicit) exchanges have the potential
to stimulate conflict and marital distress (Wills, Weiss, & Patterson, 1974).

Acute MI frequently disrupts prevailing behavioral exchange patterns in families by limiting the support the patient can give to other family members. When a patient adopts a new diet or exercise program, spouse and children may resent having to change their habits or may worry that increased activity could cause another heart attack. It is not surprising that family members frequently respond by withholding their support or by actively interfering with the diet or exercise plan (Mayou, Foster, & Williamson, 1978). These reactions tend to punish the patient's initial efforts, thereby undermining motivation to change. This probably explains the finding that the most important factor determining long-term compliance with rehabilitation exercise programs is the assistance of the patient's spouse and family in making behavior change part of the patient's daily routine (Oldridge, 1982). It is critical to develop ways to promote life-style change without disrupting important exchange patterns in the family.

Exchange disruptions can generate conflict when family members who feel shortchanged use ineffective influence strategies to redress the perceived imbalance. Conflict can become a source of chronic distress that patients may learn to avoid by abandoning their behavior-change plan. The likelihood that family conflicts will disrupt adherence depends upon the kinds of interaction processes that characterize family life from day to day. These phenomena have been examined in carefully designed behavioral observation studies by Patterson and the Oregon Social Learning Group (Patterson, 1982), as well as by Gottman, Levenson, and their associates (Gottman, 1979; Levenson & Gottman, 1983, 1985). Their work suggests that three categories of communication behavior might prove to be especially important for promoting behavior change after MI.

Recall that effective problem solving for adherence requires that people be able to recognize problems and think flexibly about them, looking at the difficulty from different angles and entertaining alternative solutions. Family interaction processes that limit family members' ability to notice problems, to express themselves, or to entertain different views and think flexibly tend to reduce the family's ability to overcome adherence threats. While the marital therapy literature is replete with varieties of family communication disorder, the three processes mentioned below describe the patterns I have most often encountered in the "normal" families attending cardiology units and rehabilitation programs. Their ubiquity in families is supported by the fact that constructs similar to these basic three are central to a variety of influential theories of family functioning (e.g., Minuchin, 1974; Olson, 1986; Reiss, 1981). They constitute widespread yet little-investigated threats to health promotion in coronary heart disease.

Problem Orientation Processes

The first and most basic communication category involves the extent to which family members tend to recognize and confront interpersonal problems openly (approach) as opposed to ignoring or trying to deny such difficulties (avoidance). Families vary greatly in their willingness to consider diverging views or share problem feelings. According to the model proposed here, families that characteristically avoid open disagreement or discourage the voicing of unpleasant feelings will be handicapped when confronted with the difficulties arising after acute MI. Couples with fears or adjustment difficulties may be reluctant to acknowledge or discuss them. In some cases it is impossible even to persuade them to discuss hypothetical vignettes used to assess couple communication styles. In fact, this avoidant pattern may be more prevalent in couples than suggested by the literature on marital adjustment. Theories of marital functioning are often derived from experience with couples who seek professional counseling (a step avoidant couples find unthinkable), thus biasing our views of marriage and family life.

The hypothesis that patients in more avoidant families will have greater difficulty adhering to life-style changes should be examined. The frequency and range of problem discussion by family members can be assessed by available self-report instruments (Bloom, 1985) as well as by behavioral role play (Grotevant & Carlson, 1987). While research on this topic is limited, there is evidence to support the hypothesis. Several studies using self-report (e.g., family environment) indices have suggested that compliance with treatment regimens for chronic diseases such as diabetes and cystic fibrosis is greater in families that encourage more open expression of feelings and opinions or foster more extensive problem discussion (Anderson, Miller, Auslander, & Santiago, 1981; Hauser, Jacobson, Wertlieb, Brink, & Wentworth, 1985; Patterson, 1985). Minuchin's well-known family systems approach to psychosomatic problems assigns processes related to Problem Orientation a prominent role (Minuchin, 1974, 1975). Indeed, Minuchin argues that excessive Problem Orientation in the form of behavior he labels "overprotectiveness" is pathogenic for anorexia nervosa (Minuchin, 1978). More extensive behavioral observation studies of family interaction are needed to clarify this issue.

Engagement Processes

A second process affecting family members' ability to recognize problems and respond flexibly involves the degree and quality of their involvement with one another. "Engagement" describes the extent to which family members take an interest in each other and enjoy being together. *Positive engagement* refers to interactions family members experience as "socially reinforcing," that is, as enjoyable, supportive, or nurturing. Observation of such interactions reveals high levels of attentive listening, frequent efforts to understand (clarify) the other person's feelings or views, and a willingness to accept one's share of responsibility for interpersonal problems (Floyd & Markman, 1984). This behavior contrasts sharply with *negative engagement*, which is characterized by frequent interrupting, ignoring what the other person is saying, criticizing, commanding, and denying responsibility. Such mutual punishment may cause families to become less engaged or to actively "disengage" as they seek to avoid each other's wrath. Disengagement can also have *non*hostile causes, such as the need to cope with demands at work or school.

These patterns have important implications for collective problem-solving effectiveness. Families whose interactions reveal high levels of positive engagement skills will tend to spend more time together and thus are more likely to notice potential adherence threats. Their listening and empathic skills make it easier for them to talk about problems and entertain different ideas about how to handle them. Their ability to understand each other's needs allows them to agree on solutions more truly satisfactory to all family members. On the other hand, families characterized by frequent or intense negative engagement will be at a disadvantage when confronting barriers to life-style change. Their tendency to disengage will make it harder to identify and frame problems. Efforts to resolve disagreements will be hampered by their inability to listen; frequent interrupting and ignoring may produce escalating arguments that lead only to frustration and mutual withdrawal (Gottman, Notarius, Gonso, & Marksman, 1976). Families that become less engaged in response to "external" occupational or other pressures are also at a disadvantage. Having little time together, they are less likely to detect potential problems or to want to spend available time discussing these difficulties.

Again, research is limited, but available data support these hypotheses. A more cohesive family environment (characterized by mutual support and cooperation) has been associated with a more nutritious diet (Kintner, Boss, & Johnson, 1983) and with more favorable long-term response to treatment for alcoholism (Finney, Moos, & Mewborn, 1980). On the other hand, frequent family conflict and a lack of organization have been found to predict early dropping out of behavioral treatment for obesity (Kirschenbaum, Harris, & Tomarken, 1984). The potential importance of Engagement processes is supported by the prominence accorded similar constructs in well-known theories of family functioning such as Olson's Circumplex Model ("Cohesion"), Minuchin's systems theory ("Boundaries," "Enmeshment"), Reiss's family theory ("Coordination"), and other approaches (Minuchin, 1974; Olson, 1986; Reiss, 1981).

Control Processes

Methods family members use to influence each other and organize family activities constitute a third major interaction variable affecting adherence. Positive control or influence is exemplified when a family member: (1) defines a problem in neutral, behaviorally specific terms that do not attack or demean (e.g.,

"When you do behavior 'X' in situation 'Y', I feel 'Z'); (2) requests a specific behavior change to correct the problem; or (3) seeks to involve the other in working out procedural guidelines or "family rules" for managing similar difficulties in the future (Ewart, Burnett, & Taylor, 1983; Ewart, Taylor, Kraemer, & Agras, 1984). Negative control is evidenced in attempts to influence others by hostile criticism, putdowns, sarcasm, or even physical attack. The latter behavior has the potential to create negatively reinforced cycles of attack and counterattack as family members try to coerce each other into compliance. Over time, the more successful "coercer" learns to become more domineering and abusive, while the "victim" is trained to terminate the abuse by becoming increasingly submissive and helpless (Patterson, 1982). In addition to the exemplary microanalytic process studies of Patterson, Gottman, and their associates, interaction constructs similar to the present Control concept are central to Olson's Circumplex Model ("Adaptability"), Minuchin's family systems approach ("Rigidity" versus "Flexibility"), and the theoretical framework proposed by Reiss (e.g., "Closure").

Families that often use negative control or coercion are expected to be less adept at solving problems because these behaviors lead to disengagement, active or passive resistance, and familial disorganization. Families whose members display positive influence skills are expected to be more engaged with one another, more competent at establishing consistent rules for behavior, and more effective at securing family support and cooperation. They thus should be more adept at overcoming adherence threats.

Intervention Guidelines

The above observations raise the question of recommending family therapy to promote adherence. Except in severely distressed families who desire help, it is my belief that intervention should probably not take the form of conventional family therapy. Few patients or their spouses will welcome the suggestion that they need counseling. An alternative approach is to develop other forms of intervention that improve family interaction without having this outcome as their stated goal.

An example of such intervention is provided by a recent study (Taylor, Bandura, Ewart, Miller, & DeBusk, 1985) my colleagues and I conducted to modify wives' perceptions of their husbands' capabilities after MI. Wives of male patients had been observed as being often worried unnecessarily about their husbands' level of physical activity, fearing that ordinary activities like climbing stairs might cause reinfarction (Croog & Levine, 1977). Husbands tended to be more confident about their capabilities, and the resulting discrepancy between husband's and wife's perceptions created tension in many families. A self-efficacy analysis suggested the possibility of removing the conflict's source (incongruent ability appraisals) by having the wife undergo a treadmill test similar to the husband's. An experiment supported our hypothesis: Wives who performed the test subsequently changed their perceptions of their husbands' capabilities to match his, whereas wives who watched the husband's test or waited outside in the lobby did not change. Involving a family member in treadmill exercise represents a comparatively simple and cost-effective way to prevent family conflict over exercise, thereby removing an important social barrier (moderator) deterring exercise participation and adherence.

Research Issues

A number of competing theories have been advanced to explain the dysfunctional interactions found in troubled families referred for psychological counseling. To date, there has been comparatively little empirical research to determine if the various theoretical approaches represent different analyses of the same underlying phenomena or if they address entirely different aspects of family functioning (Kog, Vertommen, & Vandereyken, 1987; Olson, 1986). Even less is known about the degree to which constructs developed from clinical work with severely distressed families can be applied to the broad range of more psychiatrically "normal" families with cardiovascular health problems. For example, Minuchin's extension of family systems theory to anorexia (Minuchin, Baker, Rosman, Liebman, Milman, & Todd, 1975; Minuchin, Rosman, & Baker, 1978) has not been well supported by recent empirical studies of more diverse groups of anorectic patients and their families (Kog et al., 1987; Wood & Talmon, 1983; Yager, 1982).

This writer agrees with John Gottman's assertion that the word "theory" should mean "explaining patterns in well-described phenomena" (Gottman, 1979, p. 292), and that the starting place for a theory of family interaction therefore must be the discovery and description of highly reproducible patterns or "structures" in social behavior. The three major process domains proposed here represent an initial attempt to summarize those behavioral structures that are: (1) best supported by empirical research and (2) most likely to affect patients' ability to solve adherence problems. Basic descriptive studies are needed to determine if these constructs provide reliable, valid, and useful avenues to understanding lifestyle change problems faced by patients and their families. Several hypotheses should be tested.

The present social interaction analysis predicts that patients' ability to solve adherence problems will be limited by the degree to which patient and family members share a common orientation to health problems, possess positive engagement skills, and are capable of exercising positive influence over each other's behavior. Patients in families manifesting greater problem avoidance, disengagement, and negative control patterns are expected to demonstrate less behavioral adherence, regardless of the patient's personally stated intentions. Research should be undertaken to develop "unobtrusive" interventions aimed at altering key family processes to support health behavior change. Another important area for investigation is the impact of family interaction on patient motivational processes: How and under what conditions do family interactions alter patients' reinforcement levels, self-efficacy perceptions, or self-evaluative reactions so as to influence adherence?

COPING RESOURCES AND BURDENS

When reading literature on health decision-making and adherence, I sometimes feel as if I had been lifted above mundane reality and transported to a happier world where people are free to choose and act, unhampered by financial, occupational, or other limitations. In fact, we know that socioeconomic status, sex, race, and age can have a powerful impact on patients' ability to change their behavior after MI (Oldridge, 1982). What we do not know is exactly how these influences operate to prevent change. Although the importance of macrosocial and economic influences is routinely mentioned in literature on coping, the cognitive–behavioral mechanisms through which static categories like race, sex, or class might affect problem solving and adherence receive scant attention.

The Social Problem-Solving Model addresses this need by proposing specific behavioral mechanisms capable of bridging the gap between social-demographic descriptors and individual health behavior outcomes. The present approach translates the familiar demographic categories into concrete "coping resources" available to patients. Important resources include family income, supportive social networks, work or school activities that build problem-solving skills, and personal health resources, all of which may be related to patient age, race, or sex. Coping resources also impose burdens; for example, calling on one's social network for support in a crisis creates an obligation to repay those who helped (Dressler, 1985; Riley & Eckenrode, 1986). Occupational work that creates opportunities to build problem-solving skills may also be very stressful (Karasek, Bader, Marxner, Ahlbom, & Theorell, 1981) or may reduce the time available to spend with one's family, reducing opportunities for positive engagement and constructive problem discussion.

Causal Pathways

Once social or demographic variables are defined in terms of coping resources and liabilities, they can be seen to influence adherence via their impact on patient motivational processes (reinforcement, self-efficacy, self-evaluation) and on the patients' interpersonal transactions with significant others. The model suggests that the following specific mechanisms should be investigated.

Reinforcement Effects

The consequences of dieting or exercising (Outcome Expectancies) are influenced extensively by one's financial resources. An inadequate income can limit access to needed foods, equipment, programs, or settings. Child care burdens may curtail parental involvement in health programs. People with higher incomes can create positive self-inducements by buying attractive exercise clothes, hiring babysitters, and joining health clubs.

Self-Efficacy Effects

Financial, occupational, and social resources may affect self-efficacy. People who work in low-level, menial jobs that allow little decision latitude have fewer opportunities to build confidence in their self-management and problem-solving capabilities. In fact, some occupational environments and structures may actually undermine workers' perception that they can control their lives and alter refractory behavior patterns (Frese, 1982). Prior history of illness or depression may reduce patients' confidence in their ability to comply with the health program. Individuals who are socially isolated have fewer opportunities to build self-efficacy by observing others like themselves model effective coping (Bandura, 1986).

Self-Evaluative Effects

Characteristics of a person's social network affect the type and variety of social models to which he or she is exposed. Friends, work associates, and others influence patient self-evaluation processes by modeling evaluative standards and by providing feedback that is helpful in appraising one's success at meeting valued norms. These social comparison processes influence both the type and the level of a person's reinforcement and self-efficacy goals. The present analysis suggests that the heterogeneity of respected models available in one's social network could be important for behavior change after MI. Patients whose network exposes them to a narrower range of self-evaluative standards should be less flexible in revising self-expectations or exploring new sources of self-approval and reinforcement.

Social Interaction Effects

Coping resources and burdens have a pronounced impact on family interaction. Limited financial resources, unemployment, stressful work (including child care and home management activities), or inadequate social support may adversely affect family problem orientation, engagement, and control processes. Such stressors may cause family members to be absent more often, become more self-preoccupied, or resort to anodynes such as drugs or alcohol, thus reducing their ability to recognize problems or engage in collective problem-solving. People who work in unrewarding jobs may become more negatively controlling and abusive with their families. When work is unrewarding, managers more readily resort to punishment and coercion to motivate workers (punishment is cheap and effective), thus modeling punishment as an influence technique. Moreover, stressful work may reduce workers' tolerance for frustration, causing them to resort to coercive interpersonal behavior. By increasing negative engagement, problem avoidance, and coercive interaction in the home, external stressors may greatly undermine patient problem-solving ability.

Intervention Guidelines

Counseling to help patients develop more supportive social networks, prevent or manage work stress, or control financial resources may be needed to remove threats to diet or exercise adherence. Although it may be difficult to engineer at the clinic level, greater attention should be placed on stimulating collective approaches to altering stressful working conditions affecting the adoption and maintenance of beneficial life-style changes.

Research Issues

The Social Problem-Solving Model asserts that the work environment and social support networks can influence health via their impact on patients' ability to adhere to health-promoting behaviors. Specifically, the model postulates that occupational and social influences affect health behavior via intervening motivational (reinforcement, self-efficacy, self-evaluation) and social interaction processes, which together act to enhance or undermine effect problem-solving activities. Testing these important links may suggest better ways to design work environments or foster social contacts so as to improve the health of MI patients.

COGNITIVE FUNCTION

Before concluding this discussion of model components, it is necessary to anticipate a question that a problem-solving emphasis may raise for some readers: If problem-solving skills are central to adherence, is basic intelligence then an important factor to consider when working with patients who have trouble changing? Problem solving requires that the individual be alert enough to recognize problem situations, generate alternative solutions, evaluate ways of coping, and develop an action plan. Drugs or illness may impair cognitive functioning, thus undermining problem-solving ability. Intelligence as measured by traditional IQ tests does not appear to be strongly related to social problem-solving ability, as studies investigating this relationship have reported low correlations (Spivack, Platt, & Shure, 1976). Divergent production ability, the capacity to generate many alternative uses for familiar objects, is significantly reduced in persons with low IQ but is unrelated to IQ in persons with normal or higher measured intelligence (Guilford, 1977). This is consistent with the finding that mentally retarded individuals are generally deficient both in general intelligence and adaptive social functioning, while individuals with higher IQs demonstrate greater variability in social competence (D'Zurilla, 1986).

In the Social Problem-Solving Model, intellectual functioning is presumed to affect adherence problem solving only if the patient scores in the subnormal range of general intelligence or is impaired by drugs or other effects. The dotted line in Figure 9.1 connecting Cognitive Function to Coping Resources acknowledges the relationship of intelligence to educational opportunities and other social and economic factors, while indicating that this relationship is not an important focus on the model. Specific intervention guidelines and research hypotheses concerning cognitive functioning, therefore, are not proposed for acute MI patients.

IMPLICATION FOR STAGES OF ADHERENCE

The model developed thus far specifies behavioral processes critical to establishing and maintaining long-term change. A number of researchers have argued, however, that factors affecting behavioral adherence will vary as patients move through successive stages of treatment (Kristeller & Rodin, 1984; Safer, Tharps, Jackson, & Leventhal, 1979; Suchman, 1965). These writers suggest that adherence should be viewed in a developmental perspective ranging from the initial appraisal of symptoms and decision to seek medical advice through the decision to follow the advice, undergo treatment, attempt recommended behavior changes, and, if necessary, incorporate the latter into one's usual routine. As with theories of family functioning, lack of empirical data makes it difficult to delineate these stages more precisely or specify how stages vary in the case of different health problems or diseases. The Social Problem-Solving Model offers needed guidance for this research by suggesting testable hypotheses concerning which influence processes are likely to dominate successive developmental phases.

Several investigators have proposed a three-stage framework that can be applied to a variety of health problems and should prove useful in designing descriptive studies (Kristeller & Rodin, 1984; Marlatt & Gordon, 1984). The first phase is a period of assimilation and decision making when the person evaluates the health advice and decides upon a course of action. The second stage begins when the individual tries to implement changes in his or her usual environment. The third stage occurs when the behavior change becomes a well-established part of one's routine. Kristeller and Rodin (1984) label these stages "Compliance," "Adherence," and "Maintenance," respectively.

From the social problem-solving perspective, a stage framework is useful if different causal processes influence a patient's actions at successive points in recovery. The Social Problem-Solving Model generates several hypotheses that should be examined. The first hypothesis is that Motivational processes envisioned in the model will be found to dominate the initial compliance phase of behavior change. This stage presumably occurs shortly before and after the MI patient is discharged from the hospital. Faced with advice to change problem behaviors, patients must access the credibility of the advice and its potential positive and negative consequences (reinforcement processes), appraise their ability to make needed changes (self-efficacy), and evaluate the potential consequences for self-esteem (self-evaluation). Initial compliance will be enhanced by highlighting the immediate as well as longer-term benefits of changing (reinforcement), presenting the change request in terms of a graduated series of specific behavioral steps (enhancing self-efficacy), and helping the individual identify ways the change might enhance personal views (self-evaluation).

A problem-solving focus at this stage would be contraindicated because raising potential problems might make the task seem overly difficult (e.g., by enumerating the various ways one could fail). Trying to involve other family members in the decision may also be counterproductive because the patient could experience this as coercive. Instead, the patient should be reassured by being given time to decide and encouraged not to try to change too soon or too fast. The goal is to ensure that the patient perceives the specific behaviors required and can identify important positive benefits with respect to reinforcement, self-efficacy, and self-esteem. Presentational techniques, such as graphic displays, chunking information, and repeating key points, are helpful communication aids (Kristeller & Rodin, 1984; Ley, 1976).

This initial phase might be thought to end when the patient decides to enter the cardiac rehabilitation program to implement recommended changes. An alternative view is that the decision process continues but becomes less central as the task of implementing specific behavior changes begins to occupy the patient's attention. Early in the Adoption phase (Stage II), implementation efforts uncover unexpected problems. The central issue now is feasibility; the primary task is to relabel problems as "challenges," define them in ways that render them susceptible to problem solving, and generate appropriate solutions. Additional Stage I arguments admonishing the patient to change are likely to fall on deaf ears. Instead, patients must be helped to solve practical daily problems by removing aversive consequences, setting goals that are feasible enough to build self-efficacy yet high enough to enhance self-esteem, and acquiring new self-evaluative standards by turning to other models and activities.

Self-monitoring, problem solving, and goal setting will comprise the bulk of the Stage II effort. The outcome of this phase should be a workable action plan consisting of coping alternatives for handling adherence threats and for incorporating behavior changes into daily routines in ways that are nonaversive and self-enhancing. Family interaction processes are addressed to a limited degree, as they are less critical now than they will become later. Because the spouse and family are eager to see the patient resume normal roles and wish to avoid blame, they will usually try to cooperate with initial change attempts.

Stage II could be said to end around the time the patient stops participating in active (e.g., weekly) rehabilitation sessions, often coinciding with return to work. Again, I would suggest that problem-solving and motivational appraisal processes be viewed as continuing in the *Maintenance* phase (Stage III), but gradually becoming less central as the patient develops solutions that work reasonably well much of the time. The challenge is to incorporate the new behaviors into one's fully active routine. Family processes and marcrosocial influences increasingly intrude as family members, who now view the patient as "recovered," realize that they, too, are being asked to make enduring behavior changes. Intervention must focus on helping patients use problem-solving skills to resolve family differences and cope with temptations to lapse into old ways (Jacobson & Margolin, 1979). Specific techniques to handle relapses (Marlatt & Gordon, 1984) are useful at this phase if introduced gradually as "reconditioning training." Care must be taken when presenting this topic, as patients may not have developed enough confidence in their newly acquired skills to face the possibility of "lapsing." Stage III is lifelong.

Research Issues

The full Social Problem-Solving model developed here integrates processes necessary to long-term maintenance of recommended health behaviors. Nested within the full model are component processes that influence initial compliance (Stage I) and early adoption (Stage II), as well as prolonged maintenance (Stage III). Hypotheses generated from this framework could be tested by applying a series of hierarchically integrated causal models to longitudinal data. The analysis would test the assertion that at each successive stage additional behavioral processes must be introduced as specified in the larger model. The following hypotheses represent an oversimplified but useful starting point:

1. The patient's initial decision to comply is best predicted by the Motivation components of the model, including expected reinforcement, self-efficacy perceptions, and self-evaluative reactions.
2. During Stage II implementation (e.g., program participation), the Problem-Solving components must be added to the Motivational components to account for the success or failure of initial adherence attempts.
3. The probability that the patient will achieve prolonged (Stage III) maintenance is best predicted by the full model, which introduces Social Interaction and Coping Resources as processes influencing the extent to which initial health decisions culminate in long-term success.

SUMMARY

Cardiovascular diseases and cancer have replaced infectious diseases as the leading causes of morbidity and mortality in developed nations. This change has stimulated interest in modifying individual life-style patterns now known to threaten health. Whereas the leading causes of death once could be avoided by subjecting oneself to brief screening or vaccination procedures, preventing cardiovascular disease or cancer requires a complicated and sustained struggle to alter diet, exercise, and other habits. As a result, psychological decision models developed to predict public response to health screening and inoculation programs are not always well suited to current health promotion needs.

A Social Problem-Solving Model is presented to guide the development of interventions to support long-term behavior change. This model departs from previous approaches by emphasizing factors affecting day-to-day performance of desired health behavior. Key causal components are defined in terms of modifiable behavioral processes and skills. As in traditional decision models, health knowledge and attitudes are emphasized (as reinforcement, self-efficacy enhancement, and self-evaluation processes), but their effect on adherence is seen to be mediated by cognitive problem-solving activities. Moreover, the relationship between these motivators and problem solving is moderated by ongoing social interaction with family members and significant others. Macrosocial and economic factors affect response to health promotion via their impact on motivation and on interactions within one's intimate social fields. From a developmental perspective, motivational processes dominate the early phases of decision making and initial adoption, problem-solving skills become more central when the patient tries to implement behavior changes on a regular basis, and

social interaction and macrosocial processes hold the key to prolonged maintenance. The model provides specific practical guidelines for health promotion
intervention and research.

REFERENCES

Anderson, B., Miller, J. P., Auslander, W., & Santiago, J. (1981). Family characteristics of
    diabetic adolescents: Relationship to matabolic control. *Diabetes Care, 4,* 586–594.
Baldwin, J. D., & Baldwin, J. I. (1986). *Behavior principles in everyday life, 2nd edition.*
    Englewood Cliffs, NJ: Prentice-Hall.
Bandura, A. (1973). *Aggression: A social learning analysis.* Englewood Cliffs, NJ: Prentice-Hall.
Bandura, A. (1977a). *Social learning theory.* Englewood Cliffs, NJ: Prentice-Hall.
Bandura, A. (1977b). Self-efficacy: Toward a unifying theory of behavioral change.
    Psychological Review, 84, 191–215.
Bandura, A. (1982). Self-efficacy mechanism in human agency. *American Psychologist, 37,*
    122–147.
Bandura, A. (1986). *Social foundations of thought and action.* Englewood Cliffs, NJ: Prentice-
    Hall.
Bandura, A., & Mahoney, M. J. (1974). Maintenance and transfer of self-reinforcement
    functions. *Behavior Research and Therapy, 12,* 89–97.
Bandura, A., & Whalen, C. K. (1966). The influence of antecedent reinforcement and
    divergent modeling cues on patterns of self-reward. *Journal of Personality and Social
    Psychology, 3,* 373–382.
Baron, R. M., & Kenny, D. A. (1986). The moderator–mediator variable distinction in
    social psychological research: Conceptual, strategic, and statistical considerations.
    Journal of Personality and Social Psychology, 51(6), 1173–1182.
Beck, A. T. (1967). *Depression: Clinical, experimental, and theoretical aspects.* New York:
    Hoeber.
Beck, A. T., Rush, A. J., Shaw, B. F., & Emory, G. (1979). *Cognitive therapy of depression.* New
    York: Guilford.
Becker, M. H. (1989). Theoretical models of adherence and strategies for improving
    adherence. In S. Shumaker, E. Schron, & J. Ockene (Eds.), *Handbook of health
    behavior change.* New York: Springer Publishing Co.
Belisle, M., Roskies, E., & Levesque, J. M. (1987). Improving adherence to physical activity.
    Health Psychology, 6(2), 159–172.
Black, D. R., & Scherba, D. S. (1983). Contracting to problem solve versus contracting to
    practice behavioral weight loss skills. *Behavior Therapy, 14,* 100–109.
Blechman, E. A., & McEnroe, M. J. (1985). Effective family problem solving. *Child
    Development, 56,* 429–427.
Bloom, L. (1985). A factor analysis of self-report measures of family functioning. *Family
    Process, 24*(2), 225–239.
Clausen, J. P. (1976). Circulatory adjustments to dynamic exercise and effect of physical
    training in normal subjects and patients with coronary artery disease. *Progress in
    Cardiovascular Disease, 18,* 459–495.

Croog, S. H., & Levine, S. (1977). *The heart patient recovers*. New York: Human Sciences Press.

Davidson, D. M., & DeBusk, R. F. (1980). The prognostic significance of a single exercise test 3 weeks after uncomplicated myocardial infarction. *Circulation, 61,* 236–241.

DeBusk, R. F., Kraemer, H. C., & Nash, E. (1983). Stepwise risk stratification soon after acute myocardial infarction. *American Journal of Cardiology, 52,* 1161–1166.

Dressler, W. S. (1985). The social and cultural context of coping: Action, gender, and symptoms in a southern black community. *Social Science and Medicine, 21*(5), 499–506.

D'Zurilla, T. J. (1986). *Problem solving therapy: A social competence approach to clinical intervention.* New York: Springer Publishing Co.

D'Zurilla, T. J., & Goldfried, M. R. (1971). Problem solving and behavior modification. *Journal of Abnormal Psychology, 78,* 107–126.

Epstein, S., & O'Brien, E. J. (1985). The person-situation debate in historical and current prospective. *Psychological Bulletin, 98*(3), 513–537.

Eron, L. D. (1987). The development of aggressive behavior from the perspective of a developing behaviorism. *American Psychologist, 42*(5), 435–442.

Ewart, C. K. (1989). Psychological effects of resistive weight training: Implications for cardiac patients. *Medicine and Science in Sports and Exercise, 21*(6).

Ewart, C. K., Burnett, K. F., & Taylor, C. B. (1983). Communication behaviors that affect blood pressure: An A-B-A-B analysis for marital interaction. *Behavior Modification, 7*(3), 331–344.

Ewart, C. K., Stewart, K. J., Gillilan, R. E., & Kelemen, M. H. (1986a). Self-efficacy mediates strength gains during circuit weight training in men with coronary artery disease. *Medicine and Science in Sports and Exercise, 18,* 531–540.

Ewart, C. K., Stewart, K. J., Gillilan, R. E., Kelemen, M. H., Valenti, S. A., Manley, J. D., & Kelemen, M. D. (1986b). Usefulness of self-efficacy in predicting overexertion during programmed exercise in coronary artery disease. *American Journal of Cardiology, 57,* 557–561.

Ewart, C. K., & Taylor, C. B. (1985). The effects of early postmyocardial infarction exercise testing on subsequent quality of life. *Quality of Life in Cardiovascular Care, 1,* 162–175.

Ewart, C. K., Taylor, C. B., Kraemer, H. A., & Agras, W. S. (1984). Reducing blood pressure reactivity during interpersonal conflict: Effects of marital communication training. *Behavior Therapy, 15,* 473–484.

Ewart, C. K., Taylor, C. B., Reese, L. B., & DeBusk, R. F. (1983). The effects of early post myocardial infarction exercise testing on self perception and subsequent physical activity. *American Journal of Cardiology, 51,* 1076–1080.

Finney, J., Moos, R., & Mewborn, R. (1980). Post-treatment experiences and treatment outcome of alcoholic patients six months and two years after hospitalization. *Journal of Consulting and Clinical Psychology, 48,* 17–29.

Floyd, F. J., & Markman, H. J. (1984). An economical observational measure of couples' communication skill. *Journal of Consulting and Clinical Psychology, 52*(1), 97–103.

Frese, M. (1982). Occupational socialization and psychological development: An underemphasized research perspective in industrial psychology. *Journal of Occupational Psychology, 55,* 209–224.

Friedman, H. S., & Booth-Kewley, S. (1987). The "disease-prone personality": A meta-analytic view of the construct. *American Psychologist, 42*(6), 539–555.

Friedman, M., & Ulmer, D. (1984). *Treating type-A behavior and your heart*. New York: Knopf.

Garrity, T. F. (1981). Behavioral adjustment after myocardial infarction: A selective review of recent descriptive, correlational, and intervention research. In S. M. Weiss, J. A. Herd, & B. H. Fox (Eds.), *Perspectives on behavioral medicine*. New York: Academic Press.

Gottman, J. M. (1979). *Marital interaction experimental investigations*. New York: Academic Press.

Gottman, J., Notarius, C., Gonso, J., & Marksman, H. (1976). *A couple's guide to communication*. Champaign, IL: Research Press.

Green, L. W., Kreuter, M. W., Deeds, S. G., & Partridge, K. B. (1980). *Health planning: A diagnostic approach*. Palo Alto, CA: Mayfield.

Grimm, L. G., & Yarnold, P. R. (1984). Performance standards and the type-A behavior pattern. *Cognitive Therapy and Research, 8*, 59-66.

Grotevant, H. D., & Carlson, C. (1987). Family interaction coding systems: A descriptive review. *Family Process, 26*, 49-74.

Guilford, J. P. (1977). *Way beyond the IQ: Guide to improving intelligence and creativity*. Great Neck, NY: Creative Synergetic Associates.

Hauser, S., Jacobson, A., Wertlieb, E., Brink, S., & Wentworth, S. (1985). The contribution of family environment to perceived competence and illness adjustment in diabetic acutely ill adolescents. *Family Relations, 34*, 99-108.

Homans, G. C. (1961). *Social behavior: Its elementary forms*. New York: Harcourt Brace.

Hyland, M. E. (1987). Control theory interpretation of psychological mechanisms of depression: Comparison and integration of several theories. *Psychological Bulletin, 102*(1), 109-121.

Jacobson, N. S., & Margolin, G. (1979). *Marital therapy: Strategies based on social learning and behavior exchange principles*. New York: Brunner/Mazel.

Janis, I. L., & Mann, L. (1977). *Decision making: A psychological analysis of conflict, choice and commitment*. New York: Free Press.

Karasek, R. A., Bader, D., Marxner, F., Ahlbom, S., & Theorell, T. (1981). Job decision latitude, job demands and cardiovascular disease: A prospective study of Swedish men. *American Journal of Public Health, 71*, 634-705.

Kazdin, A. E. (1984). *Behavior modification in applied settings*. Homewood, IL: Dorsey Press.

Kendall, P. C., & Fischler, G. L. (1984). Behavioral and adjustment correlates of problem solving: Validational analyses of interpersonal cognitive problem solving measures. *Child Development, 55*, 879-892.

Kintner, M., Boss, P., & Johnson, N. (1983). The relationship between dysfunctional family environments and family member food intake. *Journal of Marriage and the Family, 43*, 633-644.

Krischenbaum, D. S., Harris, E. S., & Tomarken, A. J. (1984). Effects of parental involvement in behavioral weight loss therapy for preadolescents. *Behavior Therapy, 15*, 485-500.

Kog, E., Vertommen, H., & Vandereyken, W. (1987). Minuchin's psychosomatic family revisited: A concept validation study using a multitrait-multimethod approach. *Family Process, 26*(2), 235-253.

Kristeller, J. L., & Rodin, J. (1984). A three-stage model of treatment continuity: Compliance, adherence and maintenance. In A. Baum, S. Taylor, & J. Singer (Eds.), *Handbook of psychological aspects of health*. Hillsdale, NJ: Erlbaum.

Krumboltz, J. D., & Thoresen, C. E. (1976). *Counseling methods*. New York: Holt, Rinehart, & Winston.

Langer, E., & Rodin, J. (1976). The effects of enhanced personal responsibility for the aged: A field experiment in an institutional setting. *Journal of Personality and Social Psychology, 34*, 191–198.

Leff, J., & Vaughn, C. (1985). *Expressed emotion in families: Its significance for mental illness*. New York: Guilford Press.

Lepper, M. R., & Greene, D. (Eds.). (1978). *The hidden costs of reward*. Hillsdale, NJ: Erlbaum.

Levenson, R. W., & Gottman, J. M. (1983). Marital interaction: Physiological linkage and affective exchange. *Journal of Personality and Social Psychology, 45*(3), 587–597.

Levenson, R. W., & Gottman, J. M. (1985). Physiological and affective predictors of change in relationship satisfaction. *Journal of Personality and Social Psychology, 49*(1), 85–94.

Ley, P. (1976). Psychological studies of doctor–patient communication. In S. Rachman (Ed.), *Contributions to medical psychology, Volume 1*. New York: Pergamon.

Maiman, L. A., & Becker, M. (1974). Health belief model: Origins and correlates in psychological theory. *Health Education Monographs, 2*, 336–353.

Markus, H., & Wurf, E. (1987). The dynamic self-concept: A social psychological perspective. *Annual Review of Psychology, 38*, 299–337. New York: Annual Reviews.

Marlatt, G. A., & Gordon, J. R. (1984). *Relapse prevention: A self-control strategy for the maintenance of behavior change*. New York: Guilford Press.

Mayou, R., Foster, A., & Williamson, B. (1978). Psychological and social effects of myocardial infarction on wives. *The British Medical Journal, 1*, 697–701.

Miller, N. H., Haskell, W. L., Berra, K., & DeBusk, R. F. (1984). Home versus group exercise training for increasing functional capacity after myocardial infarction. *Circulation, 70*(4), 645–649.

Minuchin, S. (1974). *Families and family therapy*. Cambridge, MA: Harvard University Press.

Minuchin, S., Baker, L., Rosman, B. L., Liebman, R., Milman, L., & Todd, T. C. (1975). A conceptual model of psychosomatic illness in children: Family organization and family therapy. *Archives of General Psychiatry, 32*, 1031–1038.

Minuchin, S., Rosman, B. L., & Baker, L. (1978). *Psychosomatic families*: Anorexia Nervosa in context. Cambridge, MA: Harvard University Press.

Mischel, W. (1968). *Personality and assessment* (p. 365). New York: Wiley.

Mischel, W. (1973). Toward a cognitive social learning reconceptualization of personality. *Psychological Review, 80*, 252–83.

Oldridge, N. B. (1982). Compliance and exercise in primary and secondary prevention of coronary heart disease: A review. *Preventive Medicine, 11*, 56–70.

Olson, D. H. (1986). Circumplex Model VII: Validation studies and FACES III. *Family Process, 25*, 337–351.

Patterson, G. R. (1982). *A social learning approach to family intervention. Volume 3: Coercive family process*. Eugene, OR: Castalia.

Patterson, J. (1985). Critical factors affecting family compliance with home treatment for children with cystic fibrosis. *Family Relations, 34*, 79–89.

Pervin, L. A. (1985). Personality: Current controversies, issues, and directions. *Annual Review of Psychology, 36,* 83–114.

Reiss, D. (1981). *The family's construction of reality.* Cambridge, MA: Harvard University Press.

Riley, D., & Eckenrode, J. (1986). Social ties: Subgroup differences in costs and benefits. *Journal of Personality and Social Psychology, 51*(4), 770–778.

Rotter, J. B. (1966). Generalized expectancies for internal versus external control of reinforcement. *Psychological Monographs, 80* (1, Whole No. 609).

Safer, M. A., Tharps, Q. J., Jackson, T. C., & Leventhal, H. (1979). Determinants of three stages of delay in seeking care at a medical clinic. *Medical Care, 17,* 11–29.

Seligman, M. E. (1975). *Helplessness.* San Francisco: W. H. Freeman.

Shephard, R. J. (1981). *Ischaemic heart disease and exercise.* Chicago: Croom Helm.

Shure, M. B., & Spivack, G. (1972). Means-ends thinking, adjustment and social class among elementary school-aged children. *Journal of Consulting and Clinical Psychology, 38,* 348–353.

Spivack, G., Platt, J. J., & Shure, M. B. (1976). *The problem-solving approach to adjustment.* San Francisco: Jossey-Bass.

Stone, L. J., & Hokanson, J. E. (1969). Arousal reduction via self-punitive behavior. *Journal of Personality and Social Psychology, 12,* 72–79.

Suchman, E. A. (1965). Stages of illness and medical care. *Journal of Health and Human Behavior, 6,* 114–128.

Taylor, C. B., Bandura, A., Ewart, C. K., Miller, N. H., & DeBusk, R. F. (1985). Exercise testing to enhance wives' confidence in their husband's capability soon after clinically uncomplicated myocardial infarction. *American Journal of Cardiology, 55,* 635–638.

Thibaut, J. W., & Kelley, H. H. (1959). *The social psychology of groups.* New York: Wiley.

Thoits, P. A. (1986). Social support as coping assistance. *Journal of Consulting and Clinical Psychology, 54*(4), 416–423.

Urbain, E. S., & Kendall, P. C. (1980). Review of social-cognitive problem-solving interventions with children. *Psychological Bulletin, 88,* 109–143.

Ward, C. H., & Eisler, R. M. (1987). Type A behavior, achievement striving, and dysfunctional self-evaluation system. *Journal of Personality and Social Psychology, 53*(2), 318–326.

Wills, T. A., Weiss, R. L., & Patterson, G. R. (1974). A behavioral analysis of the determinants of marital satisfaction. *Journal of Consulting and Clinical Psychology, 42,* 802–811.

Wood, B., & Talmon, M. (1983). Family boundaries in transition: A search for alternatives. *Family Process, 22,* 347–357.

Yager, J. (1982). Family issues in the pathogenesis of anorexia nervosa. *Psychosomatic Medicine, 44,* 46–60.

10

Dietary Intervention for Coronary Heart Disease Prevention

Barbara S. McCann, Barbara M. Retzlaff,
Carolyn E. Walden, Robert H. Knopp

Coronary heart disease is the leading cause of death in the United States, accounting for half a million deaths each year (Thom, Kannel, & Feinleib, 1985). Fortunately, there has been an impressive decline in cardiovascular disease in the past two decades, a decline that has been attributed in part to reductions in major risk factors for heart disease (Kannel & Thom, 1984). Numerous studies have consistently identified three major risk factors for coronary heart disease, which are modifiable: smoking (Kuller, Meilahn, & Ockene, 1985), hypertension (Pooling Project Research Group, 1978; Stamler, Stamler, & Liu, 1985; Szatrowski et al., 1984), and elevated plasma or serum cholesterol (Illingworth & Connor, 1985; Kannel, Castelli, & Gordon, 1979; Szatrowski et al., 1984). Individuals who quit smoking reduce their risk of coronary heart disease; those who quit prior to age 65 have half the risk for coronary heart disease of those who continue to smoke (Kannel, McGee, & Castelli, 1984); similarly, people who successfully treat

Preparation of this chapter was supported in part by the National Institutes of Health, HL28891-03, and the Clinical Nutrition Research Unit, DK35816.

their high blood pressure reduce cardiovascular disease risk (Hypertension Detection and Follow-up Program Cooperative Group, 1979a, b, 1982; Shea, Cook, Kannel, & Goldman, 1985).

Finally, recent studies have demonstrated that lowering cholesterol will prevent heart disease. That reductions in plasma total and low-density lipoprotein cholesterol levels are accompanied by a decrease in the risk of developing coronary heart disease (CHD) was established by the Lipid Research Clinics Coronary Primary Prevention Trial in 1984 (Lipid Research Clinics Program 1984a, b). The trial compared the cholesterol-lowering drug cholestyramine plus diet to placebo plus diet to test the lipid hypothesis over a 7-year investigation. The incidence of CHD was 19% lower in the cholestyramine-treated group than in the placebo group (Lipid Research Clinics Program, 1984a). Reductions occurred in both fatal and nonfatal endpoints. There was a log-linear relationship between the degree of total and low-density lipoprotein cholesterol lowering and the decrease in CHD in the group treated with cholestyramine (Lipid Research Clinics Program, 1984b); a 19% reduction in CHD risk was associated with a decrease by 8% of total cholesterol and a decrease of 11% in low-density lipoprotein cholesterol.

The release of the results of the Coronary Primary Prevention Trial in January 1984 led to the formation of the National Heart, Lung, and Blood Institute-initiated (NHLBI) National Cholesterol Education Program (NCEP) on November 15, 1985. The campaign was supported by the NIH-sponsored Consensus Development Conference "Lowering Blood Cholesterol to Prevent Heart Disease." The NCEP has been involved in disseminating to the public four "basic tenets" about cholesterol (Lenfant, 1986):

1. There is a clear association between cholesterol and coronary heart disease.
2. Cholesterol is easy to measure.
3. Everyone should know his or her cholesterol level.
4. Individuals with elevated blood cholesterol levels should do something about it.

If successful, the NCEP will greatly increase physicians' and patients' awareness of the importance of knowing one's cholesterol level and treating it if it is elevated. In this regard, recommendations of the Consensus Development Conference on Lowering Blood Cholesterol to Prevent Heart Disease included intensive dietary treatment under the guidance of a health professional in individuals with cholesterol values above the 90th percentile, with the added use of appropriate drugs if the response to diet is inadequate, and intensive dietary treatment of individuals with cholesterol levels between the 75th and 90th percentiles (Consensus Development Conference, 1985). Furthermore, the following dietary recommendations were made for all Americans (Consensus Development Conference, 1985):

1. Reduce total dietary fat intake from the current level of 40% of calories to 30% of total calories.
2. Reduce saturated fat intake to less than 10% of total calories.
3. Increase polyunsaturated fat intake to no more than 10% of total calories.
4. Reduce daily cholesterol intake to 250 to 300 mg or less.

The NCEP commitment to educating the public about cholesterol coupled with the recommendations of the Consensus Development Conference will increase the need for effective dietary interventions that can be maintained by individuals over a lifetime. Studies of the short-term effects of diets low in cholesterol and saturated fats on cholesterol levels in "captive" populations abound (e.g. Rosenthal et al., 1985), so the effectiveness of dietary changes in lowering plasma cholesterol levels is generally acknowledged. Such lowering can also be observed during intensive dietary intervention in free-living adults. For example, in an uncontrolled study in North Karelia, Finland, 30 couples kept detailed food records every other day during a 2-week baseline period, a 6-week intervention period (home visits at least twice a week by a dietitian and provision of free food items such as skim milk and lean meats), and a 6-week return-to-baseline period (Pietinen et al., 1984). During the baseline and return-to-baseline periods, couples were instructed to follow their normal diets. Changes in the percentage of calories from fat dropped from 39% to 24%; during the return-to-baseline period, it returned to 36%. The P/S ratio changed from 0.15 to 1.22, and returned to 0.16 during the return-to-baseline phase. As predicted, cholesterol dropped substantially during the intervention period, from an average of 252 mg/dl to 195 mg/dl. During the 6-week return-to-baseline period, total cholesterol increased to 247 mg/dl.

Despite such impressive short-term gains, little is understood about people's ability to remain on cholesterol-lowering diets for longer periods of time. Therefore in this chapter what is currently known about adherence to cholesterol-lowering diets in "free-living" adults will be reviewed. The focus will be primarily on adherence to diets rather than on the effects of diet on plasma or serum cholesterol reductions per se, as several good reviews on the latter subject already exist (e.g., Connor & Connor, 1985; Grande, 1980; Nichaman & Hamm, 1987; Weidman, 1980).

This chapter will begin with the presentation of a broad-based model that will serve to organize a review of efforts to date and identify gaps in current knowledge regarding the implementation of dietary recommendations. At various points we will draw upon our experience with the ongoing NHLBI-sponsored study, Dietary Alternatives for Lipid Lowering, conducted at the Northwest Lipid Research Clinic in Seattle, to highlight key points in this review. Participants in this program are men with LDL cholesterol levels above the 75th percentile who are randomly assigned to one of four diets that progressively restrict fat and cholesterol consumption. Fat restriction goals range from 30% to 26%, 22%, and 18% of calories with corresponding reductions in daily cholesterol intake (300 mg, 200 mg, 100 mg, and 100 mg, respectively). The dietary regimens are taught to participants and their spouses during 8 weekly classroom sessions attended by groups of approximately 8 to 12 couples. The dietary curriculum is taught using a combination of cognitive and behavioral techniques, including goal-setting, self-monitoring, and relapse prevention strategies. One, three, six, nine, and twelve months following the completion of the dietary classes, participants are seen individually by a dietitian in order to review their progress and turn in completed questionnaires regarding dietary adherence. Periodic monitoring of plasma lipids is provided to participants.

A MODEL OF DIETARY ADHERENCE

It is unreasonable to think that a single factor determines whether an individual will adhere to recommendations to change health-related behaviors. Over 100 different variables representing 14 different models of health behavior have been identified (Cummings, Becker, & Maile, 1980). Clearly, a multifaceted approach is needed to guide research efforts in promoting adherence to lipid-lowering diets. In our model, which is diagrammed in Figure 10.1, adherence to a prescribed regimen is affected by attributes of the individual, interactions between the individual and his or her social network (including family and community), influence from health care professionals and resources, and the compatibility between the behavior the individual must adopt in order to adhere and the environment in which the behavior must take place. Deficits in one sphere can be compensated by strengths in another. For example, a person who does not believe that a prescribed diet will lower cholesterol may still adhere reasonably well if family members committed to the program prepare most of that person's meals. Similarly, someone who is given only vague recommendations about implementing dietary changes in the physician's office may have access to more specific advice through community-wide interventions or the popular news media and hence be able to follow a lipid-lowering diet.

Evidence will be provided supporting the dietary adherence model. First, however, an examination of success to date in following cholesterol-lowering dietary regimens will be presented, along with a consideration of how one measures adherence to cholesterol-lowering diets.

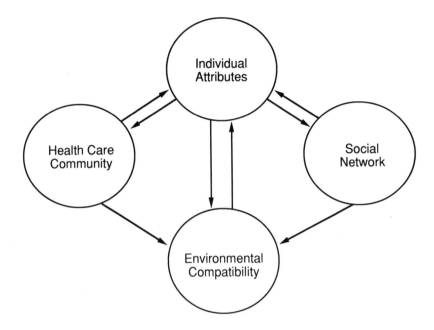

FIGURE 10.1 Interactive model of factors affecting adherence to prescribed regimens.

ADOPTION AND MAINTENANCE OF DIETARY RECOMMENDATIONS FOR CHOLESTEROL LOWERING

The recommendations of the National Cholesterol Education Program and Consensus Development Conference state that cholesterol-lowering diets should be seriously implemented by individuals whose total cholesterol level exceeds the 75th percentile and that, in addition, all Americans except children under age 2 should attempt to modify their diets for better health. What is the feasibility of persuading both healthy and hypercholesterolemic subjects to modify their diets to reduce total- and low-density lipoprotein cholesterol?

Some information on adherence to cholesterol-lowering diets among hypercholesterolemic individuals was obtained from the screening phase of the LRC–CPPT. These data demonstrate the short- and long-term effects of reductions in dietary saturated fat and cholesterol on plasma cholesterol (Gordon, Salz, Roggenkamp, & Franklin, 1982). Subjects considering participating in this clinical trial attended four monthly screening visits. During the second screening visit, which occurred 3 months prior to randomization, a moderate or "prudent" cholesterol-lowering diet was taught. The goals of this diet were to ingest 400 mg of cholesterol per day and increase the polyunsaturated-to-saturated fat ratio to

0.8 (Lipid Research Clinics Program, 1979). A specific reduction in fat intake was not specified. Thus, the 3-month interval from the diet instruction to randomization allowed an examination of this diet's effect on plasma lipoproteins in the entire cohort. In the initial 6494 men studied, total cholesterol levels dropped by 5.7% and LDL cholesterol levels dropped by 6.8% during the 1st month of dietary intervention (Gordon et al., 1982). Men whose LDL cholesterol concentrations fell below 175 mg/dl were subsequently excluded from the CPPT; subsequently, 3806 men were randomized. In men who were randomized to the placebo plus diet group, total cholesterol and LDL cholesterol concentrations decreased by 5.5% and 7.9% respectively over a 10-month period. In contrast, men randomized to cholestyramine plus diet reduced total and LDL cholesterol levels 17.8% and 25.9%, respectively, following 10 months of combined treatment (Glueck, Gordon, Nelson, Davis, & Tyroler, 1986). The conclusion from this study is that even a modest diet results in measurable cholesterol lowering. Equally importantly, it was shown that groups of dieters with incrementally larger reductions in cholesterol had incrementally larger reductions in coronary heart disease.

Adherence to the diet in the LRC–CPPT was assessed as being satisfactory. Based on 24-hour food recalls, subjects assigned to diet plus placebo decreased their intake of dietary cholesterol by 19.7%; the corresponding reduction for the medicated group was 21.1% (Lipid Research Clinics Program, 1984a). Percent reductions from prediet dietary cholesterol intakes were 17.5% for the placebo group and 18.5% for the cholestyramine group 1 year after randomization. After 7 years of study, percentage reductions in dietary cholesterol from baseline were 8.1% and 6.5% in placebo and resin groups, respectively, but this lesser restriction was partly by design, since cholesterol intake was below goal even after 7 years in the study. Percentage increases in the P/S ratios from baseline for the two treatment groups after 1 month, 1 year, and 7 years on the diet were respectively 52.1%, 43.8%, and 39.6% for the placebo group and 53.2%, 42.6%, and 40.4% for the cholestyramine group. Thus, like cholesterol intake, the P/S ratio improved from diet teaching, although it too diminished somewhat over time. Thus, while substantial improvements in diet were seen initially, a trend to revert toward predietary levels of cholesterol and fat intake was evident.

Adherence to a more restrictive diet was studied in 14 patients in Denmark who had angina and had undergone coronary arteriography (Thuesen, Henriksen, & Engby, 1986). Patients and their spouses were instructed in a diet containing only 10% of calories from fat and less than 100 mg cholesterol per day. Patients and their spouses were seen twice a week for 3 months. This very restrictive diet was associated with 33% cholesterol lowering after 3 months and 14% decrease after 12 months of follow-up during which patients were seen every 3 months. Although baseline dietary habits were not available, at 3 months patients were consuming only 10% of total calories from fat and averaged 70 mg dietary cholesterol per day. At 12 months, this had increased to 21% of calories from fat and 123 mg cholesterol per day. Only 2 of the 14 patients maintained the dietary changes evident 3 months after diet instruction.

If dietary adherence is satisfactory, sustained improvement in plasma cholesterol levels can be seen on fairly restrictive diets. Brown et al. (1984) assessed the effects of two different cholesterol-lowering diets on plasma lipid levels in 50 patients with peripheral vascular disease. One diet was the American Heart Association Hyperlipidemia Diet C diet, with goals of 50% to 55% carbohydrate, 15% to 20% protein, 25% to 30% fat, a P/S ratio of 1.7, and 25 to 30 gm dietary fiber per 1000 calories. The other diet, based on the Pritikin diet, contained 70% to 75% carbohydrate, 15% to 20% protein, only 5% to 10% fat, and 40 to 45 gm dietary fiber per 1000 calories. Patients received 4 days of intensive training in the diet and were subsequently seen after 1, 2, 4, 6, and 12 months. Participants on the AHA diet were able to maintain their percentage of calories from fat intake at around 30 to 34% during the 12 months of follow-up. Patients following the Pritikin diet were able to maintain their fat intake at around 13 to 16% of calories from fat. Both groups were able to maintain their dietary fiber intake near the targeted levels. Total cholesterol on the Pritikin diet decreased by approximately 10%. Total cholesterol decreased by 8% in subjects on the AHA diet. These reductions were sustained over 12 months by both groups.

Some efforts have been made to persuade essentially healthy individuals to adopt low-fat low-cholesterol diets. In one investigation, a dieting booklet, nutrition education, and behavior modification with nutrition education were compared in effectiveness (Foreyt, Scott, Mitchell, & Gotto, 1979). Subjects were healthy, nonhypercholesterolemic individuals who were randomized to one of three educational formats: a booklet on dieting ("Help Your Heart Eating Plan"), nutrition education, or nutrition education plus behavior modification. Subjects in both the nutrition education and nutrition education plus behavior modification conditions met in groups of 8 to 10 participants for seven weekly 60-minute sessions. In both groups, nutritional information was provided by a dietitian, and brief slide presentations covering a range of topics (eg., fats and cholesterol, dairy products) were shown. Subjects in the nutrition education plus behavior modification condition were also taught behavioral strategies, including self-monitoring, stimulus control, and contingency management techniques. The diets provided to all three groups consisted of 35% of total calories from fat, 20% from protein, and 45% from carbohydrate. Following completion of classes, subjects in the nutrition counseling and nutrition counseling plus behavior modification groups met monthly until the 12-month follow-up assessment. In these sessions, materials from the earlier weekly classes were reviewed. All groups averaged small reductions in plasma cholesterol levels of approximately 5% after the 3 months of treatment, with no differences between the groups. After 6 months, subjects who received nutritional counseling plus behavioral strategies had slightly greater reductions in cholesterol than subjects in the remaining two groups (8% reduction, compared with 3% and 4% in the booklet-only group and nutrition education only group, respectively). By 12 months, slight reductions in cholesterol for the groups receiving nutritional counseling and nutritional counseling plus behavior modification were still apparent (2% and 3%, respectively). Cholesterol levels in the group receiving a booklet only had returned to near-baseline levels. Thus, while the two treatments that included more extensive contact with participants were superior to the minimum intervention of providing a diet booklet, at 12 months follow-up the addition of behavior modification did not appear to confer any additional benefit.

To summarize, based on these studies with free-living healthy individuals and hyperlipidemic individuals, reductions in plasma or serum cholesterol levels through diet are substantial on very restrictive diets (e.g., Pietinen et al., 1984; Thuesen et al., 1986), but are otherwise modest. One could argue that these disappointing results are due to diets that are biologically ineffective in lowering cholesterol levels. However, it seems at least as likely that poor adherence to dietary recommendations accounts for the apparent failure of various dietary approaches to lowering cholesterol (Schettler, 1979). One of the reasons that so little is known about persuading people to adopt and maintain low-fat, low-cholesterol diets is that the quantification and remediation of adherence to such regimens has received little attention. Consideration of these issues follows.

MEASUREMENT OF ADHERENCE TO CHOLESTEROL-LOWERING DIETS

In the typical clinical setting, patients following cholesterol-lowering diets are often given only periodic information on changes in their plasma cholesterol levels, rather than feedback on the actual dietary changes they have made. There are several disadvantages of giving feedback only on cholesterol change. First, emphasis on cholesterol levels rather than changes in eating behaviors removes the outcome from direct control; people can alter how they eat, but they have no direct control over various blood constituents. Second, individuals vary in the extent to which they respond to low-fat, low-cholesterol diets (Katan & Beynen, 1987; Katan, Beynen, de Vries, & Nobels, 1986), so changes in plasma cholesterol levels might not accurately reflect dietary practices. A similar phenomenon has been noted in the obesity literature, where feedback to patients has generally been about changes in weight rather than changes in eating behaviors, even though people appear to be more successful at weight loss if they receive feedback based on their dietary efforts rather than on their changes in weight (Sperduto, Thompson, & O'Brien, 1986). In the Dietary Alternatives Study, described above, subjects are given feedback on their total and LDL cholesterol levels, but they also receive information about the extent of dietary change that is based on an analysis of their 4-day food record.

Some investigators have measured food intake to assess adherence to dietary recommendations. Techniques for measuring food intake include a 24-hour food recall, a food record (over a period of 3 to 7 days), or a food frequency questionnaire. In a 24-hour food recall, subjects are asked to recall everything they have eaten during the preceding 24 hours. A dietician records the information and asks specific questions about food portions and methods of food preparation. The information thus obtained is quantified in order to provide a breakdown of nutrient content. An advantage of this method is its ease of use in large-scale studies (LRC-CPPT and MRFIT). The disadvantages of the 24-hour food recall approach include susceptibility to errors in memory and uncertain representation of subjects' usual dietary intake (Block, 1982).

An example of the use of the 24-hour recall is seen in the Multiple Risk Factor Intervention Trial (MRFIT). The MRFIT was a randomized, controlled trial that compared the effects of a Special Intervention (SI) group, which received interventions to reduce smoking, blood pressure, and cholesterol, with a Usual Care (UC) group, that referred to regular physicians. Twenty-four-hour food recalls were obtained from participants in the SI group at baseline and at years 1, 2, and 3 (Caggiula et al., 1981). Enrollees in this program attended a 10-session weekly training program during which they learned to follow a diet that had these goals: reduction in percentage of calories from fat to below 35%, reduction in percentage of calories from saturated fat to less than 8%, and reduction in cholesterol intake to 250 mg/day or less. Intake of saturated fat decreased by 28.4% to 10% of total calories; the intake of dietary cholesterol decreased by 42.5% to 265 mg/dl. Thus, actual intake over approximately 2 years' time based on 24-hour food recalls corresponded reasonably well with the prescribed diet. In addition to the use of the 24-hour food recall, nutritionists made subjective ratings of participants' compliance with the dietary recommendations. The dietitians' estimates were based on interviews with the participants themselves. The advantage of using a subjective rating by a dietician is that their estimate of eating patterns may reflect more stable characteristics (e.g., long-term changes in diet) rather than whatever may have transpired during the preceding day (Caggiula et al., 1981). A surprising finding was that nutrient intake based on the 24-hour recall did not predict actual cholesterol levels, but that approximately 16% of individuals who were considered to be excellent adherers by dieticians had a more substantial change in cholesterol than participants with lower compliance ratings. Another interesting finding pertaining to the use of the 24-hour recall in MRFIT was that serum cholesterol changes and weight loss in the SI group, relative to the UC group, did not correspond well to reported differences in dietary intake (Neaton et al., 1981), suggesting that participants in the SI group either underreported dietary intake or altered their eating habits prior to their follow-up exam.

The 3- to 7-day food record is less susceptible to patients' memory distortions and obviously samples a longer, and one hopes more representative, time period. However, its primary disadvantage is susceptibility to recording errors (Block, 1982). Recording errors using the food recall method can take one of two forms. One type occurs when the subject does not accurately record what was eaten, for example, not assessing quantity appropriately or not mentioning critical ingredients. Another type of recording error is the reactive nature of recording ongoing behavior; that is, recording eating behavior actually brings about a change in that behavior. One of the therapeutic aspects of asking patients to self-monitor certain behaviors (such as smoking, drinking, or eating) is that by doing so patients invariably alter their behavior somewhat (McFall, 1977). This reactivity poses a problem when using self-monitoring to attempt an accurate assessment of people's typical diet.

The third dietary assessment technique is the food frequency questionnaire. In this technique, individuals respond to such questions as "in general, how often do you eat eggs?", subjects do not need to have good recall of what they have recently eaten, and the measure is less likely to be reactive (in contrast to food records) and may reflect more general, representative trends in dietary practices. In addition, such questionnaires can be administered quickly. However, these instruments often do not obtain sufficient detail to permit a reliable calculation of such factors as typical daily content of saturated fats and are susceptible to reporting bias. As an example, a food-frequency questionnaire was used to measure dietary changes in normolipidemic individuals who were taught a low-saturated-fat, low-cholesterol diet through a community organization (Reeves et al., 1983). In this study, 409 subjects were initially enrolled and 282 subjects completed the program through 36 months. Based on the food-frequency information obtained, dietary cholesterol intake dropped significantly at the end of 12 months, then remained fairly stable until the end of the follow-up period (36 months). Plasma cholesterol levels, which decreased initially, returned to baseline or even above baseline levels by the end of the 3-year study. The investigators noted that many of the elderly participants in the program found it difficult to complete the food frequency measure, and in general the investigators questioned the accuracy of subjects' recall.

A fourth measure of adherence is a change in the plasma fatty acid polyunsaturated/saturated fat ratio (Brown, 1968). In our own Dietary Alternatives Study, all four measures of dietary adherence are obtained. In addition, subjective estimates of dietary adherence are made by the participants, their spouses, and the dieticians. Participants and spouses make independent assessments of dietary adherence prior to the follow-up visits. Dieticians make subjective ratings of dietary adherence based on discussions with the participants at all of the follow-up visits. Participants' and spouses' ratings of adherence range from 0 to 100%. Dieticians' ratings of adherence sometimes exceed 100% when the participant is thought to be restricting intake of dietary fat or cholesterol more than required for the particular diet. A second set of dietary adherence measures is based on nutrient analysis of a 4-day food record on which participants record their total food consumption for 4 days prior to follow-up visits. The nutrient analysis of food records, using computerized food tables obtained from the Minnesota Nutrient Coding Center, yields the percentage of calories from fats and average daily cholesterol intake (mg). Percent adherence to fat and cholesterol restriction is calculated based on the targeted percentage of calories from fat and the average daily consumption of cholesterol. As with the dieticians' ratings of adherence, adherence based on fat and cholesterol intake could exceed 100% if a participant is restricting his intake of fat or cholesterol more than required for his diet. A comparison of assessment of adherence based on these two types of measures is shown in Table 10.1.

The third approach used in our study is the Diet Habit Survey developed by Sonja Connor (Hollis, Carmody, Connor, Fey, & Matarazzo, 1986), which is given to participants at 9, 10½, and 12 months of follow-up to assess reactivity and reproducibility associated with the food intake recording at 9 and 12 months of follow-up in a selected subsample. The fourth approach, measurement of plasma fatty acids, is also being employed.

ATTRIBUTES OF THE INDIVIDUAL AFFECTING ADHERENCE

In the model depicted in Figure 10.1, individual attributes are shown as central in determining the extent of adherence to prescribed regimens. A number of individual characteristics have been identified that may differentiate those who adhere to prescribed regimens from those who do not (Cummings et al., 1980). For instance, Brownell (1984) noted some important psychological characteristics that predict successful treatment of obesity. The factors include "restraint," or a person's resistance to pressures to eat, and susceptibility to the "abstinence violation effect" (Marlatt & Gordon, 1985), where violation of a rule related to dieting increases the likelihood that the individual will continue to overeat. Another characteristic that appears to predict success in achieving health-related change is an individual's perceived self-efficacy, or perception that he or she can engage in a given behavior (Strecher, DeVellis, Becker, & Rosenstock, 1986). Self-efficacy has been shown to predict a number of health-related behaviors, including smoking, weight control, contraceptive use, alcohol use, and exercise (Strecher et al., 1986).

One critical factor that bears on the treatment of hypercholesterolemia is that the disorder is usually asymptomatic. That is, individuals who do not experience

TABLE 10.1 Adherence to Dietary Goals at 1-Month Follow-Up in the Dietary Alternatives Study*

Phase	(N)	Percentage of Calories from Fat				Cholesterol Intake (mg)			
		Goal	Baseline	1 Month	% Adherence	Goal	Baseline	1 Month	% Adherence
Phase I	(145)	30	36 ± 6	27 ± 6	118	300	345 ± 151	224 ± 71	148
Phase II	(126)	26	36 ± 7	25 ± 5	108	200	315 ± 139	154 ± 40	140
Phase III	(147)	22	35 ± 6	23 ± 6	104	100	313 ± 145	116 ± 43	98
Phase IV	(64)	18	35 ± 6	21 ± 6	91	100	306 ± 131	117 ± 44	96

*% Adherence is calculated by (Goal/1 Month) × 100.

202

any symptoms are asked to make substantial changes in their behavior (Carmody, Fey, Pierce, Connor, & Matarazzo, 1982). This situation closely resembles that of hypertensives who are not motivated to take antihypertensive agents (McCann, 1987). Individuals will undoubtedly vary in the extent to which they perceive hypercholesterolemia as a threat to their health, depending on personal or family history of heart disease as an example, but identification early in life of those individuals who do not perceive that their health is yet endangered might be the most important factor in treatment.

Individual attributes also affect people's willingness to participate in preventive health programs. In the Family Heart Study, 223 of 501 families in the Portland, Oregon area who were invited agreed to participate in a 5-year nutrition education program (Hollis et al, 1984). Investigators studied the characteristics of those who joined or ultimately did not join the program. "Joiner" families tended to be professional, white-collar families with members who had attended college and included more families who dieted to lose weight. Families with members who had elevated cholesterol or a chronic disease were no more likely to join the program than other families. Families with hypertensives were less likely to join. Respondents who joined the program perceived more benefits to be associated with the diet and scored as more internal on the Health Locus of Control scale (Wallston, Wallston, Kaplan, & Maides, 1976). Joiners scored higher than nonjoiners on a test of knowledge about CHD and reported receiving more information from physicians, friends, and the media. In the Stanford Heart Disease Prevention Program (SHDPP), 33% of subjects assigned to a group receiving intensive instruction regarding cardiovascular disease prevention through behavior change did not attend all follow-up surveys (Meyer, Nash, McAlister, Maccoby, & Farquhar, 1980). Compared to subjects who remained in the program, these subjects knew less about cardiovascular disease prior to participation, smoked more cigarettes, and consumed more dietary cholesterol and saturated fats.

Based on these studies, it is concluded that individual attributes are important factors in considering who will participate in cholesterol-lowering diets as well as follow such diets faithfully. In the Dietary Alternatives Study, a number of factors potentially related to adherence are being assessed. These factors include knowledge of cholesterol-lowering diets and knowledge of strategies for maximizing dietary change and minimizing relapse, perceived self-efficacy, health locus of control, day-to-day stress, and social support.

SOCIAL SUPPORT AND ADHERENCE

Despite ample evidence that social support influences physical health (Broadhead et al., 1983), the mechanisms through which social support exerts its healthful impact remain unclear. One way in which social support may enhance physical health is by facilitating participation in behaviors that improve health, such as exercise or good eating habits (Levy, 1986). The effectiveness of interventions designed to promote weight loss is often enhanced by including a supportive spouse or family member in treatment (Murphy et al., 1982). Recent efforts have been devoted to defining the role of a supportive spouse or partner in the long-term maintenance of behavior change and the process by which such an individual influences change (e.g., Mermelstein, Cohen, Lichtenstein, Baer, & Kamarck, 1986). In addition, Brownell's study (Brownell, Heckerman, Westlake, Hayes, & Monti, 1978) would certainly suggest that the presence of a supportive individual alone is not the sole factor leading to weight loss. In their investigation, subjects who had a cooperative spouse lost more weight than subjects without a supportive spouse, but subjects whose supportive spouse received training lost even more weight.

In the Dietary Alternatives Study the importance of specific spouse behaviors in facilitating adherence to cholesterol-lowering diets is being examined (McCann, Brief, Follette, Walden, & Knopp, 1987). The Evaluation of Social Support (ESS) questionnaire was constructed for this investigation. The ESS consists of 17 questions about the spouse's assistance in dietary adherence. Parallel forms of the ESS are completed by the participant and by the spouse. The ESS asks the participant (or spouse) if the spouse is engaged in activities that may be helpful in enhancing the participants' adherence. For each activity (e.g., Did your spouse assist with food preparation?), the participant indicates whether the spouse carried out the activity. If the spouse carried out the activity, the participant is further instructed to rate the helpfulness of the activity on a 5-point scale ranging from 1 (not at all helpful) to 5 (extremely helpful). Five subscales were derived from the ESS that represent different classes of support activities: *verbal support, modeling, tangible/food support, tangible/goal-setting support*, and *support enlistment*. *Verbal support* refers to direct comments regarding the participant's dietary adherence. *Modeling* refers to adherence to the diet by the spouse. *Tangible/food support* refers to spouse's participation by purchasing and preparing foods. *Tangible/goal-setting support* refers to spouse's participation in setting regular goals for dietary adherence. The final subscale, *support enlistment*, refers to spouse's efforts to enlist support for the participant's adherence from family and friends.

The role of spouse support in adherence to diets was studied by comparing scores obtained on the ESS with measures of dietary adherence in an initial sample of 109 men (McCann et al., 1987a). Two of the aforementioned measures of adherence were used in these analyses: subjective estimates of adherence made by participants, their spouses, and the dieticians; and adherence based on nutrient analysis of a 4-day food record—average daily consumption of fats and cholesterol. Based on the prescribed intake of fat and cholesterol, calculations of percentage fat adherence and cholesterol adherence were made.

At the 1-month follow-up visit, significant correlations were observed between participants' ratings of *verbal support* and *support enlistment* and participants' estimates of their adherence. Participants' ratings of *tangible/food support* were related to dietician's estimates of adherence and to adherence to restrictions in cholesterol intake based on the food records. At this same follow-up visit, none of the spouses' ratings of social support were related to any of the adherence measures.

At the 3-month follow-up visit, participants who reported high levels of *tangible/food support* gave themselves high ratings of adherence, as did their spouses and the dieticians. Spouse estimates of adherence correlated with participants' ratings of *verbal support* and *tangible/goal-setting support*. Dieticians' estimates of adherence correlated significantly with participants' ratings of *support enlistment*. As with participants' ratings of *tangible/food support*, spouses' ratings on this support dimension were correlated with ratings of dietary adherence made by participants and dieticians.

Interestingly, at 1 month little relationship was seen between social support and adherence. However, by 3 months this relationship was evident. One possible reason for this difference is that at 3 months participants and spouses might be better able to evaluate which factors are important in maintaining adherence. By 3 months they may have had more opportunities to utilize the types of spouse support that are most effective in maintaining adherence and have learned which spouse behaviors are most important in facilitating maintenance. It will be informative to continue to follow this cohort over several months and monitor changes in perceptions of the importance of social support. A similar finding has been noted in the treatment of obesity (Brownell et al., 1978). Initially, subjects who were involved in couples training reported that mutual monitoring by their spouses was helpful. However, during follow-up they reported that spouse encouragement was most helpful. These findings also highlight a methodological point: measurement of perceptions at only one point in time might result in overlooking important factors that have not yet become evident.

It was anticipated that social support would be related to the more objective measure of adherence, namely, the dietary records and resultant calculations on fat and cholesterol consumption. However, the correlations between social support and these measures were small. It may be that social support was unrelated to these adherence measures because the measures do not account for baseline differences in consumption of fats and cholesterol and hence do not reflect the extent to which subjects had to make dietary changes. The subjective measures, on the other hand, may reflect participants' and spouses' perceptions of the effort needed for the participant to reach the dietary goal. These estimates in turn may represent a better index of the extent of change necessary. Clearly, more needs to be understood about these adherence measures.

In summary, the most consistent finding that emerged when the role of spouse support was examined 3 months following the initial intervention was that

adherence to a dietary regimen for lowering cholesterol was related to participants' and their spouses' ratings of spouse support. Specifically, tangible support
provided by the spouse in the form of purchasing and preparing food, planning
meals, and limiting the availability of inappropriate foods was related to dietary
adherence as rated by participants, their spouses, and dieticians. Other forms of
support, such as modeling, verbal support, and the enlistment of support from
others, were only marginally related to adherence ratings. In general, these
findings suggest that the provision of specific, tangible assistance in following a
program of behavior change may be the critical factor in enhancing adherence
through spouse support.

Programs implemented through clubs and organizations may be one way of
utilizing social support to facilitate adoption and maintenance of dietary
changes. A project conducted in Harris County, Texas (Reeves et al., 1983) is one
example. In this study, 409 men and women, who were members of homemaking
clubs or spouses of members, enrolled in the program. Of these, 282 completed
the 36-month program. The recommended diet consisted of 35% of total calories
from fat and a limit of 300 mg cholesterol per day. The primary intervention
period occurred during the initial 12 months of the study. Materials such as
cookbooks and pamphlets were mailed to participants monthly. In addition,
participants were invited to attend two cooking demonstrations. One-hour
nutrition programs were presented to the clubs four times during the first year of
intervention. During the nutrition programs, participants learned such behavioral principles as self-monitoring, stimulus control, and contingency management. Additional instruction was provided at 3-, 6-, 12-, 24-, and 36-month
follow-up visits. The program received considerable media coverage. The adherence measure, as noted previously, was a food frequency questionnaire. While
initial declines in plasma cholesterol were achieved, 2 years following initiation
of the program cholesterol levels reached baseline levels or even higher. By
3 years, plasma cholesterol levels exceeded baseline levels. Although long-term
maintenance of initial cholesterol reductions was not observed, the initial response of participants is encouraging.

THE ROLE OF THE HEALTH CARE COMMUNITY
IN PROMOTING ADHERENCE

Physicians, health psychologists, nurses, dieticians, health educators, and other
health care professionals will need to be able to respond to a growing demand by
the public for information and education about cholesterol. This response, in
turn, should increase the likelihood that individuals will participate in cholesterol-lowering programs. As reported earlier, individuals who are knowledgeable
about CHD and receive more information from physicians, family, and the media

(Hollis et al., 1984) or who are already practicing healthier lifestyles (Meyer et al., 1980) are more likely to participate in prevention efforts. Thus it may be particularly important for members of the health care community to make an effort to educate the public. Recent data suggest that a surprising number of individuals have many misconceptions about dietary habits and risks of CHD, including that lecithin lowers blood cholesterol and that stress is the primary cause of heart attacks (Pierce et al., 1984).

Another critical role for the health care community will be to design and test different intervention strategies to promote dietary changes. Some examples of this work already exist. For example, Crouch and colleagues (Crouch et al., 1986) compared four interventions in the treatment of hypercholesterolemia (total cholesterol level 225 mg/dl to 265 mg/dl; triglycerides < 500 mg/dl): face-to-face counseling, mail and telephone counseling, initial counseling session only, and a no-contact control group. Everyone except those in the control group attended an initial session during which participants received information on cholesterol and atherosclerosis, and behavioral recommendations were made (self-monitoring, goal-setting, and so on). Individuals in face-to-face counseling received intensive instruction during five subsequent follow-up visits. Participants in the mail and telephone follow-up group were contacted by mail on five occasions. Subjects in the initial counseling session group received behavior-change materials, but no additional counseling either in person or by telephone. Thus, all three of these groups received information on behavior change. Subjects in face-to-face counseling and mail and telephone follow-up treatment groups showed immediate substantial decreases in plasma total cholesterol levels 12 weeks following the initiation of treatment. At 1-year follow-up, the average level of cholesterol reduction achieved was a 6.2% decrease in the face-to-face group and a 4.6% reduction in the mail and phone condition. Cholesterol levels in the control group and initial counseling session only group had increased slightly at 1-year follow-up. This study demonstrated the importance of regular, sustained contact in facilitating dietary effectiveness; however, the specific role of information on behavior change cannot be evaluated in this study. The aforementioned study by Foreyt et al. (1979) is another example of an attempt to determine the best possible strategy for helping normolipidemic individuals achieve significant reductions in plasma cholesterol levels; in this case, behavioral strategies enhanced the effectiveness of a more traditional nutrition education intervention.

ENVIRONMENTAL COMPATIBILITY AND ADHERENCE TO DIETARY RECOMMENDATIONS

Henderson and Enelow (1976) provide a thoughtful description of the relationship between the extent of behavior change in the individual and the environment in which such change takes place. Specifically, they have proposed that behavior change is achieved only to the extent that it is compatible with one's environment. The implication for dietary interventions for coronary heart disease prevention is that if individuals attempt to change behavior (eat low-fat foods) in an environment that is not conducive to such change (only high-fat foods available), attempts to modify the diet will ultimately be unsuccessful.

Evidence for this phonomenon was found in the investigation of Dietary Alternatives for Lipid Lowering (McCann et al., 1987b). Men in this study kept 4-day situation logs prior to their 1- and 3-month follow-up visits. On the situation logs, participants recorded the environmental characteristics of each eating episode, including whether or not the eating episode was planned, who was present, and whether the participant was engaged in concurrent activities. In addition, participants indicated factors that contributed to or interfered with adherence to the dietary regimen. Analysis of the situation logs from the first 100 participants in this study reveal that 5 factors are consistently identified as contributing to good adherence (Figure 10.2): accurate information about the composition of foods, easy access to appropriate foods, self-perceptions about one's ability to adhere to the diet, remembering the purpose of the diet, and support from spouse. Parallel results were obtained in examining factors that interfered with good adherence (Figure 10.3). Particularly striking is the importance of intentional decisions, availability of high fat foods, and cravings. Overall, these findings illustrate the importance of *access* to low-fat, low-cholesterol food; if such food isn't readily available, or if only high fat foods are accessible, no behavioral strategies will enable an individual to adhere to a cholesterol-lowering diet.

Programs that promote dietary change in settings such as supermarkets and restaurants may facilitate behavior–environment compatibility. The NHLBI-sponsored Foods for Health program was an attempt to determine whether nutritional education provided to consumers at supermarkets could increase public awareness and knowledge of dietary means of reducing cardiovascular disease risk (Ernst et al., 1986). Ultimately, the aim of such "point-of-purchase" programs is to change consumer behavior. In addition, such programs enhance consumer access to appropriate foods by providing critical information about food content. The Foods for Health program was conducted in Washington, D.C., at Giant Food Stores. The comparison site was Baltimore, Maryland, Giant Food Stores, which received none of the general cholesterol education that was received in Washington. Information regarding reducing intake of fats, cholesterol, and calories was provided in the stores, in pamphlets, and on shelves. Analyses of the effectiveness of these programs were based on telephone surveys and food sales information. Based on the telephone surveys, participants in the D.C. area showed an approximately 6% increase in correct responses to questions regarding fat and cholesterol content in foods and the relationship between

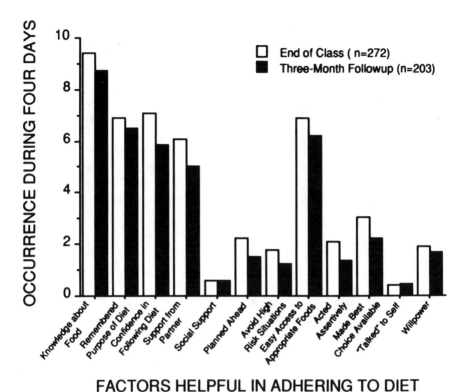

FIGURE 10.2 Factors helpful in adhering to diet.

diet and serum cholesterol. In the control city, slight decreases in the correctness of responses were noted. While the differences in food sales between the two cities were minimal, there was some evidence that the sale of low-fat milk increased in the D.C. area. The lack of an effect on actual food purchases was somewhat disappointing, but in the investigators' opinion this could have been due to inadequate monitoring of relevant food categories. Other important lessons from this project include: (1) the risk that such programs may be structured so that they reach only literate, well-educated consumers; it was estimated that only one fifth to one half of the individuals in the D.C. area read the Foods for Health materials; (2) consumer education is probably a necessary but not sufficient condition for changing consumer behavior; despite evidence that individuals exposed to the Foods for Health information had acquired greater knowledge about dietary fat and cholesterol, food purchasing behavior was not markedly affected; and (3) it may be important to determine what

characteristics of individuals modulate the effects of educational campaigns
directed toward them. It is reasonable, for example, that the individuals most
likely to put into practice information about healthy dietary habits are people
already practicing healthy life-styles. In the MRFIT, for example, smokers at
baseline reported greater intake of saturated fat and dietary cholesterol than
nonsmokers and reported less change from baseline values (Caggiula et al.,
1981). Thus such programs may be primarily "preaching to the converted."

In the statement prepared by the Atherosclerosis Study Group (Kannel et al.,
1984a), it was recommended that the food industry make changes that would
improve the quality of the American diet. The Study Group was specific in
targeting hotels, restaurants, and fast-food industries in addition to food manufacturers. They recommended a number of sweeping changes, including the
updating of packaging laws to include more information regarding the content of

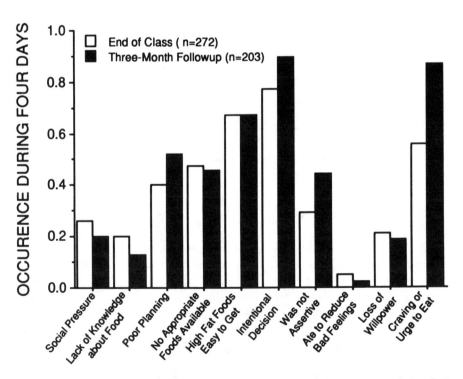

FIGURE 10.3 Factors interfering with good adherence.

packaged foods. As this is at the broadest level of intervention in our model (Fig. 10.1) and we have seen the importance of food availability, these recommendations seem appropriate and justified.

GOALS FOR FUTURE RESEARCH

Based on this review, it should be apparent that persuading large numbers of people to modify their dietary practices to prevent coronary heart disease is a potentially difficult task. The recommendations made by the Consensus Development Conference and the National Cholesterol Education Program's effort to increase physician and public awareness of elevated plasma cholesterol and its deleterious consequences will challenge health care providers to develop new means to encourage thousands of Americans to change their diets. Research to support this effort should be done in the following areas:

1. Determine which cholesterol-lowering diets are biologically most effective.
2. Develop, test, and refine measures of dietary adherence to better assess the effectiveness of interventions aimed at achieving long-term cholesterol-lowering dietary behavior change.
3. Design and test intervention strategies to implement and maintain adherence to cholesterol-lowering diets in both hyperlipidemic and normolipidemic individuals.
4. Investigate which are the most effective methods for educating the public about lowering cholesterol with diet.
5. Develop and promote the sale of cholesterol-lowering foods by the food industry to facilitate acceptance of dietary modifications.

Recent efforts to publicize the importance of knowing one's own cholesterol level and taking dietary steps to lower it should facilitate the decline of coronary heart disease morbidity and mortality. All Americans are being asked to make dietary changes, and a large number will require aggressive dietary intervention. The research goals enumerated above will need to be met in order to facilitate the adoption of and adherence to cholesterol-lowering diets.

REFERENCES

Block, G. (1982). A review of validations of dietary assessment methods. *American Journal of Epidemiology, 115*, 492–505.
Broadhead, W. E., Kaplan, B. H., James, S. A., Wagner, E. H., Shoenbach, V. J., Grimson, R., Heyden, S., Tibbin, G., & Gehlbach, S. H. (1983). The epidemiologic evidence for

a relationship between social support and health. *American Journal of Epidemiology*, *117*, 521-537.

Brown, G. D., Whyte, L., Gee, M. I., Crockford, P. M., Grace, M., Oberle, K., Williams, H. G., & Hutchison, K. J. (1984). Effects of two "lipid lowering" diets on plasma lipid levels in patients with peripheral vascular disease. *Journal of the American Dietetic Association*, *84*, 546-550.

Brown, H. B. (1968). The national diet-heart study: Implications for dietitians and nutritionists. *Journal of the American Dietetic Association*, *52*, 279-292.

Brownell, K. D. (1984). Behavioral, psychological, and environmental predictors of obesity and success at weight reduction. *International Journal of Obesity*, *8*, 543-550.

Brownell, K. D., Heckerman, C. L., Westlake, R. J., Hayes, S. C., & Monti, P. M. (1978). The effect of couples training and partner co-operativeness in the behavioral treatment of obesity. *Behavior Research and Therapy*, *16*, 323-333.

Caggiula, A. W., Christakis, G., Farrand, M., Hulley, S. B., Johnson, R., Lasser, N. L., Stamler, J., & Widdowson, G. (1981). The Multiple Risk Factor Intervention Trial (MRFIT): IV. Intervention on blood lipids. *Preventive Medicine*, *10*, 443-475.

Carmody, T. P., Fey, S. G., Pierce, D. K., Connor, W. E., & Matarazzo, J. D. (1982). Behavioral treatment of hyperlipidemia: Techniques, results, and future directions. *Journal of Behavioral Medicine*, *5*, 91-116.

Connor, W. E., & Connor, S. L. (1985). The dietary prevention and treatment of coronary heart disease. In W. E. Connor & J. D. Bristow (Eds.), *Coronary heart disease: Prevention, complications, and treatment* (pp. 43-64). Philadelphia: J.B. Lippincott.

Consensus Development Conference. (1985). Lowering blood cholesterol to prevent heart disease. *Journal of the American Medical Association*, *253*, 2080-2086.

Crouch, M., Sallis, J. F., Farquhar, J. W., Haskell, W. L., Ellsworth, N. M., Allen, B., & Rogers, T. (1986). Personal and mediated health counseling for sustained dietary reduction of hypercholesterolemia. *Preventive Medicine*, *15*, 282-291.

Cummings, K. M., Becker, M. H., & Maile, M. C. (1980). Bringing the models together: An empirical approach to combining variables used to explain health actions. *Journal of Behavioral Medicine*, *3*, 123-145.

Ernst, N. D., Wu, M., Frommer, P., Katz, E., Matthews, O., Moskowitz, J., Pinksky, J. L., Pohl, S., Schreiber, G. B., Sondik, E., Tenney, J., Wilbur, C., & Zifferblatt, S. (1986). Nutrition education at the point of purchase: The Foods for Health Project evaluated. *Preventive Medicine*, *15*, 60-73.

Foreyt, J. P., Scott, L. W., Mitchell, R. E., & Gotto, A. M. (1979). Plasma lipid changes in the normal population following behavioral treatment. *Journal of Consulting and Clinical Psychology*, *47*, 440-452.

Glueck, C. J., Gordon, D. J., Nelson, J. J., Davis, C. E., & Tyroler, H. A. (1986). Dietary and other correlates of changes in total and low density lipoprotein cholesterol in hypercholesterolemic men: The Lipid Research Clinics Coronary Primary Prevention Trial. *American Journal of Clinical Nutrition*, *44*, 489-500.

Gordon, D. J., Salz, K. M., Roggenkamp, K. J., & Franklin, J. A., Jr. (1982). Dietary determinants of plasma cholesterol change in the recruitment phase of the Lipid Research Clinics coronary primary prevention trial. *Arteriosclerosis*, *2*, 537-548.

Grande, F. (1980). Predicting change in serum cholesterol from change in composition of the diet. In R. M. Lauer & R. B. Shekelle (Eds.), *Childhood prevention of atherosclerosis and hypertension* (pp. 145-153). New York: Raven Press.

Henderson, J. B., & Enelow, A. J. (1976). The coronary risk factor problem: A behavioral perspective. *Preventive Medicine, 5,* 128-148.

Hollis, J. F., Carmody, T. P., Connor, S. L., Fey, S. G., & Matarazzo, J. D. (1986). The Nutrition Attitude Survey: Associations with dietary habits, psychological and physical well-being, and coronary risk factors. *Health Psychology, 5,* 359-374.

Hollis, J. F., Sexton, G., Connor, S. L., Calvin, L., Pereira, K. C., & Matarazzo, J. D. (1984). The Family Heart Dietary Intervention Program: Community response and characteristics of joining and non-joining families. *Preventive Medicine, 13,* 276-285.

Hypertension Detection and Follow-up Program Cooperative Group. (1979a). Five-year findings of the Hypertension Detection and Follow-up Program. I. Reduction in mortality of persons with high blood pressure, including mild hypertension. *Journal of the American Medical Association, 242,* 2562-2571.

Hypertension Detection and Follow-up Program Cooperative Group. (1979b). Five-year findings of the Hypertension Detection and Follow-up Program. II. Mortality by race-sex and age. *Journal of the American Medical Association, 242,* 2572-2577.

Illingworth, D. R., & Connor, W. E. (1985). Hyperlipidemia and coronary heart disease. In W. E. Connor & J. D. Bristow (Eds.), *Coronary heart disease: Prevention, complications, and treatment* (pp. 21-42). Philadelphia: J. B. Lippincott.

Kannel, W. B., Castelli, W. P., & Gordon, T. (1979). Cholesterol in the prediction of atherosclerotic disease: New perspectives based on the Framingham Study. *Annals of Internal Medicine, 90,* 85-91.

Kannel, W. B., Doyle, J. T., Ostfeld, A. M., Jenkins, C. D., Kuller, L., Podell, R. N., & Stamler, J. (1984a). Optimal resources for primary prevention of atherosclerotic diseases: Atherosclerosis Study Group. *Circulation, 70,* 157A-205A.

Kannel, W. B., McGee, D. L., & Castelli, W. P. (1984b). Latest perspectives on cigarette smoking and cardiovascular disease: The Framingham Study. *Journal of Cardiac Rehabilitation, 4,* 267-277.

Kannel, W. B., & Thom, T. J. (1984). Declining cardiovascular disease mortality. *Circulation, 70,* 331-336.

Katan, M. B., & Beynen, A. C. (1987). Characteristics of human hypo- and hyperresponders to dietary cholesterol. *American Journal of Epidemiology, 125,* 387-399.

Katan, M. B., Beynen, A. C., de Vries, J. H. M., & Nobels, A. (1986). Existence of consistent hypo- and hyperresponders to dietary cholesterol in man. *American Journal of Epidemiology, 123,* 221-234.

Kuller, L., Meilahn, E., & Ockene, J. (1985). Smoking and coronary heart disease. In W. E. Connor & J. D. Bristow (Eds.), *Coronary heart disease: Prevention, complications, and treatment* (pp. 65-83). Philadelphia: J. B. Lippincott.

Lenfant, C. (1986). A new challenge for America: The National Cholesterol Education Program. *Circulation, 73,* 855-856.

Levy, R. L. (1986). Social support and compliance: Salient methodological problems in compliance research. *Journal of Compliance in Health Care, 1,* 189-198.

Lipid Research Clinics Program, (1979). The coronary primary prevention trial: Design and implementation. *Journal of Chronic Diseases, 32,* 609-631.

Lipid Research Clinics Program. (1984a). The Lipid Research Clinics Coronary Primary Prevention Trial results: I. Reduction in incidence of coronary heart disease. *Journal of the American Medical Association, 251,* 351–364.

Lipid Research Clinics Program. (1984b). The Lipid Research Clinics Coronary Primary Prevention Trial results: II. The relationship of reduction in incidence of coronary heart disease to cholesterol lowering. *Journal of the American Medical Association, 251,* 365–374.

Marlatt, G. A., & Gordon, J. R. (Eds.). (1985). *Relapse prevention: Maintenance strategies in the treatment of addictive behaviors.* New York: Guilford Press.

McCann, B. S. (1987). The behavioral management of hypertension. In M. Hersen, R. M. Eisler, & P. M. Miller (Eds.), *Progress in behavior modification* (Vol. 21, pp. 191–229). Newbury Park, CA: Sage.

McCann, B. S., Brief, D. J., Follette, W. C., Walden, C. E., & Knopp, R. H. (1987a). *Spouse support and adherence in the dietary treatment of hyperlipidemia.* Paper presented at the annual meeting of the American Psychological Association, New York, NY.

McCann, B. S., Cadwallader, A., O'Leary, M., Burgher, B., Kaplan, C., Wilson, C., Brief, D., & Follette, W. C. (1987b). *Factors affecting adherence to dietary regimens in the treatment of hypercholesterolemia.* Paper presented at the annual meeting of the Society for Behavioral Medicine, Washington, D.C.

McFall, R. M. (1977). Parameters of self-monitoring. In R. B. Stuart (Ed.), *Behavioral self-management* (pp. 196–214). New York: Brunner/Mazel.

Mermelstein, R., Cohen, S., Lichtenstein, E., Baer, J. S., & Kamarck, T. (1986). Social support and smoking cessation and maintenance. *Journal of Consulting and Clinical Psychology, 54,* 447–453.

Meyer, A. J., Nash, J. D., McAlister, A. L., Maccoby, N., & Farquhar, J. W. (1980). Skills training in a cardiovascular health education campaign. *Journal of Consulting and Clinical Psychology, 48,* 129–142.

Murphy, J. K., Williamson, D. A., Buxton, A. E., Moody, S. C., Absher, N., & Warner, M. (1982). The long-term effects of spouse involvement upon weight loss and maintenance. *Behavior Therapy, 13,* 681–693.

Neaton, J. D., Broste, S., Cohen, L., Fishman, E. L., Kjelsberg, M. O., & Schoenberger, J. (1981). The Multiple Risk Factor Intervention Trial (MRFIT): VII. A comparison of risk factor changes between the two study groups. *Preventive Medicine, 10,* 519–543.

Nichaman, M. Z., & Hamm, P. (1987). Low-fat, high-carbohydrate diets and plasma cholesterol. *American Journal of Clinical Nutrition, 45,* 1155–1160.

Pierce, D. K., Connor, S. L., Sexton, G., Calvin, L., Connor, W. E., & Matarazzo, J. D. (1984). Knowledge of and attitudes toward coronary heart disease and nutrition in Oregon families. *Preventive Medicine, 13,* 390–395.

Pietinen, P., Dougherty, R., Mutanen, M., Leino, U., Moisio, S., Iacono, J., & Puska, P. (1984). Dietary intervention study among 30 free-living families in Finland. *Journal of the American Dietetic Association, 84,* 313–318.

Pooling Project Research Group. (1978). Relationship of blood pressure, serum cholesterol, smoking habit, relative weight and ECG abnormalities to incidence of major coronary events: Final report of the Pooling Project. *Journal of Chronic Diseases, 31,* 201–306.

Reeves, R. S., Foreyt, J. P., Scott, L. W., Mitchell, R. E., Wohlleb, J., & Gotto, A. M. (1983).

Effects of a low cholesterol eating plan on plasma lipids: Results of a three-year community study. *American Journal of Public Health, 73,* 873–877.

Rosenthal, M. B., Barnard, R. J., Rose, D. P., Inkeles, S., Hall, J., & Pritikin, N. (1985). Effects of a high-complex-carbohydrate, low-fat, low-cholesterol diet on levels of serums lipids and estradiol. *American Journal of Medicine, 78,* 23–27.

Schettler, G. (1979). Dietary prevention of coronary heart disease. In A. M. Gotto, L. C. Smith, & B. Allen (Eds.), *Atherosclerosis V* (pp. 209–218). New York: Springer-Verlag.

Shea, K. S., Cook, E. F., Kannel, W. B., & Goldman, L. (1985). Treatment of hypertension and its effect on cardiovascular risk factors: Data from the Framingham Heart Study. *Circulation, 71,* 22–30.

Sperduto, W. A., Thompson, H. S., & O'Brien, R. M. (1986). The effect of target behavior monitoring on weight loss and completion rate in a behavior modification program for weight reduction. *Addictive Behaviors, 11,* 337–340.

Stamler, J., Stamler, R., & Liu, K. (1985). High blood pressure. In W. E. Connor & J. D. Bristow (Eds.), *Coronary heart disease: Prevention, complications, and treatment* (pp. 85–109). Philadelphia: J. B. Lippincott.

Strecher, V. J., DeVellis, B. M., Becker, M. H., & Rosenstock, I. M. (1986). The role of self-efficacy in achieving health behavior change. *Health Education Quarterly, 13,* 73–91.

Szatrowski, T. P., Peterson, A. V., Jr., Shimizu, Y., Prentice, P. L., Mason, M. W., Fukunaga, Y., & Kato, H. (1984). Serum cholesterol, other risk factors, and cardiovascular disease in a Japanese cohort. *Journal of Chronic Diseases, 37,* 569–584.

Thom, T. J., Kannel, W. B., & Feinleib, M. (1985). Factors in the decline of coronary heart disease mortality. In W. E. Connor & J. D. Bristow (Eds.), *Coronary heart disease: prevention, complications, and treatment* (pp. 5–20). Philadelphia: J. B. Lippincott.

Thuesen, L., Henriksen, L. B., & Engby, B. (1986). One-year experience with a low-fat, low-cholesterol diet in patients with coronary heart disease. *The American Journal of Clinical Nutrition, 44,* 212–219.

Wallston, B. S., Wallston, K. A., Kaplan, G. D., & Maides, S. A. (1976). Development and validation of the Health Locus of Control (HLC) scale. *Journal of Consulting and Clinical Psychology, 44,* 580–585.

Weidman, W. H. (1980). Effect of change in diet on level of serum cholesterol. In R. M. Lauer & R. B. Shekelle (Eds.), *Childhood prevention of atherosclerosis and hypertension* (pp. 137–153). New York: Raven Press.

Commentary: Life-Style Interventions and Maintenance of Behaviors

Roger H. Secker-Walker

The five chapters concerning Life-style Interventions and Maintenance of Behaviors in this section address a spectrum of conditions that range from symptomless ones, in HIV-positive hemophiliacs and people with elevated serum cholesterols, through acute but often short-lived symptoms in children with asthma and recent acute life-threatening situations in those people recovering from a myocardial infarction, to the slowly but relentlessly progressive symptoms in people with chronic obstructive pulmonary disease. The interventions described range from special counseling for the HIV-positive hemophiliac and partner through classroom activities and parental homework to workshops and rehabilitation exercises, sometimes involving spouses. The ages of the participants in these interventions range from 8- to 11-year-olds in the school-based asthma self-management program through adolescence and young adulthood for the HIV-positive hemophiliacs to middle-aged and older people in the dietary and rehabilitation programs.

In spite of this diversity in the behaviors being addressed, the methods used to influence behavior change, and the target groups, several common themes emerge that play important roles in enhancing adherence to the life-style behaviors being sought. These common themes are the roles of self-efficacy and self-evaluation, the importance of skills training over and above appropriate knowledge and attitudes, the place of social support—more importantly from the spouse or partner for most groups, but from the parents and peer groups in the children with asthma—and recognition of the barriers to performance of the behavior. Some of these barriers may be amenable to change through advice, counseling, and skills building, but others, particularly those related to the lack of ready availability of particular foods, may not.

There are some notable distinguishing features to the life-style changes addressed in these chapters: the special need to counsel the partners of the HIV-positive hemophiliacs, the sensitive nature of this counseling, and the need to continue such support over time; the involvement of partners through homework, and the use of stories, games, and clay figures in the intervention with the asthmatic children; the involvement of spouses in cardiac rehabilitation and dietary modification interventions; the multiple behaviors that need to be addressed in patients with chronic obstructive lung disease and the use of quality-of-life measures to assess the benefit of such programs; and the importance of a supportive or compatible environment for successful dietary modification.

Each of the chapters presents areas for future research relevant to the particular behavior or behaviors being addressed. Some of these, such as the influence of stress on the immune system, the development and promotion of cholesterol-lowering foods, or the range of behaviors that need to be addressed for patients with chronic obstructive lung disease, are specific for the issues being addressed. However, others are much broader and are well summarized in the hypotheses that Ewart presents as tests of the Social Problem Solving Model. The importance of this model in identifying areas of future research lies in the manner in which it integrates three well-recognized theoretical developments: the ideas and issues associated with expectancy, self-efficacy, and self-evaluation in the decision to initiate a behavior change; the role of problem solving in implementing the behavior change; and the influence of social interactions and personal coping resources in maintaining the behavior change.

A further dimension needs to be considered in this model, and that is the broader environmental context in which the behavior change is being implemented. The broader environmental context includes several unrelated elements that influence behavior, including policies and regulations relating to the behavior, the availability or lack thereof of essential material to execute the behavior, and the social norms concerning the behavior.

Missing from the life-style interventions discussed are those related to the prevention of cigarette smoking and smokeless tobacco use and to smoking cessation and cessation of smokeless tobacco use. Much has been learned about smoking prevention and smoking cessation for the prevention of heart and lung disease. Each of these behaviors provides another area in which to test the hypotheses implicit in the Social Problem Solving Model.

SECTION III

Obstacles to Life-Style Change and Adherence

Eleanor B. Schron, Editor

Many factors can inhibit people's ability to change behaviors and to maintain healthier behavior patterns. In this section of the book, the authors address potential biological, health provider, and contextual obstacles to successful health behavior changes.

In Chapter 11, "Biological Barriers to Adoption and Maintenance of Health-promoting Behaviors," Grunberg and Lord describe a framework for the categorization of biological barriers that includes: (1) unpleasant biological side effects of healthful behaviors or therapeutic regimens; (2) interference of health behaviors with enjoyable behaviors that involve biological effects or mechanisms;

(3) biologically based physical or cognitive incompetence of individuals; (4) absence or misinterpretation of biological cues; and (5) biological effects of substance abuse that interfere with healthful behaviors. In describing each of these categories, the authors establish that biological barriers exist and are important to compliance with and adherence to health-promoting and illness-preventing behavior.

In Chapter 12, "Physician and Dentist Compliance with Smoking Cessation Counseling," Coates and colleagues describe an effective way to help physicians increase the time they take to work on smoking cessation with their patients. In addition, they provide new information on how to help physicians improve their ability to assist patients to successfully quit smoking.

Altman's focus in Chapter 13, "The Social Context and Health Behavior: The Case of Tobacco," is on policy and regulatory factors. He maintains that an understanding of why people smoke in spite of health information to the contrary can be enhanced if greater attention is paid to understanding the effects of the larger social context on health behaviors. Altman offers data suggesting that strategies employed to prevent adolescent tobacco use need to be strengthened. In addition, his review of some of the advertising and promotion tactics employed by the tobacco industry and their effects on smoking behavior and public policy decisions about tobacco use illustrate how the larger social context directly and indirectly influences smoking. Finally, his discussion of how censorship may affect consumers' smoking-related knowledge, attitudes, and ultimately behaviors is useful.

11

Biological Barriers to Adoption and Maintenance of Health-Promoting Behaviors

Neil E. Grunberg, Diana Lord

Asked to prepare a chapter on biological barriers to adoption and maintenance of health-promoting behaviors, we began in our normal way—we went to the library. Usually, as we search *Index Medicus* and *Psychological Abstracts*, we find countless numbers of studies to read. We have grown accustomed to finding comfort in watching the collection of articles grow. This time our experience was quite different. Although we found the usual abundance of writings on the general topics of interest—that is, adoption, maintenance, compliance, and

This chapter is based on a presentation made at the NHLBI Conference on Adoption and Maintenance of Behaviors for Optimal Health, Bethesda, Maryland, April 29, 1987. The opinions or assertions contained herein are the sole ones of the authors and are not to be construed as official or reflecting the views of the DoD or the USUHS.

adherence—we found almost nothing directly on target—that is, relevant biological barriers. Even in the edited volumes that provide comprehensive reviews of the general topic, we found little to examine. Analysis of two such edited volumes (Gerber & Nehemkis, 1986; Haynes, Taylor, & Sackett, 1979) revealed that less than 5% of their total pages mentioned *any* variable that could be construed as biological. Moreover, these analyses are liberal in that any mention, even if only in a sentence, was counted. Further, if we could speculate about a biological role for the point addressed (e.g., when elderly people cannot hear well, they may not understand oral instructions involving their medication), we counted it as a reference to a biological issue. This lack of discussion could mean that biological barriers to adherence and compliance (1) do not exist; (2) are not important; or (3) are not studied. Whatever the meaning, it is clear that the emphasis of the compliance literature is nonbiological.

This chapter presents our thoughts in considering whether biological barriers are relevant to the topics of compliance with and adherence to health-promoting and illness-preventing behaviors. Because we know of no programmatic research or literature that addresses this topic, we first listed everything that we could think of that fit into the general topic of biological barriers to compliance and adherence. Next we attempted to categorize the individual points and examples to determine whether larger themes emerged. In doing so, we arrived at five major themes that are offered with some supporting examples in this chapter. We believe that this exercise reveals that biological barriers exist and are important. However, we readily admit that our "editorial" offers a position without experimental evidence. We hope that our efforts stimulate empirical work in this area.

A FRAMEWORK FOR CATEGORIZATION OF BIOLOGICAL BARRIERS

We believe there are many different types of biological barriers to compliance and adherence, which may be categorized into five major groups: (1) unpleasant biological side effects of healthful behaviors or therapeutic regimens; (2) interference of health behaviors with enjoyable behaviors that involve biological effects or mechanisms; (3) biologically based physical or cognitive incompetence of individuals; (4) absence or misinterpretation of biological cues; and (5) biological effects of substance abuse that interfere with healthful behaviors. Each major category is addressed in order.

Unpleasant Biological Side Effects

When a health-promoting behavior is physically unpleasant, people are less likely to adhere to the healthful behavior. Often the unpleasantness can be extreme, while the payoffs of the health-promoting behavior are not salient or are so delayed as to reduce their incentive value. This category includes unpleasant side effects of pharmaceutical and nonpharmaceutical regimens.

Unpleasant Drug Side Effects That Are Biological Barriers to Compliance

One assumes that pharmaceutical houses wish to develop and market drugs with the widest possible therapeutic range and the fewest and weakest unpleasant side effects. Unfortunately, many therapeutically effective and lifesaving drugs have unpleasant biological effects that deter people from taking their medicine. These side effects range from mildly irritating to almost debilitating.

Unpleasant biological effects of drugs that could interfere with adherence to drug-taking therapies become clear when one consults the *Physicians' Desk Reference* (Barnhart, 1988) or more popular books about medications (e.g., Silverman & Simon, 1982). It does not require much digging to discover the plethora of unpleasant side effects of a variety of drugs. For example, tricyclic antidepressants may cause hallucinations, disorientation, delusions, anxiety, restlessness, excitement, numbness and tingling in the extremities, lack of coordination, muscle spasms or tremors, seizures, confusion, convulsions, dry mouth, blurred vision, constipation, inability to urinate, rash, itching, sensitivity to bright light or sunlight, retention of fluids, fever, allergy, nausea, vomiting, loss of appetite, stomach upset, diarrhea, agitation, inability to sleep, nightmares, feeling of panic, a peculiar taste in the mouth, stomach cramps, black coloration of tongue, yellowing eyes or skin, perspiration, flushing, frequent urination, drowsiness, dizziness, weakness, headache, and loss of hair. Who could blame the patient who stops taking medication that produces one or more of these undesired effects, or that makes an individual feel terrible?

Lifesaving antineoplastic drugs also can cause many unpleasant side effects that can interfere with a patient's willingness to undergo cancer chemotherapy. Some of these effects include nausea and vomiting, peripheral neuropathies, cerebral blindness, loss of taste and hearing, and seizures (cisplatin, Platinol); leukopenia, thrombocytopenia, anemia, anorexia, nausea, vomiting, and diarrhea (cyclophosphamide, Cytoxan); diarrhea, anorexia, nausea, vomiting, leukopenia, thrombocytopenia, and dermatitis (fluorouracil, Adrucil); ulcerative stomatitis, leukopenia, thrombocytopenia, anemia, anorexia, nausea, abdominal distress, malaise, undue fatigue, chills, fever, dizziness, skin rashes, renal failure, headaches, drowsiness, and blurred vision (methotrexate, Mexate). Thus there are a lot of reasons to stop taking lifesaving drugs on a regular basis.

Drugs taken to improve cardiovascular function can manifest a variety of unpleasant effects that may deter patients from adhering to their medication schedules, for example, abdominal discomfort, pain, and headaches (digitalis);

headaches, angina, myalgia, anthralgia, or chest pain (hydralazine); diarrhea, blurred vision, dizziness, mental lassitude, impaired concentration, and night-mares (methyldopa); insomnia or sexual impairment (propranolol); physical fatigue and dizziness (metoprolol). Certainly, when people are taking medication for an asymptomatic condition such as hypertension and the treatment produces effects that hurt, interfere with daily routines, or are embarrassing (e.g., explosive postprandial diarrhea), then these biological effects can become serious barriers to adherence to and compliance with prescribed pharmaceutical regimens.

In addition to these direct effects of drugs, there can be interactions among drugs, or between a drug and another self-administered substance, that have a resultant deleterious or unpleasant effect. For example, many drugs, which other-wise have a wide therapeutic range with few side effects, cause serious problems when taken along with alcohol. Alcohol with antianginal drugs (e.g., nitroglycerin) results in hypotension, dizziness, and syncope; alcohol with anticoagulants (e.g., Coumadin, dicumarol, Panwarfin) alters the anticoagulant action depending on acute or chronic alcohol ingestion. Also, alcohol with antidiabetic drugs (e.g., Diabinese, Dymelor, Orinase) results in unpredictable blood sugar, disulfiramlike reactions, and angina pectoris; alcohol with antihypertensive has an additive hypotensive effect; alcohol with antitubercular drugs (e.g., isoniazid, rifampin) decreases the therapeutic response and increases the likelihood of hepatotoxicity; alcohol with salicylates leads to gastrointestinal bleeding. Alcohol plus some antibi-otics (e.g., cephalosporins, furazolidone) produces disulfiramlike reactions.

Drug–drug interactions (besides alcohol) also may be dangerous or unpleasant. Even simple antacids can potentiate the effects of anticholinergics; inhibit the actions of anticoagulants; and potentiate the effects of antihistamines, antimalar-ials, and bronchodilators (e.g., atropine). Nicotine (from tobacco) has effects on catecholamines and insulin that may interfere with antidiabetic agents' effects. Also, smoking potentiates the effects of oral contraceptives on cardiovascular risk. A host of other drug interactions occur and pose a particular problem in individuals, such as elderly people, who are taking many different medications. (See Hansten, 1985, for a fuller discussion of the clinical significance of drug–drug interactions.)

There are, of course, many other undesirable side effects of drugs. This list is meant to provide an illustrative rather than comprehensive review of biological effects that are unpleasant enough to become barriers to compliance and adher-ence, particularly when weighed against the salience to the individual of the benefits of the given drugs.

Unpleasant Side Effects of Nondrug Regimens

Drugs are not the only form of treatment that can have unpleasant biological effects. Physical therapies or exercise can cause pain and unpleasant fatigue.

Skeletal muscle pain and fatigue can result from exercises performed to maintain good health, and exercise performed in a program for rehabilitation from illnesses or injuries, including heart attack, osteoporosis, and trauma to bones, muscles, or nerves.

Surgery is another nondrug treatment that results in pain, discomfort, and loss of function. Patients postpone or refuse to submit to surgery because of concerns about the risks and discomfort associated with surgery. Temporary and permanent loss of function also contribute to resistance to surgery. The biological effects of hysterectomy, oophorectomy, and mastectomy become barriers discouraging many women from undergoing critical surgical procedures. Loss of voice from a laryngectomy, loss of physical function following prostate surgery, and so on deter people from these procedures.

Diet therapies of various types also lead to unpleasant side effects because of the protective mechanism of "appetite." Restriction of caloric intake leads to hunger that can be distracting, annoying, irritating, or even painful. Avoiding certain foodstuffs because of special dietary restrictions can also lead to unpleasant feelings because of appetite. Whether we are trying to follow diets that are salt-free, low-cholesterol, low-fat, low-caloric, dairy-free, gluten-free, oxalic acid-free, low-carbohydrate, or whatever, restricting food intake to be less than our body expects translates into hunger pangs and discomfort that may range from mild to incapacitating.

In all of these cases, there is an immediate unpleasantness compared to a delayed or nonobvious gain. It does not require complex theorizing to recognize that if something feels bad, we are less likely to do it.

Interference of Health Behaviors with Enjoyable Behaviors

It does not have to hurt for us not to want to do it. Healthful behaviors also may interfere with biological pleasures, and, therefore, we may avoid these behaviors. In other words, if it interferes with something that feels good, we also are less likely to do it.

Restrictive diets designed to improve cardiovascular function (e.g., low-cholesterol diet), to decrease the likelihood of cancer (e.g., high-fiber diet), or to help us lose weight (e.g., avoidance of sweet, high-caloric foods) promote health (Grunberg, 1987) but are generally no fun. Many people would consider it a great sacrifice to give up their morning doughnut or cup of coffee. These rituals—jolts of caffeine or sugar—may have biological actions that our bodies adapt to and come to require. Undoubtedly, we miss such daily pleasures when they are unavailable or when we abstain. Perhaps the enjoyment associated with specific foods, such as salty foods or sweets, involves biologically driven hedonic preferences to consume foodstuffs needed by the body (Cabanac, 1971, 1979; Richter, 1943; Young, 1936, 1955). In this context, it is interesting to note that cigarette smokers prefer and consume more sweets after cessation of smoking (Grunberg, 1985, 1986a). Anecdotal reports indicate that similar phenomena accompany abstinence from habitual use of alcohol or narcotics. Perhaps the enjoyment derived from eating specific foods taps similar biological processes involved in self-administration of some drugs of dependence (Grunberg, in press). It has been proposed, for example, that the unpleasantness associated with withdrawal from habitual drug use is attenuated by consumption of sweets and carbohydrates (Grunberg, 1986b; Grunberg & Baum, 1985). Whether or not this hypothesis linking drugs of dependence to food preferences is correct, it is clear that we enjoy consuming certain foods and that restrictive diets are not enjoyable. Therefore, we tend to cheat on these diets.

In addition to eating, people enjoy drinking, smoking, and using "recreational" drugs. Consumption of alcohol, nicotine, marijuana, cocaine, and other psychotropic drugs is reportedly enjoyable—in some cases calming, in other cases exhilarating, and in many cases perceived as necessary by the users. But the health message for these substances is loud and clear: don't smoke at all; don't drink in excess; don't get hooked on other drugs, especially if they are illegal. In addition, it is often important not to engage in these behaviors (especially drinking and smoking) when taking medications because of the potentiating aversive drug interaction effects. Whether motivated by the pleasurable effects of psychotropic drugs or by the discomfort of abstinence or withdrawal, people who use these substances often choose to continue recreational drug use rather than to adopt more healthful behaviors.

Another example of behaviors that promote health but interfere with biologically based enjoyable behaviors is safe sex practices. To avoid AIDS, men are told to use condoms. This advice is sound and could save lives. But condoms can decrease the sensuality and pleasures of sexual intercourse. They also require time and trouble that interrupts intimate, arousing moments.

As another example of health behaviors that interfere with biologically based enjoyable behaviors, consider medication schedules. Some medications require administration in the middle of the night or during a sleep period. This inconvenience also pits the health-promoting behavior against a biologically necessary and pleasant state.

As a final example in this category, it is noteworthy that many people find specific physical activities to be enjoyable. Medications that are accompanied by the instruction "Do not operate a motor vehicle or other large equipment" are at least a nuisance and in some cases a restriction that interferes with pleasures and daily routines. Instructions to avoid strenuous exertion (including physical activity, lifting, exercise, and sexual activity) may interfere with our jobs, hobbies, and general fun.

In all of these cases, the interference of healthful behaviors with enjoyable behaviors is not insurmountable. But the incompatible relationship of these behaviors and the intensity of the pleasures lost must be reckoned with and not ignored. For example, most people agree that safe sex practices are important. Yet the fact that condoms reduce physical pleasure may offset concerns about venereal diseases or AIDS, especially when the likelihood of contracting those diseases is viewed as infinitesimal. To optimize adherence to healthful behaviors, we must address and balance the biological and psychological aspects of the healthful behaviors with their effects that interfere with strong pleasure.

Physical or Cognitive Incompetence

Another category of biological barriers to adherence and compliance involves incompetence or deficiencies in physical or biologically based cognitive abilities of patients. For example, deafness interferes with understanding oral instructions about prescribed health behaviors. Impaired vision interferes with written instructions about prescribed health behaviors. Color deficiencies in vision interfere with one's ability to adhere to medication regimens that require taking different-colored pills on different days or at different times. These types of problems have been identified in the elderly but also apply to the general population. Physical barriers to adherence and compliance also include some allergies. For example, food allergies may interfere with nutrition, drug allergies may prevent administration of effective pharmacologic agents, and contact-dermatologic reactions may interfere with use of.some soaps and may prevent safe sex practices. Biologically based cognitive impairments or incompetencies that interfere with healthful behaviors include mental retardation, Alzheimer's disease, and senile dementias.

Absence or Misinterpretation of Biological Cues

Another factor that may affect compliance and adherence but that does not receive appropriate attention in the research literature is the patient's failure to experience or correctly interpret symptoms of underlying disorders. Simply put, I feel fine, so I am fine. That means, if I feel fine, I don't need medication, I don't need bed rest, I don't need to restrict my activities. Yet premature discontinuation of therapy because of improvement or absence of symptoms can be dangerous. For example, a course of antibiotics to treat bacterial infections will usually extend well beyond fever, aches, and weakness. Symptomless diseases such as hypertension require treatment whose effects will not be perceived by the patient. Misinterpretation of symptoms (e.g., I get headaches whenever my blood pressure is high) may lead to inappropriate self-dosing or abstinence (e.g., I don't have a headache, so I don't need to take my pills).

A variant of the "feel fine so no treatment is necessary" problem is "I feel fine so I don't have to do anything special to promote or improve health." For example, I feel fine, so I don't have to exercise, I don't have to watch my cholesterol intake, I don't have to quit smoking, I don't have to avoid too much exposure to the sun.

Adherence and compliance also are reduced when a given healthful behavior has no noticeable positive effects that are obvious to the individual. I've been exercising for weeks, yet I don't feel any better; in fact, I feel worse. I've given up eggs at breakfast, mayonnaise on my sandwiches, butter on my dinner rolls, yet I feel the same as before. I take my pills religiously, yet I feel the same as before—I bet the doctor gave me sugar pills. These experiences and the lack of awareness of bodily state, therapeutic effects, or preventive effects should be addressed and explained to patients.

What a patient expects will happen with a treatment or illness may be wrong. But this expectation, compared to the reality experienced, affects confidence in a given healthful behavior, the credibility of the care provider, and the likelihood of adhering to and complying with healthful behaviors.

Substance Abuse as a Biological Barrier

Today, cigarette smoking is on the top of everyone's list as the single most preventable cause of premature death and illness. The health message is clear: Don't smoke. To put this simple message into practice, however, is far from simple, as most habitual smokers and their families are well aware. Use of tobacco products is an addictive behavior involving powerful psychological and biological reinforcers. Therefore, for habitual smokers to abstain from smoking requires cessation of self-administration of an addictive psychopharmacologic agent, namely nicotine. Cessation of smoking may be accompanied by irritability, irascibility, anxiety, sleep disturbances, inability to concentrate, and body weight gains (Grunberg & Bowen, 1985; Shiffman, 1979). These biologically based abstinence effects are powerful barriers to adopting and maintaining a healthful life-style. In addition, abstinence means that the smoker will no longer receive effects of the drug that are considered positive, such as decreased body weight, increased concentration, and decreased anxiety.

Other abused substances, including alcohol, opiates, and sympathomimetics, similarly have biological effects that are reinforcing and abstinence effects that are unpleasant. Therefore, abstinence from use and abuse of these substances clearly is blocked by well-known biological barriers.

Moreover, some substances (e.g., alcohol, some tranquilizers), when used in excess, reduce motivation or competence to comply with instructions involving other healthful behaviors. All of the prodding, helpful hints, or coercion in the world cannot get someone who is in a dazed, apathetic state to exercise, eat right, or take medication on schedule.

CONCLUSIONS AND RECOMMENDATIONS

Biological factors are important and must be considered if we are to make headway in increasing compliance with and adherence to healthful behaviors. The other chapters in this book clearly establish that it is critical to understand psychological and behavioral factors in order to deal with lack of compliance and adherence. In addition, these factors have been the focus of attention in the compliance and adherence literature. However, we merely have to reflect on our own daily routines to realize that no matter how sophisticated the psychological theory or model, it leaves a lot out. Biological and behavioral variables must both be addressed. We don't floss our teeth regularly because it takes time, it's boring, it hurts, and there's no immediate gain. We don't eat right all the time because the "unhealthy" foods taste great and are accessible. We don't engage in safe sex practices regularly because they are troublesome, there are no immediate gains, and there are immediate losses.

We have compiled extensive theoretical and research literature addressing compliance and adherence issues. Unfortunately, their approaches have been unidisciplinary. We are not going to make much progress on this problem until *all* of the major variables—biological, behavioral, psychological, and sociological—are considered. The fact that the editors of this volume decided to include this chapter on a topic that has received so little theoretical or empirical attention reflects the growing appreciation of biobehavioral, multidisciplinary approaches to the study of health and behavior. We hope that this brief chapter encourages systematic and comprehensive investigations of biological as well as psychological variables that may affect adoption and maintenance of health-promoting behavior.

REFERENCES

Barnhart, E. R. (Ed.). (1988). *Physicians' desk reference* (42nd Ed.). Oradell, NJ: Medical Economics.

Cabanac, M. (1971). Physiological role of pleasure. *Science, 173*, 1103–1107.

Cabanac, M. (1979). Sensory pleasure. *Quarterly Review of Biology, 54*, 1–29.

Gerber, K., & Nehemkis, A. (Eds.). (1986). *Compliance: The dilemma of the chronically ill.* New York: Springer Publishing Co.

Grunberg, N. E. (1985). Nicotine, cigarette smoking, and body weight. *British Journal of Addiction, 80*, 369–377.

Grunberg, N. E. (1986a). Behavioral and biological factors in the relationship between tobacco use and body weight. In E. S. Katkin & S. B. Manuck (Eds.), *Advances in behavioral medicine, volume 2* (pp. 97–129). Greenwich, CT: JAI Press.

Grunberg, N. E. (1986b). Nicotine as a psychoactive drug: Appetite regulation. *Psychopharmacology Bulletin, 22*(3), 875–881.

Grunberg, N. E. (1987). Behavioral factors in preventive medicine and health promotion. In W. Gordon, A. Herd, & A. Baum (Eds.), *Perspectives on behavioral medicine, volume 3*. New York: Academic Press.

Grunberg, N. E. (in press). The inverse relationship between tobacco and body weight. In L. T. Kozlowski et al. (Eds.), *Research Advances in Alcohol and Drug Problems, 10,* 273–315. New York: Plenum Press.

Grunberg, N. E., & Baum, A. (1985). Biological commonalities of stress and substance abuse. In Saul Shiffman & Thomas A. Wills (Eds.), *Coping and substance use* (pp. 25–62). New York: Academic Press.

Grunberg, N. E., & Bowen, D. J. (1985). Coping with the sequelae of smoking cessation. *Journal of Cardiopulmonary Rehabilitation, 5,* 285–289.

Hansten, P. D. (1985). *Drug interactions: Clinical significance of drug–drug interactions.* Philadelphia: Lea & Febiger.

Haynes, R. B., Taylor, D. W., & Sackett, D. L. (Eds.). (1979). *Compliance in health care.* Baltimore: Johns Hopkins University Press.

Richter, C. P. (1943). Total self regulatory functions in animals and human beings. *Harvey Lecture Series, 38,* 63–103.

Shiffman, S. M. (1979). The tobacco withdrawal syndrome. In N. A. Krasnegor (Ed.), *NIDA research monograph 23: Cigarette smoking as a dependence process* (pp. 158–184). Rockville, MD: DHEW, ADAMHA.

Silverman, H. M., & Simon, G. I. (1982). *The pill book* (2nd ed.). New York: Bantam Books.

Young, P. T. (1936). *Motivation of behavior.* New York: Wiley.

Young, P. T. (1955). The role of hedonic processes in motivation. In M. R. Jones (Ed.), *Nebraska symposium on motivation* (pp. 193–238). Lincoln: University of Nebraska Press.

12

Physician and Dentist Compliance with Smoking Cessation Counseling

Thomas J. Coates, Rachel Vander Martin,
Barbara Gerbert, Robert R. Richard,
Steven R. Cummings

"Compliance" is usually used to describe how well patients follow physicians' prescriptions to take medication or advice regarding life-style modification. We present in this chapter an additional important perspective: the degree to which physicians and dentists themselves comply with strategies that will help their patients modify life-styles. This analysis is important because medical practitioners may be in a powerful position to influence health by motivating patients for life-style change (Wells, Lewis, Leake, Schleiter, & Brook, 1986). This is true for several reasons:

1. Physicians and dentists see a large proportion of the population on a regular basis. About 70% of the American population visit a physician at

This work was supported by Grant #CA38374A from the National Cancer Institute.

least once per year (USDHEW, 1979), while 54% (Graves, 1984) visit a dentist at least once a year. Those who are sicker, and therefore more in need of life-style change, are likely to see physicians and dentists more frequently.

2. Physicians and dentists also have an opportunity to develop an ongoing relationship with their patients through follow-up visits. This gives them the opportunity to use health-related concerns to motivate patients to change their behavior. They may be able to catch patients at "points of vulnerability" and thus maximize motivation for behavior change (Eraker, Becker, Strecher, & Kirscht, 1985).

3. Physicians and dentists also represent a credible source of information about health-related issues. Patients frequently look to their health care providers for up-to-date information about how to manage illness and preserve health (Wells et al., 1986).

4. Physician and dentist counseling can be effective in reducing patient smoking (Russell, Stapleton, Hajek, Jackson, & Belcher, 1988). But this requires that patients be counseled more than once using different intervention modalities (Kottke, Battista, DeFriese, & Brekke, 1988).

Whether or not physicians and dentists use their position to engage actively in disease prevention and health promotion in primary care practice is of great importance to health professionals interested in behavior change. To better understand physician behavior regarding health promotion, we use three recent University of California, San Francisco (UCSF) studies. The first studies report physician and dentist responses to a mailed survey on their reported smoking cessation preventive health practices. The second study discusses the results of a randomized controlled trial on physician counseling for smoking cessation. The final study analyzed the conditions under which patients received advice about their smoking.

Using data from these studies, we will discuss the extent to which physicians and dentists engage in smoking cessation counseling activities, barriers to use of prevention activities, and some proposed solutions. This analysis becomes important because one solution to poor patient compliance may lie in more persistent and effective efforts to motivate patient behavior change (Martin & Coates, 1987).

STUDY 1: SELF-REPORTED PHYSICIAN AND DENTIST SMOKING CESSATION COUNSELING PRACTICES

A random sample of internists and family practice specialists (Cummings et al., 1989a) and a random sample of dentists (Gerbert, Coates, Zahnd, Richard, &

Cummings, 1989), all practicing in San Francisco, were selected by picking every sixth physician and dentist in the San Francisco telephone directory. Each health care provider thus chosen was mailed a six-page questionnaire regarding their smoking cessation counseling practices. Responses were received from 208 physicians (92% response rate, median age 40–49, 83.8% white) and 82 dentists (82% response rate, median age 30–39, 65.7% white, 27.1% Asian). Four physicians were currently smokers, 43.3% were former smokers; three dentists were currently smokers, 38.2% were former smokers. While we have no comparable data on dentists, a recent analysis done by the authors on physician respondents and nonrespondents to the Quit for Life Project (Study 2) showed no significant differences in counseling attitudes or practices between the two groups (Cummings et al., 1989b).

Physicians and dentists were surveyed on the following items:

- Time spent on various procedures during a typical work week.
- The extent to which they engage in smoking cessation activities with patients.
- Their opinion and use of nicotine chewing gum.
- Their attitudes toward and compliance with smoking cessation-related activities.
- A composite description of their counseling effectiveness and skill.
- Important barriers to smoking cessation counseling in their practice.

Physicians and dentists surveyed agreed strongly that the major barriers to smoking cessation counseling were that smokers are not interested in quitting and that they perceived their advice to be ineffective (Figure 12.1). Other barriers endorsed were the fact that dentists and physicians were not skilled in counseling and did not have the time to do it, that they were not paid by insurance to counsel, that they forgot to bring it up, and that they felt that patients might leave their practice.

As Study 2 will show, many of these barriers can be remedied by training and education. Efficacy and skills can be enhanced by effective continuing medical education (CME) programs. Forgetting to counsel might be remedied by reminders (Cohen, Stookey, Katz, Drook, & Smith, 1989); lack of time to counsel might be remedied by effective methods for counseling.

STUDY 2: QUIT FOR LIFE

Quit for Life was a randomized controlled trial of a brief intervention with physicians in general practice. The intervention was designed to help physicians counsel their patients more effectively to quit smoking. Two separate, parallel

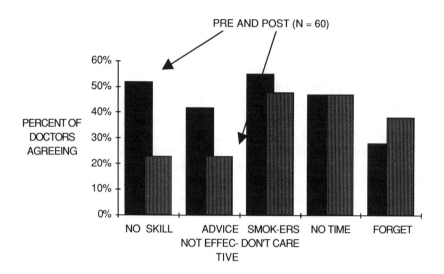

FIGURE 12.1 Barriers to smoking counseling.

studies were conducted: one in 38 private practice offices (Cummings et al., 1989b) and the other at four Kaiser Permanente sites (Cummings et al., 1989a). Physicians who volunteered to participate were randomly assigned to experimental or control groups by workplace unit. In private practice, workplace unit meant one solo or group practice; in Kaiser the workplace units were medical stations. In private practice, 44 physicians (female 12%, white 95%, current smokers 5%, former smokers 27%) were recruited and randomized (24 experimental, 20 control) from 38 offices. In Kaiser 81 physicians (female 28%, white 80%, current smokers 5%, former smokers 29%) from 22 medical stations were recruited and randomized (40 experimental, 41 control).

After randomization, the experimental physicians participated in two 45-minute small-group training sessions. These sessions included lectures on how to counsel smokers to quit, using a brief, stepwise approach (ask, motivate, set a date), videotapes illustrating the approach, and role-playing among participants to practice using the technique. The training was done by either a physician or psychologist from UCSF. Models of variations (relapse, failure, resistance) were discussed, and follow-up visits with counseled patients were encouraged. Experimental group physicians were also trained in the selective use of nicotine gum. Participants received a syllabus that outlined and supplemented the seminars and were given the option of using project-designed booklets, quit-date RX pads, and posters for their offices. Six to eight weeks after initial training, a 45-minute follow-up session was held that included a short lecture and discussion. Physicians were asked to complete a baseline questionnaire on knowledge, behavior, efficacy, and barriers regarding smoking cessation counseling before they were randomized into control and experimental groups. Three months after the intervention both groups were asked to complete an abbreviated version of the baseline questionnaire to measure changes in attitudes and compliance.

In addition to the physician training, the physicians' staffs were also trained by project research staff. Registered nurses, L.P.N.s, medical assistants, and receptionists were given an overview of the project and instructed on how to attach project-supplied "reminder" stickers to smoking patients' charts. Staff compliance in attaching the reminders varied from site to site. The project staff monitored and encouraged the medical staff and kept the physicians supplied with booklets and other requested materials.

For each participating physician, a consecutive sample of patients who smoked was drawn by screening every patient who saw the physician and inviting all smokers to participate until either a maximum sample size of 30 patients per physician was met or a maximum data collection time of 16 weeks had passed. A total of 907 private practice patients were thus enrolled, with an average of 20.6 patients per physician.

Patients completed a self-administered baseline questionnaire in the office prior to being examined by the physician to determine smoking history and attitudes. Patients were subsequently interviewed by telephone as soon as possible after the visit to determine what was said about smoking during the visit. The completion rate for the telephone "exit survey" was 91%.

Approximately 84% of the original patients were interviewed by telephone 1 year after their visit with the physician. They were asked about their current smoking status and other smoking-related variables. Self-reported quitters were validated biologically using both carbon monoxide and saliva cotinine.

The Quit for Life program was effective in reducing the experimental group physicians' perceptions that patients were not interested in learning about smoking cessation and in increasing physicians' personal efficacy with regard to smoking cessation counseling (Table 12.1). The program had no impact on physicians' perceptions that time, insurance reimbursement, and forgetting to bring up the subject were barriers to smoking cessation counseling.

Tables 12.2a and 12.2b (private practice physicians) present the immediate outcomes of the degree to which physicians followed the counseling protocols with their smoking patients. The Quit For Life (QFL) program was successful in increasing the extent to which physicians brought up the topic of smoking in general medicine encounters. In the Kaiser experimental group (Table 12.2a) the subject came up 50% of the time, in the control group 45% of the time. In the private practice experimental group (Table 12.2b) the subject of smoking came up 64% of the time with the experimental group while in the control group it came up 44% of the time. Once the topic was brought up, experimental physi-

TABLE 12.1 Changes in Physicians' Responses to Questionnaire*

	Before training (%)	After training (%)	change (95% C.I.)**
"I am effective"	32.4	58.8	+26.5 (+3.5 to +37.9)
"I have skills"	78.4	100	+21.6 (+5.6 to +21.6)
Sometimes or often suggest setting a date to quit (%)	48.7	100	+51.3 (+34.0 to +51.3)
Using gum, smokers should stop smoking first (% correct)	51.4	85.7	+34.3 (+10.6 to +44.3)

*Experimental group physicians only. Largest $n = 39$ and smallest $n = 34$ because of missing data.
**By exact binomial test for difference between paired proportions.
(From Cummings et al., 1989. Used with permission.)

TABLE 12.2a Results of Telephone Interviews with Patients After Visits with their Physicians, Kaiser Group

	Control	Experimental	Difference (95% C.I.)
All Visits* Smoking discussed (%)	44.9	50.1	5.2 (+0.7 to +9.7) 16.5 (+13.2 to +19.8)
Visits in which smoking was discussed† Mean time discussing smoking (min)	4.2	5.4	1.1 (+0.5 to +1.8)
Physician asked for quit date (%)	11.1	37.6	26.5 (+21.2 to +31.8)
Smoker agreed to set quit date (%)	5.4	24.7	19.3 (+14.8 to +23.8)
Written prescription for quit date (%)	1.2	16.1	14.9 (+11.4 to +18.4)
Prescription for nicotine gum (%)	10.4	10.2	−0.2 (−4.2 to +3.8)

*Smallest sample sizes: 940 for experimental group and 942 for control group due to missing data.
†Smallest sample sizes: 466 for experimental group and 417 for control group due to missing data.
(From Cummings et al., 1989a. Used with permission.)

TABLE 12.2b Private Practice Physician Counseling About Smoking During Visits*

	Control	Experimental	Difference (95% C.I.)
All Visits*			
Smoking discussed (%)	44.4	64.4	20.1 (+13.2 to +27.0)
Received self-help booklet (%)	36.7	9.3	27.4 (+21.7 to +33.1)
Visits in which smoking was discussed†			
Mean time spent discussing smoking (min)	5.2	7.5	2.3 (+1.0 to +3.5)
Physician asked for quit date (%)	12.4	38.4	26.5 (+21.2 to +31.8)
Smoker agreed to quit date (%)	5.1	29.2	24.1 (+17.2 to +30.9)
Written reminder of quit date (%)	1.1	16.8	15.7 (+10.4 to +20.9)
Nicotine gum prescribed (%)	19.4	13.2	−6.2 (−13.7 to +1.4)
Given follow-up appointment about smoking (%)	10.6	19.1	10.2 (+6.3 to +14.1)
Physician suggested a treatment program (%)	13.3	14.4	1.1 (−5.8 to +8.1)

*Based on telephone interviews with patients after visits with their physicians.
**Smallest sample sizes: 411 for experimental and 407 for control group due to missing data.
†Smallest sample sizes: 261 for experimental and 177 for control group due to missing data.
(From Cummings et al., 1989b. Used with permission.)

cians implemented the intervention protocol with significantly more patients than the control physicians.

STUDY 3: WHO GOT COUNSELED

From another perspective, however, the results were discouraging. In the Kaiser group, 50% of the smoking patients did not have the topic raised for them, and in the private practice group, 36% of the smoking patients were not asked about smoking. Of particular interest is the tendency of physicians to bring the subject up with some groups of people and not with others. We, therefore, completed the following analysis to investigate more completely the conditions under which the topic of smoking was likely to come up with smoking patients.

The subject of smoking cessation was more likely to come up with patients who were white than with patients who were black or Hispanic. More patients who had some college received counseling than those with no college. Patients who smoked more than a pack of cigarettes per day, smoked their first cigarette within 15 minutes of awakening, and who answered yes to "I am addicted to cigarettes" were also more likely to receive counseling.

In addition, smoking was more likely to come up if the patient had a smoking-related symptom or illness, if their family and friends wanted them to quit, and if the patient wanted to quit and was confident she or he could quit. Patients reported having smoking mentioned more often during a first visit and physical exam than during routine follow-up and urgent care visits. Ironically, few of these variables predicted who would stay off cigarettes for at least 3 months following their physician's advice. Those most likely to quit were those who wanted to quit and expressed the confidence to do so and who delayed their first cigarette-beyond 15 minutes of waking up. Blacks were more likely than white to achieve 3-month cessation.

This analysis suggests that physicians may engage in smoking counseling due to cues in the environment rather than perceiving the activity as a routine part of primary practice. Thus the topic may come up when the physician is reminded by the patient's symptoms or by the fact that the patient raised the topic. Based on this assumption, programs designed to enhance smoking cessation counseling need to look at the observed behavior along with self-reports on what physicians see as barriers to counseling. For example, if physicians are only counseling heavy smokers with smoking-related symptoms and illnesses, they may be missing opportunities to use the same skills with lighter, asymptomatic smokers who may be less addicted and therefore more open to the idea of quitting (Li, Coates, Ewart, & Kim, 1987).

HOW CAN PHYSICIANS BE MOTIVATED TO INCREASE PRIMARY AND SECONDARY PREVENTION EFFORTS?

The Quit for Life program demonstrated that a brief intervention using a stepwise approach was effective in educating physicians, increasing their perception that they could be effective cessation counselors, and motivating them to bring up the subject of smoking in general medicine encounters. However, much more needs to be done to increase physician compliance with smoking cessation counseling practices (see Ockene et al., 1987). Programs like Quit for Life need to be amplified with strategies that will cue and reinforce physicians to raise the topic of smoking (Demak & Becker, 1987).

Especially important may be materials that are aimed at modifying the practice environment and the norms of the practice community with regard to smoking cessation counseling. It appears that lack of time is a very difficult barrier to overcome, especially if the physician is part of an HMO, where patient load is often very heavy. It would appear that modifications may have to be made in the system to allow more time per visit if smoking counseling is to become a regular part of routine care.

The extra time may need to be compensated for by reimbursement. This involves pressing insurance companies to be more open to the idea of reimbursement for smoking counseling. At the present time very few insurers are willing to pay for extra visits on smoking cessation. If more individual practices and HMOs instituted smoking counseling as part of routine care this problem would be addressed.

Other options involve instituting systems to educate patients to ask for help on smoking, using the medical support staff to both remind the physician to do the counseling, and supplementing the physician's efforts with stop smoking programs, support groups, and literature. Patients do not perceive that physicians are or want to be involved in their smoking cessation efforts (Anda, Remington, Sienko, & Davis, 1987). Educating patients that this is an appropriate and proper role for physicians may be crucial. The key seems to be in coordinating the system, staff, physician, and patient efforts to all work in the same direction. An integrated approach may be needed to ensure steady and consistent application of effective smoking cessation counseling.

The research implications are also clear. We know that physicians think that counseling about smoking cessation is important and will do so when cued. Studies are needed, especially experimental investigations, that will demonstrate how systems such as we have suggested can be put in place and the impact that these systems have on smoking cessation counseling.

REFERENCES

Anda, R. F., Remington, P. L., Sienko, D. G., & Davis, R. M. (1987). Are physicians advising smokers to quit? The patient's perspective. *Journal of the American Medical Association*, 257, 1916–1919.

Cohen, S. J., Stookey, G. K., Katz, B. P., Drook, C. A., & Smith, D. M. (1989). Encouraging primary care physicians to help smokers quit. *Annals of Internal Medicine*, 110, 648–652.

Cummings, S. R., Coates, T. J., Richard, R. J., Hansen, B. H., Zahnd, E. G., Vander Martin, R., Duncan, C., Gerbert, B., Martin, A. R., & Stein, M. J. (1989). Training physicians in counseling about smoking: A randomized trial of the "Quit for Life" program. *Annals of Internal Medicine*, 110, 640–647.

Cummings, S. R., Richard, R. J., Duncan, C. L., Hansen, B., Vander Martin, R., Gerbert, B., & Coates, T. J. (1989). Training physicians about smoking cessation: A controlled trial in private practice. *Journal of General Internal Medicine*, 4, 482–489.

Demak, M. M., & Becker, M. H. (1987). The doctor-patient relationship and counseling for preventive care. *Patient Education and Counseling, 9,* 5-24.

Eraker, S. A., Becker, M. H., Strecher, V. J., & Kirscht, J. P. (1985). Smoking behavior, cessation techniques, and the health decision model. *The American Journal of Medicine, 78,* 817-825.

Gerbert, B., Coates, T. J., Zahnd, E., Richard, R. J., & Cummings, S. R. (1989). Dentists as smoking cessation counselors. *Journal of the American Dental Association, 118,* 29-32.

Graves, R. C. (1984). Dental health needs and demands in American society: Current trends. *Health Values, 8,* 13-20.

Kottke, T. E., Battista, R. N., DeFriese, G. H., & Brekke, M. L. (1988). Attributes of successful smoking cessation interventions in medical practice: A meta analysis of 39 controlled trials. *Journal of the American Medical Association, 259,* 2882-2889.

Li, V. C., Coates, T. J., Ewart, C., & Kim, N. (1987). The effectiveness of smoking cessation advice given during routine medical care: Physicians can make a difference. *American Journal of Preventive Medicine, 3,* 81-86.

Martin, A. R., & Coates, T. J. (1987). A clinician's guide to helping patients change behavior. *Western Journal of Medicine, 146,* 751-753.

Ockene, J. K., Hosmer, D. W., Williams, J. W., Goldberg, R. J., Ockene, I. S., Biliouris, T., & Dalen, J. E. (1987). The relationship of patient characteristics to physician delivery of advice to stop smoking. *Journal of General Internal Medicine, 2,* 337-340.

Russell, M. A. H., Stapleton, J. A., Hajek, P., & Jackson, P. H. (1987). District programme to reduce smoking: Effect of clinic supported brief intervention by general practitioners. *British Medical Journal, 295,* 1240-1244.

Russell, M. A. H., Stapleton, J. A., Hajek, P., Jackson, P. H., & Belcher, M. (1988). District programme to reduce smoking: Can sustained intervention by general practitioners affect prevalence? *Journal of Epidemiology and Community Health, 42,* 111-115.

U.S. Department of Health, Education, and Welfare. (1979). Smoking and health: A report of the Surgeon General. Public Health Service (*DHEW* Publication NO. (PHS) 79-50066). Washington, DC: U.S. Government Printing Office.

Wells, K. B., Lewis, C. E., Leake, B., Schleiter, M. K., & Brook, R. H. (1986). The practices of general and subspecialty internists in counseling about smoking and exercise. *American Journal of Public Health, 76,* 1009-1013.

13

The Social Context
and Health Behavior:
The Case of Tobacco

David G. Altman

In recent years a great deal has been learned about factors that influence the initiation, maintenance, and cessation of smoking, and progress has been made in the design and implementation of smoking cessation programs (Schwartz, 1987). A wide variety of approaches has been developed, including self-care, education, medication, nicotine chewing gum, hypnosis, acupuncture, physician counseling, risk factor preventive trials, community programs, and behavioral programs (Schwartz, 1987). The overall downward trend in smoking rates in the United States is probably due in part to the successful design and implementation of these and other smoking control programs. The bad news is that almost one third of the U.S. population still smokes, the adolescent smoking rate did not change from 1984 to 1987, and some ethnic minority groups are smoking at increased rates. This chapter presents data illustrating that this bad news may be partially attributed to the influence of the larger social context.

The author thanks Irwin Altman, Ph.D., Abby C. King, Ph.D., Robert Klesges, Ph.D., Sally Shumaker, Ph.D., and Richard A. Winett, Ph.D. for their helpful comments.

Smoking is a complex behavior, rooted in biological, social, environmental, historical, and cultural contexts. To adequately understand it, therefore, one must account for how it is influenced at multiple levels of analyses. This chapter focuses on: (1) how regulatory and policy factors influence smoking behavior, a largely neglected area of analysis in comparison with the role of personal and social factors, and (2) prevention of smoking. The main body of the chapter reviews topics in the regulatory and policy domains that have been or might be targets of public policy and legislation at local, state, or federal levels. Specifically, these topics include cigarette advertising and promotion, the 1971 broadcast ban on tobacco advertising, media practices relative to the modeling of smoking, self-censorship in the popular press, cigarette taxation, access to cigarettes by minors, regulation of smoking in public settings, and government price supports of the tobacco industry. Before these topics are reviewed in depth, however, the philosophical perspective taken in the chapter is discussed.

While this chapter focuses on regulatory and policy factors, it is important to note that a comprehensive biopsychosocial analysis would attend to the important influences of biological factors (e.g., nicotine addiction) and psychosocial factors (e.g., peer pressure) (Benowitz, 1988; DHHS, 1988; Engel, 1977; Schwartz, 1982) as well. The points raised in this chapter, therefore, are not meant to minimize the fact that tobacco use is a drug addiction that goes beyond personal choice and interpersonal influence.

The focus taken in this chapter is perhaps best illustrated by examining a well-researched topic from the perspective to be taken here. Research on the effects of interpersonal influences on smoking has in recent years attracted considerable research attention (Perry, Murray, & Klepp, 1987; DHHS, 1987). One of the more widely studied variables has been peer pressure, with many programs successfully designed and implemented to increase the ability of adolescents to practice social resistance skills (Best, Thomson, Sanit, Smith, & Brown, 1988; Botvin, 1986; Evans, 1980; Harken, 1987; Klepp, Halper, & Perry, 1986; Schwartz, 1987). While there has been a great deal of research and successful programs mounted on this topic, most of it is done with minimal consideration to the larger social context. Yet one way to increase our understanding of adolescent peer pressure to smoke is to consider the effects of regulatory and policy variables.

For example, easy access to cigarettes by minors, low tax rates (and therefore relatively cheaper cigarettes), and advertisements portraying the positive interpersonal relationships that result from smoking may all increase the opportunities and motives for young people to adopt smoking and may enhance their ability to serve as influences on others. Peer pressure can succeed only if the substances around which pressure is exerted (i.e., tobacco) are available at a certain time and place and are viewed desirably. Thus preventing adolescent tobacco use is not simply an issue of equipping individuals with resistance skills.

Moreover, when and where peer pressure occurs and the developmental stage of pressured (and pressuring) individuals are also important variables to consider. It is likely, for example, that the opportunities to exert peer pressure are enhanced after school and before parents return home from work, during social events, on weekend nights, and during summer months.

Our approach is influenced by ecological and systems theory, which view behavior as a function of the surrounding context. These theories are guided by the principle that the whole is more than the sum of its parts (Kuhn, 1975; Stein, 1974; Stokols, 1980; Wicker, 1979). Through interaction and feedback, each component in a system is affected by other components and by the larger environment in which it exists. Through transactions with their environments, systems grow, differentiate, change, and become more complex over time (Stein, 1974). Thus behavior and environment are interdependent rather than independent domains (Wicker, 1979). Furthermore, an ecological perspective considers different levels of analysis like the layers of an onion, each system nested within another, with each system constrained both by the system it surrounds and the system that surrounds it (Wicker, 1979).

The ultimate goal of all interventions directed at smoking behavior, regardless of the level of analysis, is to improve the health status of individuals since individuals, not systems or environments, experience illness and health. The focus of macrolevel interventions (e.g., increasing the tax on cigarettes) may also influence the actions that individuals take (e.g., not purchasing cigarettes). Similarly, a goal of many microlevel interventions (e.g., teaching worksite employees how to quit smoking) may influence actions taken at higher levels of analysis (e.g., implementation of a worksite smoking policy). There are interactional and synergistic connections among levels of analysis. The means by which individuals are reached and influenced, however, can vary as a function of the level at which one intervenes. In more cases than not, there is a reciprocity of influence between levels of analysis (Winett, King, & Altman, 1989). Furthermore, individuals and systems are not "mutually exclusive or opposite ends of a political or theoretical continuum" (Green, 1986, p. 29). In the case of smoking, for example, focusing on one level has its concomitant costs and benefits. Curtailing and eventually eliminating smoking in the workplace may require changes in organizational policies that are mutually agreeable to management and labor, implementation of co-worker support programs, and availability of cessation programs for individuals attempting to quit smoking. Some of the variables that affect smoking behavior, by level of analysis, are listed in Table 13.1. As noted previously, the focus of this chapter will be on the policy and regulatory level of analysis.

There is a relative scarcity of studies on health behavior that specify the sequence or causal linkages by which individuals influence, and are influenced by, the larger social context (Altman & King, 1986; Winett et al., 1989). Even

TABLE 13.1 Factors Related to Smoking Behavior

Personal	Interpersonal	Community	Regulatory/Policy
Nicotine addiction	Peer pressure	Worksite smoking policy	Advertising /promotion
Stress	Family stress		
Knowledge of hazards	Role models	Social reinforcement	Excise tax
Attitudes re: smoking	Physician advice	Access to vending machines	Laws re: legal age and access
Socioeconomic status		Behavior settings conducive to smoking	Modeling in movies
Self-efficacy		Free distribution	1971 broadcast ban
Age			Censorship in press
Gender			Federal price supports
			Lobbying by tobacco industry
			Warning labels

analyses of smoking behavior from a sociocultural perspective do not carry the multilevel analogy to its fullest (e.g., Syme & Alcalay, 1982). In a review article on relapse with addictive substances, for example, Brownell, Marlatt, Lichtenstein, and Wilson (1986) propose an organizing framework for understanding the determinants and predictors of lapse and relapse. They classify variables on the basis of individual and interpersonal factors, physiological factors, and environmental and social factors. Environmental and social factors, however, are defined narrowly as social support and immediate environmental stimuli and external contingencies (e.g., social pressure, cues from situations previously associated with the addictive behavior). While their review highlights the many achievements made in the prevention of relapse, it does not review how the *larger* social context may affect relapse.

Similarly, the 1987 report on smoking and health submitted to Congress (DHHS, 1987) reviews four factors affecting smoking behavior: physiological, psychological, cognitive, and social and demographic. The social and demographic factors discussed were social support, socioeconomic status, occupational status, age, race, and gender. Later in the volume, communitywide and worksite smoking programs are reviewed. Likewise, a review on the prevention of smoking among schoolchildren suggests that the primary antecedents of adolescent smoking are demographic, social–environmental, personality, intrapersonal and psychosocial, and biological, with the influence of the social environment (e.g., prevalence of smoking among peers, family) being the most important (Best et al., 1988). While the factors highlighted in this review are important contributors to smoking behavior, we propose that our understanding of smoking behavior can be enhanced if greater attention is paid to understanding the effects of the larger social context.

For the most part, therefore, the dominant perspective on smoking control gives relatively little attention to the direct or indirect influence of macrolevel variables. In notable exception, Iverson (1987) uses a general multilevel perspective to review worksite, school, community, physician, policy, and economic smoking control programs and argues that all must be considered in a comprehensive smoking control effort. This chapter will not review the many accomplishments of smoking control worksite programs, physician-based programs, clinical trials (e.g. Multiple Risk Factor Intervention Trial [MRFIT]), and community programs (e.g., Stanford Three Community Study and Five City Project, Minnesota Heart Health Project, Pawtuckett Heart Health Project, North Karelia Project). Reviews of these programs exist elsewhere (c.f., Altman & King, 1986; Iverson, 1987; Schwartz, 1987; Winett et al., 1989).

REGULATORY AND POLICY CONTEXT AND SMOKING BEHAVIOR
Overview

The American Public Health Association (APHA) has recognized the important influence of macrolevel variables on cigarette smoking by issuing policy statements on the taxation, advertising, and promotion of tobacco products (APHA, 1987). They note that taxation is an effective deterrent to smoking adoption and cessation; the social costs of smoking far exceed the excise taxes imposed on cigarettes; the federal government provides large subsidies to the tobacco industry; fixed tobacco taxes encourage its future use, since inflation erodes the impact of taxes on consumption; and tobacco is imported cheaply. Based on these factors, the Association proposes increasing the import duty on tobacco products, increasing federal taxes on tobacco by at least a factor of five, increasing state taxes on tobacco products, and indexing the tobacco tax rate to inflation or to increases on the wholesale price of tobacco products. They also note that cigarettes are the most heavily promoted product in the U.S., advertising is deceptive, the tobacco industry and the media have not voluntarily controlled deceptive advertising, the industry continues to market tobacco to young people and women, smokeless tobacco advertising has increased dramatically (particularly among young males), and print media's reliance on tobacco advertising revenues diminishes the coverage of the health effects of smoking. As a result, the Association proposed a ban on all media advertising and promotion of all tobacco products. Similarly, the American Heart Association has called for an increase in the federal excise tax, elimination or restriction of tobacco advertising and promotion, assurance of nonsmokers' rights, and identification of methods to assist tobacco farmers in the transition to farming other crops or to other professions (Warner, et al., 1986).

While the consumption of tobacco has been dropping about 2% a year, it still remains at high levels. In 1987, the following levels of consumption in the U.S. were recorded (Tobacco Institute, 1988): 575 billion cigarettes, 2.7 billion large cigars and cigarillos, over 1 million little cigars, 23 million pounds of pipe and roll-your-own tobacco, 76 million pounds of chewing tobacco, and 45 million pounds of snuff. Tobacco products were distributed in 939,000 retail outlets, including almost 619,000 vending machines (Tobacco Institute, 1988).

The tobacco problem is not limited to the United States. In recent years the American tobacco industry has made major inroads into the international marketplace. Tobacco leaf and tobacco products now set export records each year and as an export category outperform most of the other American exports (Anonymous, 1987a). Over 100 billion cigarettes were exported in 1987 to other countries, an increase of 36% from the previous year (Tobacco Institute, 1988). While Americans use about 600 billion cigarettes each year, Chinese consume well over 1 trillion (Stoffman, 1987)—about one in four Chinese children will die from smoking-related illnesses (Advocacy Institute, personal communication, June 14, 1988). If current trends continue, four million people worldwide per year will die from tobacco-induced illness by the year 2000 (Advocacy Institute, personal communication, June 14, 1988).

Tobacco growers are a strong political constituency and are able to influence tobacco policy because tobacco holds great value as an economic cash crop, tobacco farming occurs within restricted and well-defined geopolitical areas, and there are large numbers of farmers and tobacco production employees (Bell & Levy, 1984). In 1988, Philip Morris attempted to capitalize on the potential political influence of smokers and the tobacco industry by placing advertisements in the popular press emphasizing the economic clout of the 54 million people who smoke (e.g., "$1 trillion is too much financial power to ignore. America's 55.8 million smokers are a powerful economic force. If their household income . . . were a Gross National Product, it would be the third largest in the world."). Further evidence of tobacco industry aggressiveness is seen in the proliferation of smokers' rights groups in recent years (e.g., Smokers' Rights Alliance, The Great American Smoker's Club, Inc., Committee for Airline Passengers' Rights, Smokers, People United for Friendly Smoking, Tobacco Users Fight for Fairness, and Smokers' Rights). Many of these groups are supported financially by the tobacco industry.

Cigarette Advertising and Promotion

The tobacco industry spent $2.4 billion dollars in 1986 on advertising and promotion (FTC, 1988). These expenditures have increased rapidly in the past few decades, climbing from about $261 million in 1964 to their current level. In contrast, public and private counteradvertising totalled about $5 million in 1985, a 400-fold difference (Warner, 1986a, b). Among all products, expenditures for cigarette advertising are first in outdoor media, second in magazines, and third in newspapers (Davis, 1987). The tobacco companies continue to disseminate aggressively their messages through advertising. For the first time in 24 years, Proctor and Gamble was dislodged by Philip Morris in 1987 as the number one advertiser in the U.S. In 1987, Philip Morris spent $1.7 billion advertising its products, a 7.9% increase from 1986.

An analysis of eight popular magazines in 1985 found that the average number of tobacco advertisements *in each issue* was approximately six (Albright, Altman, Slater, & Maccoby, 1988).

The targets of magazine tobacco ads have also changed since 1960, with more attention in recent years going to youths, women, and minorities (Albright et al., 1988; Davis, 1987; Ernster, 1985). In addition, the tobacco industry targets different demographic groups with customized ads. Magazines with large youth readerships, for example, receive disproportionately more ads with recreation and risk and adventure themes, while women's magazines receive disproportionately more ads with romantic and erotic themes (Altman, Slater, Albright, & Maccoby, 1987). Headlines from the *U.S. Distribution Journal*, the trade magazine for the tobacco and candy industries, echo this approach: "Cigarette companies target growing female segment—New brands, line extensions designed to appeal to women's tastes."

In another advertising vehicle, Lippman (1986) reports that there are over 40,000 tobacco billboards in this country. While the brand name and imagery of billboard and taxicab tobacco advertisements are easily identifiable, under normal driving conditions a large majority of people cannot read the Surgeon General's warning on them (Davis & Kendrick, 1989).

Some aspects of tobacco advertising are regulated by states. Utah is probably the state with the most restrictive policy toward cigarette advertising (due in large part to the influence of the Latter-Day Saints (Mormon) religion, which discourages smoking). The state prohibits advertising on billboards, streetcars, buses, and any other public displays. It does, however, allow cigarette dealers to post signs indicating that cigarettes can be purchased at a given location (DHHS, 1987).

How Ads Affect Behavior

The mechanisms by which advertising influences smoking-related behavior could have direct or indirect effects (Warner, 1986b). The potential direct effects include enticing children and teens to experiment with tobacco, reducing current smokers' resolve to quit or to consider quitting, increasing smokers' daily consumption of cigarettes, and encouraging former smokers to resume smoking. The indirect mechanisms by which advertising could influence smoking include discouraging an open discussion in the media of the hazards of tobacco because of a dependence on advertising revenues for economic survival and contributing to an environment in which smoking is perceived as socially acceptable. Warner (1986b) concluded that advertising and promotion almost certainly have both indirect and direct effects on consumption, although the evidence for indirect effects is more conclusive.

Brand Switching

The tobacco industry continues to maintain, despite a great deal of public and professional protests to the contrary, that their advertising strategies are designed to influence current smokers to switch brands rather than to attract nonsmokers such as women and youths. Several individuals familiar with the tobacco industry contradict this position, For example, Emerson Foote, former chairperson of the board of McCann-Erickson, the world's second largest advertising agency and once responsible for $20 million in cigarette accounts, said in this regard: "I am always amused by the suggestion that advertising, a function that has been shown to increase consumption of virtually every other product, somehow miraculously fails to work for tobacco products" (Foote, 1981 p. 1667).

Examining the brand-switching argument of the tobacco industry by using simple mathematical logic also raises questions about the intent of cigarette advertisers. Each year, about 1 million smokers die and another 1.5 million smokers quit smoking. Therefore, the tobacco industry must recruit about 2.5 million new smokers each year just to maintain (not increase) the current smoking prevalence rate (Warner, 1986b). Since 60% of smokers begin smoking by the age of 14 and 90% by the end of their teenage years (Johnston, O'Malley, & Bachman, 1987), 5000 children and teenagers would have to start smoking each day of the year for the tobacco industry to maintain the smoking prevalence rate (Warner, 1986b). Although there is some evidence that tobacco companies recognize their inability to increase or even to maintain the present smoking rate in the U.S. (as is evidenced by their increased attention to the international market and to the diversification of their product line to include, among other products, large food operations), it is reasonable to assume that they will continue to engage in activities to enhance the likelihood that the U.S. prevalence rate is maintained. In this regard, it must be recognized that tobacco continues to be a highly profitable product in this country, more profitable than most other consumer products. In 1986, for example, RJR–Nabisco had $3.8 billion in U.S. cigarette assets, with a return on assets of $1.4 billion (37%). In contrast, their food business had assets of $9.8 billion but only earned shareholders $820 million, an 8.4% return (Stoffman, 1987). Likewise, with the acquisition of Kraft by Philip Morris, food will account for 60% of total Philip Morris sales but only 37% of total income (Orr, 1988a). The Marlboro brand alone accounts for $5.4 billion in sales. Overall, the six major tobacco companies in the U.S. have pretax profit margins of about 30%, a figure extraordinarily high for a mature industry (Seligman, 1987).

There are additional facts that negate the tobacco industry's position on the role of advertising being limited to brand loyalty and brand switching: (1) only 10% of smokers switch brands each year (FTC, 1985); (2) over two thirds of existing cigarette brands are owned by Philip Morris and R. J. Reynolds, indicating that most brand switching occurs among brands owned by the same company (Tye, Warner, & Glantz, 1987); (3) assuming a brand-switching argument, in 1983 the tobacco industry would have spent about $346 for every smoker who switched brands at the same time that the after-tax profit generated by the average smoker was about $80.00, thereby resulting in significant monetary losses (Tye et al., 1987); and (4) expenditures for cigarette advertising in magazines with large young male and female readerships are high (Davis, 1987; Hutchings, 1982). In addition, several studies have found that adolescents are quite aware of specific cigarette advertisements and of the promotional tactics used by tobacco companies to support sporting and other promotional events (Chapman & Fitzgerald, 1982; Goldstein, Fisher, Richards, & Creten, 1987; Ledwith, 1984).

Warning Labels

Cigarette warning labels have been required on packages since 1964 and illustrate that cigarettes are one of the only consumer products in which "correct" use, that is, smoking, leads to harmful effects. Citing FTC data, Syme and Alcalay (1982) report that less than 3% of all adults exposed to warning labels on cigarettes actually read them. These data suggest that warning labels may not have much of a direct effect on smoking behavior, and it is unclear whether the rotating labels now used on cigarette packages are more or less likely to be noticed. It is conceivable, however, that labels, along with a variety of other influences in the regulatory and policy context, contribute to a norm that smoking is undesirable and unhealthy.

Interestingly, the tobacco industry uses the warning labels to their advantage in liability suits. In essence, tobacco industry attorneys have argued successfully that labels provide sufficient warning to consumers about the potential dangers of tobacco use. Basically, the industry argues that smoking is a matter of free choice and personal responsibility. In a document on tobacco litigation, Philip Morris representatives suggest that one of the fundamental issues raised by tobacco litigation cases centers around "the implications for society of permitting recovery for injuries allegedly caused by products with claimed risks that are well-known" (Murray Bring, Senior Vice President and General Counsel, Philip Morris Companies, Inc., personal communication, August 30, 1988).

Promotion

Promotion of cigarettes in social, educational, artistic, and athletic events is also a major activity of the tobacco industry and is important to the tobacco industry's efforts to attract new smokers and maintain brand loyalty among current ones (Davis, 1987; Warner et al., 1986a). Citing data from the FTC, Davis (1987) notes that promotional expenditures (e.g., promotional allowances, sampling distribution, distribution bearing name, distribution not bearing name, public entertainment) have increased rapidly, from 26% in 1975 to 48% in 1984, in comparison to advertising expenditures. These data may represent a subtle change in the tactics of tobacco advertisers away from obvious promotional strategies to more subtle ones.

It is estimated that corporate sponsors invest hundreds of millions of dollars in special-event promotions with a yield in terms of audience exposure in the billions of dollars (Felgner, 1987). Examples of such promotions include the Virginia Slims tennis tournaments, Winston rodeo series, Marlboro country music series, Kool Jazz Festival, John Player Special motor racing, Kool Achiever Awards (for adults who improve the quality of inner-city communities), Philip Morris sponsorship of national art exhibits and museums, and the omnipresent cigarette billboards in stadiums and public arenas.

Philip Morris sponsors a writing contest with a $15,000 first prize that asks people to write an essay "that explores and questions censorship of expression . . . that defines and defends the First Amendment's application to American business; and that specifically questions the ramifications of a tobacco advertising ban on the future of free expression in a free market economy." RJR–Nabisco alone sponsors over 1600 events each year and is so committed to sponsorship that it created RJRN Golf as a separate business unit within the company (Felgner, 1987). As a sign of the importance of promotion, *Sport* magazine in 1988 awarded Philip Morris with a grand prize for its creativity in sports marketing for its Virginia Slims and Marlboro campaigns. There have been several reports of cigarette companies distributing free cigarettes to youth as young as elementary school students (Davis & Jason, 1988; Whelan, Sheridan, Meister, & Mosher, 1981).

The head of the Smokeless Tobacco Institute outlined the importance of tobacco company promotions and provided a perspective different from that taken by tobacco control advocates:

> Few industries I know of have compiled a more impressive record of economic, scientific, social and cultural contributions to American life than ours. You can't go to

a museum, attend a rodeo, NASCAR race, fishing tournament or other special event—sporting or cultural—without benefitting from the tobacco industry's continuing commitment to these American traditions. (Kerrigan, 1988, p. 21)

The effects of these promotions on the knowledge and attitudes of children and adolescents were examined in the United Kingdom (Aitken, Leathar, & Squair, 1986). The authors report that most children understand the concept of sponsorship, and many are actually able to associate specific brands with sponsored sports by the time they are in late elementary and early junior high school. In a 1987 column in the San Francisco Chronicle, Glenn Dickey noted some of the economic, political, and ethical challenges that the Women's International Tennis Association (WITA) faces as it considers dropping from cigarette company sponsorship. The issues he raises with regard to women's tennis certainly apply to other athletic, musical, and social events:

- The contract. The cigaret[te] company has the right to match any other offer that is made for sponsorship, which makes it very difficult for the tennis association to sell to another company . . .
- The fragile nature of the women's tennis association. Women's tennis has prospered partially because their organization, unlike the men's, has been very tightly organized. . . . They have put together strict rules about participation in tournaments, and they have prohibited players from participating in exhibitions at the time of a sanctioned tournament.
- Loyalty. Those who have been involved for a long time with women's tennis, either playing or in an executive role—or both—remember that the cigaret[te] company financed the tour at a time when no other sponsor would touch it. . . . The cigaret[te] company is so tied to women's tennis that people refer to the tournament by the company's name. What sponsor would willingly give up that kind of identification? (Dickey, 1987, p. 51)

The Affect of the 1971 Ban on Television and Radio Cigarette Advertising

During the years 1967 to 1970, television and radio broadcasters were required under the FCC Fairness Doctrine to donate air time to antismoking media in order to balance advertising sponsored by the tobacco industry. The FCC ruled that the ratio of antismoking ads to smoking ads had to be no less than one to five (Abernethy & Teel, 1986). The effects of the resulting media antismoking campaign showed that it was effective in countering tobacco advertising (Hamilton, 1972; Teel, Teel, & Bearden, 1979; Warner, 1986a; Warner et al., 1986a). One analysis suggests that the antismoking messages reduced per capita consumption about two times as much as cigarette advertising increased it (Hamilton, 1972). An econometric study by Lewitt, Coate, and Grossman (1982) (reviewed by Warner et al., 1986a) suggests that the advertising ban reduced the teenage smoking prevalence rate by 0.6% from 1970 to 1974.

When legislation was passed in 1971 banning tobacco advertising on television and radio, antismoking advocates hoped that per capita consumption of cigarettes would fall sharply. Interestingly, however, overall per capita consumption did not start dropping until the mid-1970s. One explanation was the effectiveness of the antismoking campaign, that is, the banning of tobacco ads on television and radio, which eliminated any rights to equal broadcast time for health messages (except for public service announcements), produced a dramatic increase in tobacco advertising and promotion expenditures in other venues (e.g., outdoor, magazines, sponsorship of events) and may have contributed to an increase in the overall consumption of tobacco products (Teel et al., 1979). The ban, then, may not have accomplished what health advocates had hoped; indeed, a major effect was to reduce access of antismoking advocates to public media (Teel et al., 1979). Moreover, because print media readerships are more loyal than television viewers and it is more cost-effective to deliver messages through print channels than through broadcast channels, the ban may have benefited the tobacco industry (Teel et al., 1979). Teel et al. (1979) go on to suggest that the ban, by diverting tobacco advertising money to print media, may be the primary explanation for the appearance, growth, and economic prosperity of special-interest magazines as well as newspapers.

Since the early 1960s, antismoking compaigns, events, and messages have occurred in numerous forums—broadcast media, narrowcast media (pamphlets, brochures, flyers, etc.), and community events. In an analysis of the effects of the overall antismoking campaign (beginning with the Surgeon General's report in 1964), Warner illustrates that in the absence of this broad-based campaign, per capita consumption of cigarettes would have been 20 to 30% higher by 1975 and 40% higher by 1978 (Warner, 1977, 1981).

In recent years there has been an effort in the U.S. to extend the broadcast ban of cigarettes to all forms of advertising and promotion, not just to radio and television. There is precedence for this action in that Canada, Norway, Finland, Iceland, and Singapore have already passed such legislation (Sternberg, 1988). The Canadian law, passed in 1988 (Tobacco Products Control Act), bans all tobacco advertisements in newspapers, magazines, and at point-of-purchase, prohibits promotion of tobacco in sporting or cultural events, and requires the tobacco industry to include a listing of the health hazards of tobacco on each package.

Experiences in Norway suggest that a total ban on cigarette advertising and promotion, as *one* component of a broad-based tobacco control effort, may be an effective strategy for preventing the adoption of smoking (Lochsen, Bjartveit, Hauknes, & Aaro, 1983). The campaign in Norway includes a ban on all advertising as well as other strategies designed to restrict smoking (e.g., establishment of governmental bodies dealing with smoking, intensification of public education efforts, use of mass media). The data indicate that in the absence of this national effort, smoking rates would have been 23% higher over about a 20-year period.

Short of a total advertising and promotion ban in this country, other options exist (Warner et al., 1986). These include allowing only tombstone advertising (e.g., restricting ad content to pictures of cigarette packages or the brand name, and disallowing models, slogans, scenes, or colors); strict enforcement of an advertising and promotion code to remove false and misleading imagery; counteradvertising paid for by the federal excise tax or tobacco company contributions; changes in tax laws to eliminate tax deductions for cigarette advertising and promotion expenditures; and banning ads in magazines and other outlets with large youth exposure.

Media Practices Relative to Modeling of Smoking

The modeling of smoking behavior also occurs widely in television and movies, although it is less recognizable than advertising and promotion in print media. The promotion of tobacco in motion pictures is increasingly a problem, even in movies directed to children and adolescents (Tobacco and Youth Reporter, 1988c). While the prevalence of smoking actors is less now than it was during the period from the 1930s to the 1960s, it is still an important issue to many tobacco control advocates.

Cruz and Wallack (1986) conducted a content analysis of routine prime time television shows in the fall of 1984 (116 hours of programming) and found that there was about one act of smoking during each hour of programming, almost two thirds of the smokers were lead characters, males were three times more likely to be smoking than females, and 70% of smokers were in "strong or enduring roles" (as opposed to "bad or outside the law"). Moreover, there was only one instance in which the potential desire to quit smoking was portrayed. The rate of smoking acts per hour varied by the type of television show as follows: situation comedies, .36; movies made for TV, .83; dramas, 1.01; movies made for theatres, 1.62. This study illustrates vividly the social norms surrounding smoking among television writers, producers, and actors.

In the movie industry, related incidents have been reported. Evidence that consumer products advertised implicitly in movies results in increased sales is evident from the movie *ET*, in which the promotion of Reese's Pieces® candy resulted in an 85% increase in sales. In the movie *Superman II*, Philip Morris paid to have Marlboro displayed prominently throughout the movie. In the Walt Disney movie *Baby*, the lead character is a smoker (Tobacco and Youth Reporter, 1986, p. 11). And finally, smoking was associated with God in the adolescent movie *Two of a Kind*, in which, for example, one of God's assistants drives a bus with a huge Camel cigarette advertisement on the side. The promotion of cigarettes in movies is planned and strategic rather than coincidental. While the effects of these promotions on actual smoking behavior are difficult to determine, they contribute along with other advertising and promotional strategies to a norm that smoking is desirable.

While tobacco advertising and promotion in print and electronic media contribute significantly to shaping public attitudes and behaviors toward tobacco, it is not the only source of influence. Coverage of smoking in the popular press is also a key medium through which tobacco messages are disseminated. The next section of the chapter illustrates how the popular press covers smoking and health.

Self-Censorship in the Popular Press

There is now a great deal of evidence that magazines accepting cigarette advertisements are less likely to cover tobacco and health issues (Warner, 1985; Warner & Goldenhar, 1989; Weis & Burke, 1986). Popular women's magazines that accept cigarette advertisements generally do not cover the harmful effects of tobacco. It is not an issue of these magazines not being interested in health-related topics, as they do cover nutrition, stress, contraception, and mental health (Warner, 1985; Whelan et al., 1981). In fact, these magazines cover these nonsmoking health topics from 12 to 63 times more than they cover smoking. For example, analysis of 12 women's magazines during a 12-year period from 1967 to 1979 found that the mean number of antismoking or smoking cessation articles published per year was 2 (range 0 to 11). In contrast, these magazines ran an average of 4.5 articles on stress, 8.6 on nutrition, 9.3 on contraceptives, and 21.5 on mental health (Whelan et al., 1981). The one magazine that did not accept cigarette advertising, *Good Housekeeping*, ran a total of 11 articles on smoking during this time period. The blatant inattention to the hazards of smoking was evident in several articles appearing in these magazines. One of these, entitled "The ABC's of Preventive Medicine," ran through the alphabet providing health advice for each letter. Smoking or tobacco was not mentioned. Another article entitled "Seventy-Six Ways to Save Your Life" did not suggest quitting smoking (Whelan et al., 1981). The March 1987 issue of *Working Mother* magazine had as the lead story "What Every Pregnant Woman Should Know" and discussed healthy foods and preparing for a safe delivery. It did not mention that pregnant women should not smoke, and it included six full pages of cigarette advertising (Tobacco and Youth Reporter, 1988a). The lack of attention by many popular magazines to the potential health effects of smoking data fly in the face of the Surgeon General and other health professionals who have noted that smoking is the single most preventable cause of premature death and disability.

One of the more interesting cases of censorship appeared in *Newsweek* magazine (Warner, 1985). In the November 7, 1983 supplement on "Personal Health Care" prepared by the American Medical Association with support from the magazine, the article noted that the supplement provided information on good health from the most dependable source, the medical profession. It would discuss "the most important things" related to health. It then went on to devote 16 full pages to diet, exercise, weight control, and stress and gave smoking coverage in only four sentences, none of which identified it as a health hazard. In the same issue, the magazine had 12 pages of cigarette advertisements worth about $1 million in revenue. When questioned about the lack of attention to smoking, *Newsweek* responded: "we naturally share concerns regarding smoking . . . but hope that you understand that there is just not enough space sometimes to do justice to all subjects involved" (Warner, 1985). As one could imagine, there was considerable uproar among health professionals about this attitude, enough so that in October 1984, *Newsweek* published a brief but strong statement about the negative effects of smoking. This issue of *Newsweek* contained only four cigarette advertisements.

More recently, the August 15, 1988 issue of *Newsweek* had a cover article that explored the "medical mystery" of miscarriages. The article failed to mention cigarette smoking as a potential cause even though one of the four rotating Surgeon General warnings states: "Smoking by pregnant women may result in fetal injury, premature birth, and low birth weight" (Tobacco and Youth Reporter, 1988b). In fact, a Marlboro ad in this issue of *Newsweek* had this warning label printed on it!

When magazines that accept cigarette advertisements cover the smoking and health issue, the tobacco industry plays hardball. The magazine *Mother Jones* is a case in point. When it decided to run a series of articles on smoking, the tobacco advertisers dropped their ads permanently and almost put the magazine out of business (Whelan et al., 1981). Clearly, journalists, magazines, and publishers are placed in a difficult economic position if they decide to cover the smoking and health topic without the support of the majority of other magazines. Smaller magazines with less financial stability are at even greater risk of bankruptcy if their income from cigarette advertisements is lost (Warner, 1985).

The tobacco industry has positioned itself and its policies as standing for freedom of speech. The research cited above and the related issues raised in the next few paragraphs illustrate that freedom of speech is compromised by tobacco industry efforts to censor coverage of smoking and health.

One of the most disturbing cases related to censorship is the 1988 decision by RJR–Nabisco to fire its longtime advertising agency, Saatchi & Saatchi DFS Inc., after the agency prepared a television ad for Northwest Airlines showing passengers applauding the airline's decision to ban smoking on all flights. The

Nabisco account, which had been held by Saatchi & Saatchi for 16 years and was worth $84 million, sent a clear message to advertising and other businesses that the tobacco industry will exert its considerable economic strength to protect its product. As tobacco companies continue to purchase nontobacco companies (e.g., General Foods, Del Monte, Nabisco, Kraft), this influence will become greater and more worrisome to tobacco control advocates and others interested in an honest presentation of the facts on smoking and health.

Censorship in research is a related problem to self-censorship in the popular press. From 1954 to 1986, the Council for Tobacco Research, an industry-sponsored organization, provided over $110 million to 600 "independent" scientists for almost 1000 research projects (Anonymous, 1987b). The industry cites this support of research as an example of its unbiased attitude toward the effects of tobacco. Not surprisingly, the tobacco industry fails to acknowledge the 50,000-plus studies linking tobacco use to ill health. In essence, their research program, which now focuses predominantly on basic science far removed from smoking and health, has a public relations goal rather than a scientific one (Tye, Townsley, & Hanks, 1988).

Another related censorship issue emanates from California, where the tobacco industry spent over $16 million dollars in an attempt to defeat a 1988 state proposition that would increase the state tax on tobacco by 25 cents, with the money being used in part to support health education and research (the tobacco industry lost, 58 to 42%, despite spending so much money and hiring George Bush's advertising media wizard Roger Ailes. In expensively produced television ads and slick, mass-distributed newspaper-like publications sent out to various groups in California, the tobacco industry claimed the following: "Prop 99 means more crime . . . ;" "Wealthy doctors profit at expense of California taxpayers;" and "Proposition 99 fuels gang violence warns law enforcement."

The main point to this discussion is how censorship may affect consumers' smoking-related knowledge, attitudes, and ultimately behaviors. Survey data indicate that the typical citizen in this country does not know about the specific health risks of smoking (literature reviewed in Shiffman, 1986; Warner, 1985). The conventional belief is that both smokers and nonsmokers are well aware of the dangers of smoking. How can they not be, when each package of cigarettes is labeled with a warning describing some of the dangers, and the U.S. Surgeon General issues routine reports summarizing the health hazards of tobacco use?

Survey data about the knowledge of smoking, however, suggest an alternative viewpoint (Shiffman, 1986; Warner, 1986b). Most people recognize that smoking causes cancer. This knowledge, however, appears to be superficial—many do not realize that smoking reduces life expectancy, is the *principal* cause of lung cancer, and that lung cancer is usually fatal. Moreover, knowledge that smoking is related to heart disease, chronic obstructive lung disease, and problems during pregnancy is "soft" (Warner, 1986b). A 1984 Harris poll found that, although experts rated smoking cessation as the best thing to do to improve health, the public rated it at the bottom of a list of 10 options, below even taking vitamins and minerals (Shiffman, 1986). National survey data suggest further that one third of American adolescents do not believe that smoking poses a great risk to their health (Johnston et al., 1987). In summary, Warner notes that smoking is rated by the public as a threat on a par with toxic dumps, saccharine, and obesity, and that smokers do not personalize the threats of smoking. In an environment of responsible media coverage of the health risks of smoking, it is probable that fewer people would adopt smoking and more people would quit smoking (Warner, 1985).

As reviewed in the previous sections, smoking behavior is influenced by advertising and promotion, and by coverage of smoking and health in the popular press. As with any consumer product, however, use of the product is in part influenced by its cost. In the case of tobacco, its cost to consumers is influenced by state and federal tobacco taxes. The effects of these taxes are reviewed in the next section.

Taxation of Cigarettes

The taxation of cigarettes is regulated federally and by states (DHHS, 1987). As of 1987, North Carolina had the lowest tax rate per pack (2 cents) while Maine had the highest (28 cents). Including North Carolina, there are five states with tax rates between 2 and 8 cents (the other four are Kentucky, South Carolina, Virginia, and Wyoming). In contrast, eight states (including Maine) have tax rates above 25 cents per pack (Connecticut, Hawaii, Iowa, Massachusetts, New Jersey, Oregon, and Wisconsin are the others). Across all states, taxes averaged 31% of the average retail price (1984 figures). This is down considerably from the 1965 figure of 51% and down from the average of over 40% for each year between 1954 and 1976. Only four states prohibit the sale of clove cigarettes (Florida, Idaho, Nevada, and New Mexico).

The tax rates on cigarettes and the impact on the retail price of a pack of cigarettes are strongly related to smoking behavior. Warner (1986c) estimates that an 8-cent decrease in the federal cigarette excise tax would encourage about one million young people aged 12 to 25, and several hundred thousand adults to become smokers. Conversely, an 8- to 16-cent increase in the tax would encourage 1 to 2 million young people, and 800,000 to 1.5 million adults to either quit or not take up the habit. Sensitivity to cigarette prices is inversely related to age, due in part to the fact that young people tend to be less addicted to nicotine and on average have less disposable income than older adults (Warner, 1986c). Thus increasing the price of cigarettes through increasing taxes on tobacco may be one of the most effective ways to prevent or stop smoking among large groups of people, especially those under the age of 25. This strategy is a persuasive example of the effects that regulatory and policy variables have on individual behavior.

Income generated by taxes on tobacco can be earmarked specifically for health-related research or for school health education programs. Unfortunately, however, only six states use money generated from taxes on tobacco to support health-related programs (Alaska, Idaho, Kentucky, Louisiana, Nebraska, and New Jersey). Moreover, only 18 states require elementary and secondary schools to instruct students on the dangers of tobacco, and only 3 states implement in-service training programs for school staff on the effects of tobacco (DHHS, 1987).

The author knows of no empirical data examining the effects on smoking behavior, or on social norms of earmarking tobacco taxes to health-related research or school health education programs. The topic seems ripe for investigation, and perhaps the 1989 enactment of Proposition 99 in California (a 25-cent increase in the tax on tobacco), and the earmarking of some of these funds for health education, will allow for an interesting case study. An interpretation of current state policies toward this issue is that the minimal state support for health concerns sets a tone that could influence social norms. Moreover, it would be interesting to examine whether states that use tobacco tax revenue for health research and intervention programs would, overall, be committing more money to negating the negative health effects of tobacco than states that do not use tax revenue for these purposes.

One policy alternative is to earmark a few pennies of the federal excise tax on tobacco for an antismoking media campaign. One penny per pack would generate about $300 million in annual revenue, enough for a sizeable campaign. For the typical smoker who consumes a pack and a half per day, this would add about $5.50 more each year to the cost of cigarettes. If 5 cents were earmarked, $1.5 billion would be generated, and each smoker would pay about $27 each year (Warner, 1986b). Warner (1986a) noted persuasively:

> The beauty of this proposal, in addition to its independence from tobacco advertising per se, is that the revenue to combat tobacco use would shrink automatically as the campaign worked and hence as the need for it diminished: as tobacco use fell, the tax yield would decrease proportionally. The campaign would self-destruct as Americans ceased their self-destructive tobacco habits.

Federal income tax policy also relates to smoking (at least under tax laws in the early 1980s). An interesting medical tax deduction allowed by the Internal Revenue Service is for meals and lodging provided during treatment for substance abuse (drugs, alcohol). The IRS does not allow, however, deductions for smoking cessation programs (or other preventive measures) (Syme & Alcalay, 1982).

Smoking behavior is influenced both by consumer demand and by tobacco supply. The next section of the chapter focuses on the supply of tobacco. In particular, it examines how access to tobacco by minors affects smoking behavior.

Access to Cigarettes by Minors

Access to cigarettes is a critical determinant of whether people (particularly children and adolescents) experiment with or maintain smoking behaviors. Since few smokers begin smoking after high school (Johnston et al., 1987), and one third to two thirds of adolescents who smoke two or more cigarettes in their lifetimes become habitual smokers (Benowitz, 1988), efforts to prevent the adoption of smoking must focus on preventing children and adolescents from becoming addicted. One way to do this is to limit their access to tobacco. Unfortunately, minors currently have easy access to tobacco (Altman, Foster, Rasenick-Douss, & Tye, 1989; Anonymous, 1988c; Forester, Klepp, & Jeffery, 1989; Kirn, 1987; Naidoo & Platts, 1985; Stanwick, Fish, Manfreda, Gelskey, & Skuba, 1987).

There is wide variability in how states define minors. Ten states do not regulate the sale to or use of tobacco to minors (Colorado, Georgia, Kentucky, Louisiana, Montana, New Hampshire, New Mexico, Virginia, Wisconsin, and Wyoming), and two states permit its towns, cities, and municipalities to enact such ordinances (Missouri, South Dakota). Hawaii defines a minor as anyone under the age of 15, while Utah and Alabama are the most restrictive with minors being those under the age of 19. The percentage breakdown states use to define minor status is as follows: no age, 20%; age 15, 2%; age 16, 20%; age 17, 8%; age 18, 46%; age 19, 4% (DHHS, 1987).

Access to cigarettes for adults has been treated by states in some rather strange ways. For example, in South Carolina, cigarettes confiscated from dealers who failed to pay taxes are donated to mental patients residing in state facilities. Conversely, it is a misdemeanor to sell tobacco to reformatory inmates in the state of New Jersey. And as a measure of the power of nicotine addiction (or of prison officials!), prison officials in Pennsylvania and Kentucky have the authority to grant or withhold cigarettes from inmates so as to control inmate behavior (DHHS, 1987).

Enforcing existing laws regulating access to cigarettes among underage youth has recently become a key strategy in the armamentarium of tactics used by tobacco control advocates. A large study conducted in 441 California stores found that minors could purchase cigarettes over-the-counter in 73% of stores and from 100% of vending machines. Tobacco was available in a wide variety of store types. After a 6-month community and merchant education campaign, minors were only able to purchase cigarettes in 39% of stores (and 100% of vending machines) (Altman et al., 1989). These educational programs, combined with legislative and regulatory approaches (e.g., requiring a license to sell tobacco, banning the sale of tobacco vending machines, increasing enforcement of access laws, and strengthening the penalties for selling tobacco to minors), could do much to reduce this problem (Altman et al., 1989; DiFranza, Norwood, Garner, & Tye, 1987). The social norms surrounding cigarette access can encourage the adoption of smoking behavior among underage youth. As an example of the extent of this problem, tobacco industry reports acclaim in headlines that "Drug Chains Evolve into Today's Smokeshops" and "Suppliers See Gold in C-Store [convenience store] Tobacco Sales" (Anonymous, 1988a, p. 42). In the case of convenience stores, sales of cigarettes have increased dramatically in recent years—from 17.5% of sales in 1980 to 34% in 1988. Excluding gasoline, tobacco products are the number-one-selling category in convenience stores (Orr, 1988b).

In contrast to the lack of attention given to laws around tobacco access, many communities have taken a keen interest in regulating smoking in public settings.

Regulation of Smoking in Public Settings

The regulation of smoking in public places has become a principal strategy in the tobacco control movement. According to Americans for NonSmokers' Rights, an advocacy group in California, there now exist about 350 city and county ordinances restricting smoking in public places, and to date no nonsmokers' rights bill has been repealed. This group estimates that almost 50% of the population of California live in areas that protect the rights of nonsmokers (Bureau of National Affairs [BNA], 1986). A review of each state's limitations on smoking in public places is contained in DHHS (1987). In a nationwide Gallup poll conducted in the mid-1980s, 88% of all respondents and 80% of respondents who smoked thought that some type of worksite smoking policy was advantageous, although only 12 and 4% respectively thought that smoking should be banned (BNA, 1986).

Examples of nonsmokers rights' policies include the Interstate Commerce Commission restricting smoking to the back 30% of buses, the Civil Aeronautics Board requiring airplanes to provide nonsmoking areas, the recent ban of smoking on flights of less than 2 hours, and many cities and counties banning smoking in public places (e.g., by 1986 in California, over 73 cities had passed ordinances restricting smoking in workplaces) (BNA, 1986; Glantz & Stromberg, 1988; McManus, Taylor, & Patrick, 1988). The nonsmokers' rights movement has even extended into casinos—traditional havens of smoking. Caesar's Casino in Lake Tahoe Nevada advertises their Cleopatra Casino, the "world's only nonsmoking casino."

As just one example of the powerful effect of social norms, when a large worksite in the northwest passed a smoking ban, 8% of smokers quit, consumption of cigarettes among smokers decreased by six cigarettes per day, and the percentage of smokers attending smoking cessation programs at the worksite increased thirteenfold (Martin, 1987, personal communication). It is unlikely that the cost-effectiveness of a skills training worksite intervention would be better than a smoking ban. However, the ban worked synergistically with personal and group smoking cessation interventions, with the overall effect being greater than those for a ban or smoking classes alone.

The tobacco industry has been aggressive in its attempts to influence public opinion about nonsmokers' rights. In 1983, for example, the tobacco industry spent over $1 million in an effort to prevent passage of a San Francisco ordinance regulating smoking in the workplace. This was 15 times more than what was spent by groups supporting the ordinance (Martin & Silverman, 1986; McManus et al., 1988). The tobacco industry lost the battle as the ordinance passed narrowly (50.4% to 49.6%).

Government Price Supports of the Tobacco Industry

Price supports for tobacco have historically been high in order to ensure that farmers' profits from growing tobacco exceeded profits from other crops. Due to intense world competition and higher prices of U.S.-grown tobacco, by 1984 there were over 1.4 billion pounds of tobacco stored in warehouses throughout the U.S. In effect, the price support program, by preventing a free market, maintained the price of tobacco at artificial levels and caused public relation problems for the government in the sense that they were paying for a product that caused health problems for which they also had to pay indirectly (e.g., through Medicare and disability insurance).

It is likely that government policy keeps the price of raw tobacco grown in this country higher than the world market, thereby limiting supply. Leigh and Gonzalez (1987) suggest that the artificial inflation of tobacco prices through price supports may actually promote public health because consumption is inversely related to price. Even so, it is ironic that the government pays for such a public health nuisance, and as Warner (1988) notes, these subsidies may serve to promote tobacco use, be it indirectly, through their influence on tobacco decisions made by politicians. He suggests that subsidies illustrate the ambivalence of the U.S. government toward tobacco and, because of their high visibility, may diminish the effectiveness of tobacco control programs funded or supported by the government.

The tobacco industry not only receives widespread legislative support for tobacco subsidies but also for a variety of other issues that come before Congress. A partial explanation of support of the tobacco industry lies in the financial contributions of the industry to politicians. In an article published in *The Nation*, Corn (1987) states that Senator Robert Dole has become the "point man" for the tobacco industry, despite the fact that tobacco is not grown in his home state of

Kansas. Corn suggests that Dole's support of the tobacco industry can be traced to campaign contributions and honoraria financed by the tobacco industry, Dole's desire to become majority leader (and his need for support from Jesse Helms and other legislators from tobacco states), his interest in maintaining a Republican majority in the Senate, and corporate gifts made to a tax-exempt charitable organization for the disabled that was established by Dole.

In an analysis of Congressional voting patterns for an amendment to the 1985 farm bill that would abolish the federal tobacco price support program, Haas and Marek (1987) report that legislators who voted protobacco received almost three times the amount of money from tobacco industry PACs than did legislators who voted antitobacco. The magnitude of tobacco industry contributions to legislators is large. For example, in one year Philip Morris contributed over $613,000 to members of Congress (Haas & Marek, 1987).

Another variable to consider in this regard is the amount of money the government spends on smoking prevention and cessation efforts compared to the contribution that smoking makes to the overall health care burden. While the discrepancy appears to be narrowing, it has a long way to go. In 1987, for example, the U.S. Public Health Service spent $45 million on smoking control programs and research, as compared to the $2.4 billion the tobacco industry spent in 1986 advertising and promoting its product. Given that cigarette smoking is the single most important contributor to death and disease, $45 million is hardly enough money to understand and control tobacco use (cf. Cormier, Prefontaine, Mac-Donald, & Stuart, 1980). In terms of economics, the tobacco industry wields the strength of Goliath while the tobacco control advocates have resources consistent with David. As highlighted throughout this chapter, however, there is more to tobacco policy and consumption than economics alone.

Any analysis of the economic effects of tobacco must be carefully conducted. As Warner (1987) notes, reducing or eliminating tobacco-related disease would alter dramatically the health and social welfare systems and would probably have less of an economic effect than is thought by both sides of the debate—the huge savings cited by the tobacco control movement and the huge costs cited by the tobacco industry. Moreover, Warner identifies serious limitations in the commonly taken positions of tobacco and antitobacco groups with respect to the economic effects of tobacco use. Warner concludes by suggesting that the major effect of a tobacco-free society is not necessarily an economic one. Rather, it is an improved quality and quantity of life.

SUMMARY

Smoking control interventions presently focus predominantly on increasing the skills of smokers (e.g., to quit or prevent relapse) and the skills of nonsmokers at risk of smoking (e.g., social resistance skills training to decrease the effects of peer pressure to smoke). Great progress has been made in the design and implementation of these interventions, and they should certainly be part of any tobacco control effort. That over one quarter of the population still smokes (with higher rates among subgroups) and the best cessation programs generally do not achieve more than a 25% sustained quit rate indicates that the tobacco control movement still has much to accomplish. In this chapter, we outline some of the regulatory and policy factors that may affect smoking behavior and suggest that attention to these factors in the larger social context may advance efforts to prevent the initiation of tobacco use.

Relative to programs directed at individuals or groups, there are fewer examples of smoking control programs that address the influence of the larger social context. For example, few programs address the fact that youth have ready access to cigarettes in local stores; work with store merchants to enforce access laws already on the books; put pressure on their local newspapers, magazines, and billboard companies to ban tobacco advertising; pressure local government to pass nonsmokers' rights bills or ordinances; or encourage worksites to establish nonsmoking policies in public settings. The skills required to engage in such advocacy and policy research are not usually within the repertoire of professionals involved in community health promotion, although the American Cancer Society (1987a, b) has published the first manuals to specifically help people to learn these skills. It is likely that learning these advocacy skills would increase the effectiveness of other more traditional approaches to smoking prevention and cessation.

Another theme of this chapter is that smoking behavior and the settings in which such behavior occurs are interdependent. Recognizing this point would help tobacco control advocates attend to the settings in which tobacco use is most encouraged and salient (e.g., free distribution of cigarettes at neighborhood events, tobacco billboards in settings frequented by children, cigarette vending machines near schools). This is in contrast to the traditional approach, which assumes that the physical and policy environments are background variables to the beliefs and behaviors of individuals.

Attending to the influence of the social context on smoking behavior poses a number of challenges to researchers and interveners. First, it is difficult to partial out the relative contributions of multiple levels of influence on specific smoking-related knowledge, attitudes, and behaviors. Similarly, assessing the interrelationships and potential synergistic effects between levels is extremely difficult. While there are multivariate data analytic strategies that can model complex relationships such as these (e.g., LISREL), it is more than a statistical problem. The critical issue is how behavior is influenced by, and influences, multiple levels of analysis in a complex web of place and time. A thesis of this chapter is that smoking behavior cannot be understood adequately if it is viewed as influenced by personal-level variables alone, irrespective of where and when the behavior occurs or of the surrounding social context. In short, interventions that are effective at certain times, in certain settings, and with certain people may not be effective in other places, times, or with different people. If these assumptions about the multiple levels of influence on smoking behavior are accepted, then interventions designed to prevent the adoption or promote the cessation of smoking should ideally be designed with consideration of the social context.

The ideas in this chapter point to a number of future research questions in need of concentrated attention. First, the larger field of health psychology and the specific issues of adherence to health-related behaviors discussed throughout this book would benefit from incorporating a multilevel, social context perspective into research. In addition to simply cataloging and measuring variables in the larger social context, it is important to study how the different levels interact or link with each another through amplification or counteracting forces.

Second, methodological advances are needed. While the armamentarium of methodological tools to measure the social context of health phenomena is perhaps less developed than are the tools to measure intrapsychic variables, their development is essential to an adequate understanding of health-related behaviors. It is important to recognize that health behaviors do not occur within a contextual vacuum devoid of historical, current, and anticipated and unanticipated future events.

Third, health behavior researchers should reach out to other social and health scientists for complementary theories, concepts, and methodologies. In particular, researchers and practitioners interested in adherence would benefit enormously from examining and using theories and concepts beyond the personal and interpersonal levels of analysis (Winett et al., 1989). Using multilevel and contextually valid approaches could add further insights into the complex analysis of the influences on health-related behaviors such as smoking.

Much has been accomplished in the tobacco control movement, and there is reason to maintain optimism about future progress (Iglehart, 1986). The rate at which progress is made in reducing tobacco use and in understanding other health behaviors, however, is critically dependent upon attending to the influences of the larger social context.

REFERENCES

Abernethy, A. M., & Teel, J. E. (1986). Advertising regulation's effect upon demand for cigarettes. *Journal of Advertising, 15*(4), 51–55.

Aitken, P. P., Leathar, D. S., & Squair, S. I. (1986). Children's awareness of cigarette brand sponsorship of sports and games in the UK. *Health Education Research, 1*(3), 203–211.

Albright, C. L., Altman, D. G., Slater, M. D., & Maccoby, N. (1988). Cigarette advertisements in magazines: Evidence for a differential focus on women's and youth magazines. *Health Education Quarterly, 15*(2), 225–233.

Altman, D. G., Foster, V., Rasenick-Douss, L., & Tye, J. B. (1989). Reducing the illegal sale of cigarettes to minors. *Journal of the American Medical Association, 261*(1), 80–83.

Altman, D. G., & King, A. C. (1986). Approaches to compliance in primary prevention. *Journal of Compliance in Health Care, 1*(1), 55–73.

Altman, D. G., Slater, M. D., Albright, C. L., & Maccoby, N. (1987). How an unhealthy product is sold: Cigarette advertising in magazines, 1960–1985. *Journal of Communication, 37,* 95–106.

American Cancer Society. (1987a). *Smoke fighting.* New York: Author.

American Cancer Society. (1987b). *Smoke signals.* New York: Author.

American Public Health Association. (1987). Taxation of tobacco products: Advertising and promotion of tobacco products. *American Journal of Public Health, 77*(1), 102–103.

Anonymous. (1987a). Tobacco's record exports set trade balance example. *The Tobacco Observer, 12*(5), 1.

Anonymous. (1987b). Tobacco research council's grants exceed $110 million. *The Tobacco Observer, 12*(5), 5.

Anonymous. (1988a). Drug chains evolve into today's smokeshops. *United States Distribution Journal, 215*(4), 42.

Anonymous. (1988b). Minors easily buy tobacco. *DOC News and Views, Spring,* 10.

Bell, C. S., & Levy, S. M. (1984). Public policy and smoking prevention: Implications for research. In J. D. Matarazzo, S. M. Weiss, J. A. Herd, N. E. Miller, & S. M. Weiss (Eds.), *Behavioral health: A handbook of health enhancement and disease prevention* (pp. 775–785). New York: Wiley.

Benowitz, N. L. (1988). Pharmacologic aspects of cigarette smoking and nicotine addiction. *New England Journal of Medicine, 319*(2), 1318–1330.

Best, J. A., Thomson, S. J., Sanit, S. M., Smith, E. A., & Brown, K. S. (1988). Preventing cigarette smoking among school children. *Annual Review of Public Health, 9,* 161–201.

Botvin, G. J. (1986). Substance abuse prevention research: Recent developments and future directions. *Journal of School Health, 56*(9), 369–374.

Brownell, K. D., Marlatt, G. A., Lichtenstein, E., & Wilson, G. T. (1986). Understanding and preventing relapse. *American Psychologist, 41*(7), 765–782.

Bureau of National Affairs. (1986). *Where there's smoke: Problems and policies concerning smoking in the workplace.* Washington, DC: Author.

Chapman, S., & Fitzgerald, B. (1982). Brand preference and advertising recall in adolescent smokers: Some implications for health promotion. *American Journal of Public Health, 72*(5), 491–494.

Cormier, A., Prefontaine, M., MacDonald, H., & Stuart, R. B. (1980). Lifestyle change on the campus: Pilot test of a program to improve student health practices. In P. O. Davidson & S. M. Davidson (Eds.), *Behavioral medicine: Changing health lifestyles* (pp. 222–255). New York: Brunner/Mazel.

Corn, D. (1987). Bob Dole and the tobacco connection. *The Nation,* March 28, (1, 396–399).

Cruz, J., & Wallack, L. (1986). Trends in tobacco use on television. *American Journal of Public Health, 76*(6), 698–699.

Davis, R. M. (1987). Current trends in cigarette advertising and marketing. *New England Journal of Medicine, 316*(12), 725–732.

Davis, R. M., & Jason, L. A. (1988). The distribution of free cigarette samples to minors. *American Journal of Preventive Medicine, 4*(1), 21–26.

Davis, R. M., & Kendrick, J. S. (1989). The Surgeon General's warnings in outdoor cigarette advertising: Are they readable? *Journal of the American Medical Association, 261*(1), 90–94.

Department of Health and Human Services, Public Health Service. (1988). *The health consequences of smoking: Nicotine addiction: A report of the Surgeon General* (DHHS Publication No. CDC 88-8406). Washington, DC: U.S. Government Printing Office.

Dickey, G. (1987). Time for tennis to say no to cigaret ads. *San Francisco Chronicle,* February 17, p. 51.

DiFranza, J. R., Norwood, B. D., Garner, D. W., & Tye, J. B. (1987). Legislative efforts to protect children from tobacco. *Journal of the American Medical Association, 257,* 3387–3389.

Engel, G. L. (1977). The need for a new medical model: A challenge for biomedicine. *Science, 196,* 129–136.

Ernster, V. L. (1985). Mixed messages for women: A social history of cigarette smoking and advertising. *New York State Journal of Medicine, 85,* 335–340.

Evans, R. I. (1980). Behavioral medicine: A new applied challenge to social psychologists. In L. Bickman (Ed.), *Applied social psychology annual* (Vol. 1, pp. 279–305). Beverly Hills, CA: Sage.

Federal Trade Commission. (1985). *Report to Congress: Pursuant to the Federal Cigarette Labeling and Advertising Act 1984.* Washington, DC: U.S. Government Printing Office.

Federal Trade Commission. (1988). *Report to Congress: Pursuant to the Federal Cigarette Labeling and Advertising Act 1986.* Washington, DC: U.S. Government Printing Office.

Felgner, B. (1987). Marketers pursue special events for niche in consumer lifestyle. *United States Tobacco and Candy Journal, 214*(17), 16–18.

Foote, E. (1981). Advertising and tobacco. *Journal of the American Medical Association, 245,* 1667–1668.

Forester, J. L., Klepp, K. I., & Jeffery, R. W. (1989). Sources of cigarettes for tenth graders in two Minnesota cities. *Health Education Research, 4*(1), 45–50.

Glantz, S. A., & Stromberg, D. (1988). Public attitudes regarding smokefree airlines. *American Journal of Public Health, 78*(10), 1366.

Goldstein, A. O., Fischer, P. M., Richards, J. W., & Creten, D. (1987). Relationship between high school student smoking and recognition of cigarette advertisements. *Journal of Pediatrics, 110*(3), 488–491.

Green, L. W. (1986). Individuals vs. systems: An artificial classification that divides and distorts. *HealthLink,* September, 29–30.

Haas, E., & Marek, C. (1987, September). *Smoking them out: Tobacco dollars/tobacco votes.* Washington, DC: Public Voice for Food and Health Policy.

Hamilton, J. R. (1972). The demand for cigarettes: Advertising, the health scare, and the cigarette advertising ban. *Review of Economics and Statistics, 54,* 401–411.

Harken, L. S. (1987). The prevention of adolescent smoking: A public health priority. *Evaluation and the Health Professions, 10,* 373–393.

Hutchings, R. (1982). A review of the nature and extent of cigarette advertising in the

United States. In proceedings of the *National Conference on Smoking and Health: Developing a Blueprint for Action* (pp. 249-262). New York: American Cancer Society.

Iglehart, J. K. (1986). The campaign against smoking gains momentum. *New England Journal of Medicine, 314*(16), 1059-1064.

Iverson, D. C. (1987). Smoking control programs: Premises and promises. *American Journal of Health Promotion, 1*(3), 16-30.

Johnston, L. D., O'Malley, P. M., & Bachman, J. G. (1987). *National trends in drug use and related factors among American high school students and young adults, 1975-1986.* Washington, DC: National Institute on Drug Abuse.

Kirn, T. F. (1987). Laws ban minors' tobacco purchases, but enforcement is another matter. *Journal of the American Medical Association, 257,* 3323-3324.

Klepp, K. I., Halper, A., & Perry, C. L. (1986). The efficacy of peer leaders in drug abuse prevention. *Journal of School Health, 56*(9), 407-411.

Kuhn, A. (1975). *Unified social science: A system-based introduction.* Homewood, IL: Dorsey.

Ledwith, F. (1984). Does tobacco sports sponsorship on television act as advertising to children? *Health Education Journal, 43*(4), 85-88.

Leigh, J. P., & Gonzalez, R. A. (1987). Government policies toward tobacco growing promote health. *Journal of the American Medical Association, 258*(4), 471.

Lippman, M. (1986). The moral imperative to correct deceptive cigarette billboard ads. *Tobacco and Youth Reporter, 1*(1), 10.

Lochsen, P. M., Bjartveit, K., Hauknes, A., & Aaro, L. E. (1983). *Trends in Tobacco Consumption and Smoking Habits in Norway. Report of the Norwegian Council on Smoking and Health.* Presented at the fifth world conference on smoking and health, Winnipeg, Canada, July.

Martin, M. J., & Silverman, M. F. (1986). The San Francisco experience with regulation of smoking in the workplace: The first twelve months. *American Journal of Public Health, 76*(5), 585-586.

McManus, J., Taylor, C. B., & Patrick, C. (1988). *Community approaches to the prevention and cessation of smoking.* Palo Alto, CA: Health Promotion Resource Center, Stanford University.

Naidoo, J., & Platts, C. (1985). Smoking prevention in Bristol: Getting maximum results using minimum resources. *Health Education Journal, 44,* 39-42.

Orr, A. M. (1988a). Philip Morris uses tobacco cash to buy Kraft. *U.S. Distribution Journal, 215*(12), 6.

Orr, A. M. (1988b). Suppliers see gold in c-store tobacco sales. *U.S. Distribution Journal, 215*(12), 17.

Perry, C. L., Murray, D. M., & Klepp, K. I. (1987). Predictors of adolescent smoking and implications for prevention. *Morbidity and Mortality Weekly Review, 36*(4S), 41S-47S.

Schwartz, G. E. (1982). Testing the biopsychosocial model: The ultimate challenge facing behavioral medicine? *Journal of Consulting and Clinical Psychology, 50*(6), 1040-1053.

Schwartz, J. L. (1987). *Review and evaluation of smoking cessation methods: The United States and Canada, 1978-1985.* Washington, DC: U.S. Government Printing Office.

Seligman, D. (1987). Don't bet against cigarette makers. *Fortune,* August 17, 70-76.

Shiffman, S. (1986). Psychosocial factors in smoking and quitting: Health beliefs, self-efficacy, and stress. In J. K. Ockene (Ed.), *The pharmacologic treatment of tobacco dependence: Proceedings of the world congress, November 4-5, 1985* (pp. 48-62). Cambridge, MA: Institute for the Study of Smoking Behavior and Policy.

Stanwick, R. S., Fish, D. G., Manfreda, J., Gelskey, D., & Skuba, A. (1987). Where Manitoba children obtain their cigarettes. *Canadian Medical Association Journal, 137*, 405-408.

Stein, I. (1974). *Systems theory, science, and social work.* Metuchen, NJ: Scarecrow Press.

Sternberg, K. (1988). Canada severely limits means for conveying tobacco companies' messages to potential users. *Journal of the American Medical Association, 260*(17), 2480-2481.

Stoffman, D. (1987). Where there's smoke. *Report on Business Magazine, 4*(3), 20-28.

Stokols, D. (1980). The use of intrapersonal and contextual theories in social psychology. In R. F. Kidd & M. J. Saks (Eds.), *Advances in applied social psychology* (Vol. 1) (pp. 198-211). Hillsdale, NJ: Erlbaum.

Syme, S. L., & Alcalay, R. (1982). Control of cigarette smoking from a social perspective. *Annual Review of Public Health, 3*, 179-199.

Teel, S. J., Teel, J. E., & Beardon, W. O. (1979). Lessons learned from the broadcast cigarette advertising ban. *Journal of Marketing, 43*, 45-50.

Tobacco Institute. (1988). *Tobacco industry profile 1987.* Washington, DC: Author.

Tobacco and Youth Reporter. (1986). R. J. Reynolds reaches kids with "Moviegoer." *1*(1), 13-14.

Tobacco and Youth Reporter. (1988a). Cigarettes for a working mom. *3*(1), 8.

Tobacco and Youth Reporter. (1988b). Newsweek again censors smoking hazards. *3*(1), 8.

Tobacco and Youth Reporter. (1988c). Pushing smokes in kids' movies. *3*(1), 3.

Tye, J. B., Townsley, W. E., & Hanks, D. (1988). Tobacco industry research effort reveals corporate evil. *Tobacco and Youth Reporter, 3*(1), 10.

Tye, J. B., Warner, K. E., & Glantz, S. A. (1987). Tobacco advertising and consumption: Evidence for a causal relationship. *Journal of Public Health Policy, 8*(4), 492-508.

U.S. Department of Health and Human Services. (1987). *Smoking and health: A national status report. A report to Congress* (DHHS #87-8396). Washington, DC: U.S. Government Printing Office.

Warner, K. E. (1977). The effects of the anti-smoking campaign on cigarette consumption. *American Journal of Public Health, 67*(7), 645-650.

Warner, K. E. (1981). Cigarette smoking in the 1970s: The impact of the antismoking campaign on consumption. *Science, 211*, 729-731.

Warner, K. E. (1985). Cigarette advertising and media coverage of smoking and health. *New England Journal of Medicine, 312*(6), 384-388

Warner, K. E. (1986a). Selling health: A media campaign against tobacco. *Journal of Public Health Policy, 7*(4), 434-439.

Warner, K. E. (1986b). *Selling smoke: Cigarette advertising and public health.* Washington, DC: American Public Health Association.

Warner, K. E. (1986c). Smoking and health implications of a change in the federal cigarette excise tax. *Journal of the American Medical Association, 255*(8), 1028-1032.

Warner, K. E. (1987). Health and economic implications of a tobacco-free society. *Journal of the American Medical Association, 258*(15), 2080-2086.

Warner, K. E. (1988). The tobacco subsidy: Does it matter? *Journal of the National Cancer Institute, 80*(2), 81-83.

Warner, K. E., Ernster, V. L., Holbrook, J. H., Lewit, E. M., Pertschuk, M., Steinfeld, J. L., Tye, J. B., & Whelan, E. M. (1986a). Promotion of tobacco products: Issues and policy options. *Journal of Health Politics, Policy and Law, 11*(3), 367-392.

Warner, K. E., Ernster, V. L., Holbrook, J. H., Lewit, E. M., Pertschuk, M., Steinfeld, J. L., & Whelan, E. M. (1986b). Public policy on smoking and health: Toward a smoke-free generation by the year 2000—A statement of a working group to the subcommittee on smoking of the American Heart Association. *Circulation, 73*(2), 381A–395A.

Warner, K. E., & Goldenhar, L. M. (1989). The cigarette advertising broadcast ban and magazine coverage of smoking and health. *Journal of Public Health Policy, 10*(1), 32–42.

Weis, W. L., & Burke, C. (1986). Media content and tobacco advertising: An unhealthy addiction. *Journal of Communication, Autumn,* 59–69.

Whelan, E. M., Sheridan, M. J., Meister, K. A., & Mosher, B. A. (1981). Analysis of coverage of tobacco hazards in women's magazines. *Journal of Public Health Policy, 2,* 28–35.

Wicker, A. W. (1979). *An introduction to ecological psychology.* Monterey, CA: Brooks-Cole.

Winett, R. A., King, A. C., & Altman, D. G. (1989). *Health psychology and public health: An integrative approach.* New York: Pergamon Press.

Commentary: Individual and Environmental Constraints to Health Behavior Change

Jeffrey V. Johnson

Although the three articles in this section represent relatively distinct conceptual approaches to the examination of obstacles to life-style change, a common theme does emerge: Health behavior change frequently lies outside the simple volitional control of the individual. Moreover, implied in this position is a subtle critique of conventional behavior change strategies that place the major emphasis on reeducating the individual to transform his or her own behavior. According to the articles in this section, a cognitive-individualistic orientation ignores both the relatively unconscious physiological mechanisms that elicit and reinforce certain adverse health behaviors as well as elements in the environmental context or "behavioral setting" that serve to explain the formation and maintenance of life-style behavior.

Grunberg and Lord, in reviewing what little is known concerning the biological barriers to compliance and maintenance of healthy behaviors, point out that many individuals do not "do what is good for them" for a very simple reason: The unpleasant or even painful effects stemming from a change to positive health behaviors are often not compensated for by a subsequent increase in positive feelings or sensations. For example, in the case of smoking cessation, the authors note that an individual who stops smoking experiences immediate feelings of nicotine deprivation, combined with the loss of a valued aid to concentration, anxiety reduction, and appetite suppression. In other words, the negative physiological aspects of a major behavioral change often outweigh the relatively abstract concept of improved health. As Grunberg and Lord point out, ". . . the interference of health behaviors with enjoyable behaviors is not insurmountable. But the incompatible relationship of these behaviors and the intensity of the pleasures lost must be reckoned with and not ignored."

Coates and his colleagues address a rather different type of impediment to life-style change: the degree to which health care providers actively deal with the health behaviors of their patients. They point out that physicians are of strategic importance in the overall effort to encourage life-style change due both to their credibility and because they have regular contact with patients, especially during critical junctures when intervention might be most effective. However, many physicians do not consider life-style issues an integral part of their medical routine.

Coates et al. discuss their own intervention study, which provided training sessions to physicians on how to counsel their smoking patients on how to quit. Although the program appeared to be useful in improving the counseling ability of physicians, it was less successful in breaking down certain environmental barriers outside of the individual physician's control. No matter how motivated a physician might be in regard to changing his or her own medical practice to incorporate health behavior concerns, the structure of the workday often does not permit the time for such patient involvement. Moreover, as the authors note, the lack of reimbursement from insurance carriers for this type of prevention-orientated activity was another aspect of the overall context of a physician's practice that served to impede time reallocation.

The centrality of context to an understanding of health behavior change is the major focus of Altman's contribution to this section. According to Altman, there is currently a bias toward attributing human behavior to "personal or dispositional factors rather than to environmental or situational factors." However, in order to understand and change a behavior that is practiced by millions, such as smoking, a macrolevel strategy is necessary. Using smoking as an example, Altman provides a multilevel analysis of the social context of lapse and relapse and argues that societal-level influences such as regulatory activity, taxation, and advertising are probably of much greater importance than has previously been recognized.

As Altman notes, little research to date has focused on the linkage between social structure, behavioral settings, and individual health behavior. However, the relationship between the structure of the social environment and individual experience and behavior has been a classical theme in social science. Recently investigators have focused on specific behavioral settings, such as the workplace, that promote structured patterns of activity that contribute to adult socialization and learning (Frese, 1982). Research findings indicate that workers in jobs that permit occupational self-determination and control tend to take a more active and creative approach to life in general (Kohn & Schooler, 1982). By contrast, those with restricted possibilities for self-determination tend to exhibit a more inflexible and passive orientation (Karasek, 1981; Kohn & Schooler, 1983). Although this approach is only now being applied to the study of health behavior, there is some indication that those with constrained environments exhibit more adverse health behaviors (Johnson & Hall, 1989).

In conclusion, the chapters in this section provide a necessary reminder that change is usually more difficult and complex then we first anticipate. In the study of health behavior, we must be careful not to place too much of the burden of responsibility on the individual's conscious willingness to change while underestimating the effects of physiological impediments and situational and environmental constraints.

REFERENCES

Frese, M. (1982). Occupational socialization and psychological development: An underemphasized research perspective in industrial psychology. *Journal of Occupational Psychology, 55,* 209–224.

Johnson, J. V., & Hall, E. M. (in press). Social support in the work environment and cardiovascular disease. In S. Shumaker & S. Czajkowski (Eds.), *Social support and cardiovascular disease.* New York: Plenum Press.

Karasek, R. A. (1981). Job socialization and job strain: The implications of two related psychosocial mechanisms for job design. In B. Gardell & G. Johansson (Eds.), *Working life: A social science contribution to work reform* (pp. 75–93). London: Wiley.

Kohn, M., & Schooler, C. (1982). Reciprocal effects of the substantive complexity of work and intellectual flexibility: A longitudinal assessment. *American Journal of Sociology, 84,* 24–52.

Kohn, M., & Schooler, C. (1983). *Work and personality: An inquiry into the impact of social stratification.* Norwood, NJ: Albex.

SECTION IV

Life-Style Change and Adherence Issues within Specific Populations

Christine T. Parker, Editor

Theory and measurement of behavior change, life-style intervention and maintenance of behaviors, and obstacles to life-style changes and adherence have all been dealt with in prior sections of this volume. However, these sections have not addressed the potentially serious problems that present obstacles to adherence in specific populations. The chapters in this section describe adherence issues associated with minority populations, the young, and the elderly in an attempt to determine if specific subpopulations within the United States have unusual problems that negatively affect their ability to adhere to medical regimens.

In Chapter 14, Lewis and colleagues address health care utilization by minorities, describe a conceptual framework for consideration of health care patterns among minority patients, illustrate associations between sociocultural factors and adherence, and recommend treatment strategies that could improve adherence in minority patients. As the Black population is a significant minority in the United States, both in terms of size and in terms of morbidity and mortality, much of the chapter is devoted to cultural, economic, and sociological obstacles to adherence in this population. Lewis et al. describe research performed by the Howard University Center for Sickle Cell Disease on health care needs, perceptions of health care, and methods to improve adherence in young Blacks with sickle cell disease.

In Chapter 15, Aledort and colleagues describe determinants and correlates of adherence in the young that have been garnered from the literature. An examination of family therapy in chronic disease as a framework for improving patient adherence in the young is proffered; an adherence intervention for young hemophiliacs that is being tested at the Mount Sinai Medical Center is based on this model and is described in depth. Obstacles to research in the young are described and recommendations for future research identified.

In Chapter 16, Roth describes many of the problems the elderly face in adhering to medical regimens, particularly to medication regimens. Roth examines drug use in the elderly and the difficulty they exhibit with dosages of prescription drugs. He gives examples of adherence problems in common disorders in the elderly and describes adverse drug reactions and reasons for nonadherence in this population. Also, suggestions for improving adherence in this population are delineated.

The discussant for this section, Dr. Merwin Greenlick, takes an adversarial position in discussing the need to emphasize the problems in adherence of specific populations. His contention is that adherence problems are, for the most part, the same for all populations and that these problems stem more from lack of patient belief in the efficacy of treatment regimens than manipulation of the regimens themselves. Greenlick provides the refreshingly simple view that the problems facing adherence researchers are more a result of lack of empathy with patients in the design of interventions than from patient resistance to complying with regimens that will improve their health or extend their life spans. Although this view may have merit, reality may be that cultural differences and *access* by researchers to specific populations, or of these populations to health care, may influence adherence behaviors differentially.

The authors of these chapters have identified some potential causes for lack of adherence in specific populations that give researchers much food for thought.

In their description of minority populations, Lewis et al. present some interesting recommendations for future research with minority populations. Roth mentions some little-known factors that could have immense impact on the efficacy of interventions used with the elderly. Aledort et al. describe just a few of the plethora of problems associated with research on the young. And Greenlick takes a totally different tack on research by indicating that perhaps emphasizing differences among populations may not be as important as increasing patient belief in the efficacy of their treatment regimens. These chapters should provide researchers in the adherence field with much to discuss in development of their study methods.

14

Patient Adherence in Minority Populations

Deborah Lewis*, Faye Z. Belgrave,
Roland B. Scott

Adherence to medical treatment is a subject that continues to be widely discussed in health care facilities; however, health decision making in minority populations has received far less attention by investigators. By focusing on a research and clinical program conducted at the Howard University Center for Sickle Cell Disease (HUCSCD) in Washington, D.C., this chapter examines several aspects of minority health care utilization; describes a framework in which to consider health care patterns among minority patients; and illustrates factors that are associated with adherence patterns. Finally, this chapter presents recommendations related to treatment strategies. Because the Black population is the largest minority group in this country and comprises most of the participants studied in this project, observations and experiences related to this specific population will be the primary focus of discussion.

REVIEW OF THE LITERATURE

Although the compliance literature is inconsistent with respect to several issues, there is a consensus that minority populations in this society manifest dispro-

*Deborah Lewis is now a senior clinical psychologist at the National Rehabilitation Hospital.

portionately greater amounts of health problems and encounter unique obstacles when attempting to seek and use health care services (U.S. Dept. of Health and Human Services [DHHS], 1985a). This can be better understood when statistics of minority groups are compared with statistics for the rest of the population.

Morbidity and Mortality in Minority Populations

Although mortality rates are not a comprehensive measure of health status, a decrease in the death rate provides a good measure for assessing overall improvements in the health status of a population. In general, nonwhites have experienced greater decreases in mortality than whites (DHHS, 1985b); however, despite these decreases, nonwhites have a higher mortality rate. For example, in 1980 the mortality rate for nonwhites was 37.5% higher than for whites.

When the death rates of the Black population are assessed, the disparity is even more pronounced; life expectancy and infant mortality rates are good examples of this. In 1983, life expectancy reached a new high of 75.2 years for whites and 69.6 years for Blacks, a gap of 5.6 years. Blacks today have a life expectancy already reached by whites in the early 1950s—a lag of about 30 years. In 1981, Blacks suffered 20 infant deaths per 1000 live births, twice the level of 10.5 infant deaths for whites and similar to the rate of infant deaths for the white population in 1960 (DHHS, 1985a).

In analyzing mortality data from 1970 through 1981, a DHHS report identified six causes of death that accounted for more than 80% of the mortality observed among nonwhite minorities in excess of that of the white population. These causes included: cancer, cardiovascular disease and stroke, chemical dependency (including death due to cirrhosis), diabetes, homicides or accidents, and infant mortality.

Table 14.1 presents the leading causes of excess mortality and the percentage that each cause contributed to the total excess deaths in Blacks for the years 1979 through 1981. For Black males and females combined, excess deaths accounted for 47% of the total annual deaths in those 45 years old or less and 42% of deaths in those 70 and older.

Utilization of Health Care by Minority Populations

Given the health disparity between whites and minority populations, and more specifically the Black population, it is important to consider the possible differences that may exist in utilization patterns that are demonstrated by these groups. In a study by DHHS, the author noted that utilization of health services and health status of minorities were not as high as for the white population. A study of utilization patterns in several major categories of health care

TABLE 14.1 Average Annual Total and Excess Deaths in Blacks Selected Causes of Mortality, United States, 1979-1981

Causes of excess death	Excess deaths males and females cumulative to age 45		Excess deaths males and females cumulative to age 70	
	Number	Percentage	Number	Percentage
Heart disease and stroke	3,312	14.4	18,181	30.8
Homicide and accidents	8,041	35.1	10,909	18.5
Cancer	874	3.8	8,118	13.8
Infant mortality	6,178	26.9	6,178	10.5
Cirrhosis	1,121	4.9	2,154	3.7
Diabetes	223	1.0	1,850	3.1
Subtotal	19,749	86.1	47,390	80.4
All other causes	3,187	13.9	11,552	19.6
Total excess deaths	22,936	100.0	58,942	100.0
Total deaths, all causes	48,323		138,635	
Ratio of excess deaths to total deaths	47.4%		42.5%	
Percentage contribution of six causes to excess death	86.1%		80.4%	

Source: US Department of Health and Human Services (1985a). *Black and Minority Health*. Washington, DC: U.S. Government Printing Office.

—ambulatory care, inpatient care, and extended care—indicated the following:

1. A smaller proportion of nonwhites see a physician during the year.
2. The average number of physician visits per year is lower for nonwhites.
3. Outpatient department utilization is higher among minority groups; despite this, outpatient rates of nonadherence among such groups remain significantly high.
4. Fewer minorities report using physicians as a regular source of health care.
5. A larger proportion of minorities report no regular source of health care. (DHHS, 1985b, pp. 231–235)

It was based on data such as these that an investigation of issues that involve adherence patterns in minority groups was undertaken at the Howard University Center for Sickle Cell Disease (HUSCD). The primary research question was: What factors have an impact on health care compliance of Blacks at this facility? A related question was: What factors have led to discrepancies in access to adequate health care between this group and the wider society?

Framework for Improving Minority Access to Care

There has been extensive documentation on the multitude of variables that affect health-seeking behaviors, as well as the process that involves such behaviors. However, attempts to study this phenomenon in minority patients have been limited, and to date there have been few specific investigations that describe the various processes, stages, and types of decisions that are made by these groups when seeking medical care.

Investigators such as Becker and Maiman (1975) and Haynes (1976) have discussed the limitations of traditional approaches to studying adherence. Descriptions of the patient's personality and sociodemographic characteristics are enumerated, rather than providing an adequate understanding of the patient. Little attention is given to those values, beliefs, and perceptions that individuals may bring to the health setting.

The tendency is to utilize the traditional medical model of diagnosis and curing or, as McGoldrick (1982, p. 5) states, a "systematic inattention to illness" when we consider health issues. In essence, the patient becomes the root of the nonadherence and treatment difficulty rather than considering the person's cultural and societal frames of reference when seeking help. A host of studies, including those by Tseng and McDermott (1981), Harwood (1981), and Rakel (1977), posit that people differ in their experience of pain, what they label as a symptom, how they communicate about their pain or symptoms, their beliefs about the cause of their illnesses, their attitude toward health professionals, and the treatment they desire or expect. More specifically, decisions to utilize the health care system are strongly influenced by cultural norms. Zola (1966) points out that although more than 90% of the population experience physical symptoms of illness at any given time, the vast majority (i.e., 70–80%) choose to manage their problems outside the formal health care system.

Such limitations observed in traditional approaches to health care issues may be applied to the minority individual's experience; that is, issues surrounding minority health status encompass larger areas than specific illness dynamics. In a critique of traditional study of Black families, Allen (1978) asserts this point in the following statement:

> Clarity of these elaborate analyses of dyadic interactions or individual attributes often suffers, due to the failure of researchers to place these processes in a larger sociohistorical context . . . Black families are treated as autonomous entities apart from the social, economic, historical, and political contexts in which they are located and which largely determine their internal relationship. (p. 123)

An appreciation of cultural variability therefore suggests that a comprehensive framework is needed to address the health experiences of minority patients. A psychosocial-cultural approach should be used to conceptualize such experiences. This is based on an ecological perspective of the interrelatedness of the individual and his or her social environment. Among factors that are believed to be especially significant in influencing health care status within the minority environment are (1) psychological factors; (2) family factors; (3) community factors; and (4) societal or institutional issues. A brief description of how each of these factors relates to the experience of the Black population, and more directly, health issues, provides further understanding of the need for this framework.

Psychological Factors

Unique patterns of exposure to stressors and ways of dealing with stress and adversity in the Black population play a significant role in health decision making and health outcomes. An increasing body of research suggests that the way an individual copes with stress and the resources available to resolve situations, rather than the stressor itself, play important roles in health outcomes. For Blacks, however, the available resources have been extremely limited, and such restrictions have existed for many years. Thus there has emerged a life-style that has been characterized by economic and legal powerlessness, resulting in a negative influence on health status.

Experiences related to such stressors have left emotional scars on the lives of many Black individuals. Such consequences have included feelings of helplessness, hopelessness, isolation, anger, and apathy. Feelings of lack of control over life outcomes, including health consequences, may be another byproduct of such stressors. Although many Blacks have addressed such obstacles with positive coping patterns, it is important to recognize the prevalence and disruption of such factors in the lives, and particularly the health care environments, of others.

More directly, the onset of the illness experience coupled with the stressors of the medical care system highly exacerbated such psychological distress. It is not an uncommon reaction, therefore, for minority individuals in the midst of other obstacles to deny the presence of illness symptoms. Whether they seek medical care is influenced by past and present interactions with the health care system. In some instances, as will be described, it is perceived that other support systems—such as a family member or a minister—are more "trusted" to give appropriate care.

Family Factors

The Black family has been the focus of investigations for decades. While the past literature has focused on deficiencies felt to exist in this unit, such as the matriarchal system, more recent studies have recognized the positive influence of the family on the individual and the larger community.

In Robert Hill's (1972) *Strength of Black Families*, the nurturing quality of the family, both in history and in the present day, is cited as being the impetus for the survival of many individuals. Martin and Martin (1978) refer to the particular predominance of the Black extended family:

> The Black extended family is a multigenerational independent kinship system which is welded together by a sense of obligation to relatives; is organized around a family base household; is generally guided by a dominant family network; and has a built in mutual aid system for the welfare of its members and the maintenance of the family as a whole. (p. 1)

Anderson and Hildreth (1982), in a study on intergenerational relations in the Black family, found that reciprocal sharing and support were very common between adult children and their elderly parents. McAdoo (1983) found that even among middle-class Blacks a strong extended family network exists. She reports that child care was the most important help given in the family exchange system. Other researchers, such as Billingsly (1968), Hill (1972), Stack (1974), and Aschenbrenner (1975), have also pointed out the high level of cooperation and sharing found in the Black family. In particular, Aschenbrenner suggests that the extended kin network of the Black family in part defines its cultural uniqueness.

The concept of the Black extended family has application to involvement in the health care system. In general, there has been extensive documentation in the literature that focuses on the role of the family and other social support systems in the health care environment. According to Travis (1976), chronic illness among children affects every family in such a way that the sick child and its family members are intertwined in a dynamic changing constellation. To accommodate and adjust to the stress in caring for such children, Travis states that many families attempt to create support systems and networks within and outside the family. Help is sought to cope with demands on family relationships, financial problems, housing adaptation, and the unpredictability of acute episodes related to the child's disease that disturb the family's life-style.

Shontz and Fink (1961) describe the range of personal reactions that occur in families where there is a chronic illness. They outline stages that occur upon the family's receipt of the initial diagnosis. There is often shock, followed by panic, and a gradual realization of the crisis. Second, feelings of denial may occur, as well as later periods of depression and anxiety as the diagnosis becomes more of a reality. As resources are found and coping patterns are developed, such emotional consequences are less severe.

Many of the above dynamics related to health issues have application to Black families. For example, Slaughter and Anderson (1983) and Dilworth-Anderson and Slaughter (1985) have done work on families with sickle cell disease. They state:

There are many ways in which the known symptoms of childhood sickle cell anemia may influence family functioning. If the child's illness is perceived to connote "bad blood" in the family, shame, or even guilt, may be experienced by family members. If the child's pain and necessary dependency during such times connote deficiency or "weakness," a subtle resentment of the child may develop. If independence and school achievement are highly valued, but children cannot compete as expected and desired, the family members may turn from the child as symbol of their parents and future success, collective well-being, and unity. If it is generally preferred that the child's life center around relationships within home and family, the child's illness may exacerbate predispositions by family members to "overprotect" and insulate it from extrafamilial contacts, including peers and other adults. (p. 22)

A resulting direct consequence within the Black family system may be the manner in which health concerns are addressed and acted upon. A parallel may be drawn between what is known about Black families and compliance with mental health treatment: Black Americans also consult extended family and kin and their minister when faced with stress and problems. They are reluctant to seek mental health care since reliance on the extended kin is easier and less humiliating; but when their resources are depleted, they have to seek other services including mental health. They initially mistrust the therapist as an outsider and experience him or her as an intruder. . . . They also have a basic concern about being discriminated against in the treatment chosen for them. (Singer, 1967; Yamamoto, James, & Palley, 1968)

The Black family, then, carries a number of issues and experiences into the health care environment. The obstacles encountered in the inherent pressures and frustrations that arise have an impact on the nonadherence patterns that may develop.

Community Factors

According to Caplan (1974, pp. 4–5), a support system is defined as a "continuing social aggregate that provides individuals with opportunities for feedback about themselves and for validation of their expectations about others, which offset deficiencies in these communications within the larger community context." In the Black community there are several support systems that have an impact on involvement in the health care system. These support systems complement the inability of traditional social services or mental health facilities to adequately address the obstacles faced by this group. For instance, several writers have pointed to the significant role played by the Black church in helping Blacks to cope with societal pressures and stress (Franklin, 1974; McQueen, 1977; Staples, 1971). This community support system provides a maintenance of family solidarity, status conferral, leadership development, expressive function or release of tension, and a place for social interaction.

A final point relating to the community involves its relationship to the Black extended family. Investigators such as Allen (1978) note that if the strengths and weaknesses of Black family functioning are to be assessed accurately, it is important to assess how kin networks operate in the broader community context. Allen specifically states:

> Just as the recurring behaviors of individual family members have meaning and purpose in the life of the total family, so the recurring behavior of the total family system has meaning and purpose in the life of that family's significant social community. More specifically, for example, the parent–child dyadic relationship influences, and is certainly influenced by, both other relationships within the household as well as those with significant kin and non-kin outside of the household. (p. 123)

This point supports the previously discussed need to adopt a more global perspective when considering Black individuals and related health functioning.

Larger Social System or Institutional Factors

There are many organizations in the larger social system that influence involvement of the minority individual in the health care system. These include political, employment, housing, and educational systems in addition to health care systems. Racial discrimination and inequities impact negatively on opportunities and outcomes for minorities within our institutions.

It is well established that Blacks have more difficulty entering the medical care system (DHHS, 1985a). Factors relating to financial assets (e.g., insurance), quality of initial care, transportation to facilities, and staff or bed availability determine whether individuals enter medical treatment. Blacks are more likely to live in neighborhoods that are not accessible to medical care. Furthermore, public transportation to medical facilities is not as available in many Black neighborhoods. Blacks are more likely to be covered by public insurance or to be uninsured than nonblacks. In fact, Long (1987) reported that Blacks are about 1.5 times more likely than nonblacks to be uninsured (22% versus 15%).

Often the patient has been discouraged by the experiences of other family or community members. The message given regarding patient treatment involvement may be negative. If the individual is able to enter the system, he or she may be faced with long clinic waits, communication barriers, lack of clarity about illness symptoms, and difficulties with recommended treatment regimens. If the patient is hospitalized, the ongoing pressures of the treatment environment must be faced. In addition to the possibility of unsatisfactory treatment, further obstacles may include negative interactions with health care professionals.

Many minority individuals have experienced obstacles similar to those described. The reception that a Black patient may receive in a given health setting is uncertain. As previously described in the discussion on psychological factors, a certain amount of anticipatory anxiety is likely as the patient approaches the health care setting. Most certainly, then, adherence patterns are affected.

The Minority Individual Within the Health Care System

Given the presence of the above-mentioned factors that can have an influence on the minority individual, experiences within the health care system are varied and complex. Psychological stressors may lead the individual to question his or her place in the system. The cumulative effect of not only one health problem but many illnesses and other stressors can cause additional turmoil.

For the minority individual who has to endure such experiences, a relevant question may be posed: Where do I place this illness in relationship to those other difficulties I am having? Other questions often follow: What does this illness mean in my life? Is it such a severe interruption that it cannot be overcome? Will I die from the illness, or the stress from having it? Will some of the symptoms subside or go away completely? Do I have any control over the stressors in my life? Can the medical care system really help? More importantly, does the medical care system care about me? Will the medical staff understand my fears and concerns? How can I best involve my family and community in my health concerns? Can my family and community address the overwhelming stressors that are prevalent?

HOWARD UNIVERSITY CENTER
FOR SICKLE CELL DISEASE

The extent to which such issues have an influence on specific health decision making was examined at Howard University Center for Sickle Cell Disease. Sickle cell disease is a genetic disorder of the red blood cells and affects primarily those of African descent in this country. Several aspects of the factors described above were identified by Howard University researchers. They included psychological, family, community, and institutional factors.

Psychological factors included those related to self-esteem, perception of control of the health environment, and perceptions of the disease such as the perception of the severity of the illness. Family and community factors were those that assessed the availability of social support, including the frequency of supportive and helpful behaviors performed by others. Finally, institutional factors related to issues in treatment environments.

The results of this research point to the need for carefully designed treatment interventions when working with minority patients. At the Howard Center for Sickle Cell Disease, a treatment program known as the "compliance clinic" was developed to address this problem. A comprehensive description of this effort is beyond the scope of this chapter; however, in summary, the goals of the compliance clinic were to: (1) provide counseling and educational services for nonadherent individuals; (2) to provide consultation to medical care staff; and (3) to monitor and improve the effectiveness of the clinic through ongoing research and evaluation. In the compliance clinic, ongoing emphasis was placed on the patient's total environment. Thus the intervention encompassed several of the economic, cultural, familial, and community factors discussed earlier. For instance, a frequently utilized technique was home contact by health care providers.

METHOD

Sample

The sample consisted of 70 patients or parents of patients attending the Center for Sickle Cell Disease at Howard University in Washington, D.C. Forty-five of the subjects were patients, and 25 of the subjects were parents. Parents of patients were included in the study sample, as they were responsible for appointments of their children. The sample included 28 males and 42 females; age ranged from 17 to 56.

Procedures

Subjects were approached while attending regularly scheduled outpatient appointments at the clinic. Their cooperation was enlisted for participation in a study of the health care needs of patients with sickle cell disease. They were informed that refusing to participate would not affect in any way their treatment services. Honest reponses were requested and confidentiality was assured.

Measures

The questionnaire was comprised of demographic items with the scales and items described below.

Social Support

Social support provides information that tells individuals that they are loved, valued, and part of a network of communication and mutual obligation (Cobb, 1976). This support may be emotional, cognitive, instrumental, or a combination of these. Involvement of significant others can facilitate or impede movement toward positive health behaviors by providing information on appropriate behaviors, by aiding or hindering the behavioral process, and by providing feedback on the behaviors themselves. The results of a number of studies point to the positive relationship between social support and adherence (Levy, 1980).

The social support scale used in this study was developed by Wilcox (1981) and was used to determine the frequency of supportive and helpful behaviors performed by others. The scale measures the availability of emotional, cognitive, and instrumental support. Respondents were asked to indicate how available each type of help was by circling frequently available, sometimes available, or rarely available support. Examples of scale items included "Someone who will listen to you carefully and talk over problems with you" and "Someone who will lend you their car for a few hours." The reliability and validity of this scale were found acceptable.

Feelings about Treatment Environment

A positive perception of the treatment environment is associated with greater adherence to health care recommendations. A positive treatment environment includes professional, caring, and courteous health care providers. Other factors include an accessible facility with convenient scheduling.

A 13-item Likert-type scale was developed to obtain information on how subjects felt about their treatment environment. Subjects indicated their degree of agreement or disagreement with a series of statements such as "Patients' requests are frequently ignored at the Sickle Cell Center" and "When I call or come to the Center, I am greeted warmly and made to feel comfortable." A Chronbach's alpha coefficient of .89 was computed, indicating that the internal consistency of the scale was acceptable.

Health Locus of Control

The degree to which persons feel that they have control over health outcomes has been found to be related to adherence. Health locus of control is the generalized expectancy that health outcomes are determined by one's actions (internal locus of control) or by external forces that are beyond one's control (external locus of control). Persons with an internal locus of control are more likely to feel that they can influence health outcomes, while persons with an external locus of control may be more likely to feel that health outcomes are beyond their control. Individuals with an internal orientation are expected to exhibit more positive health behaviors, including adherence, as these individuals feel they make a difference in their health outcomes.

The health locus of control scale used in this study was an 18-item scale used to assess the degree to which subjects felt they had control over their health outcomes (Wallston, Wallston, Forsberg, & King, 1984). The scale had acceptable reliability and validity.

Self-Esteem

Self-esteem is the way one feels about oneself. A positive feeling about oneself has been correlated with adherence. Individuals with positive self-esteem are more likely to engage in positive health behaviors. Rosenberg's (1965) self-esteem scale was used in this study. This instrument is a 10-item Likert-type scale. Subjects were asked to indicate the extent of agreement or disagreement with statements such as "At times I feel useless." This instrument has been used in a number of studies and has satisfactory reliability and validity.

Perception of Disease Severity

Disease severity and adherence has been investigated in a number of studies; one was performed by the authors (Moorman & Belgrave, 1984). The results of the authors' study, using a population of patients with sickle cell disease, indicated perception that one's disease as severe was associated with higher levels of adherence. The three measures of disease severity used in this study are described below.

Perception of Interference of Disease. This scale was developed to determine the degree to which patients perceived that their disease interfered with routine activities. Subjects were asked to respond to statements about the extent to which the disease interfered with activities such as employment, social activities, and sports, on a scale ranging from "interferes greatly" to "does not interfere at all." The reliability coefficient (Cronbach's alpha) of the scale was .85 for the study sample.

Symptom Checklist. Frequency of symptoms is another index of disease severity; the one used here was a list of symptoms associated with sickle cell disease. Subjects were asked to indicate the degree to which symptoms (e.g., weakness and sluggishness, jaundice, irritability, nausea, depression, excessive pain, loss of appetite, anxiety) were a problem by responding to a scale ranging from "not a problem" to "a very serious problem."

Perception of Disease Severity. A global measure of the perception of disease severity was obtained by asking subjects to respond to the following question: "In general, how serious do you think your (or your child's) illness is?" The scale was a 4-point scale ranging from "extremely serious" to "not serious."

Measure of Adherence

A measure of appointment-keeping behavior was obtained by asking subjects the following question: "In general, how would you rate your appointment-keeping pattern?" A 5-point scale ranging from "always keeps appointments" to "never keeps appointments" was used. Some validity information was collected using this item and other measures of adherence. Data pertaining to the actual percentage of appointments kept were available on a subsample of patients ($n = 25$). Patients' rating of appointment behavior correlated ($p < .01$) with the percentage of appointments actually kept for this subsample of patients. The self-rating measure of appointment-keeping behavior also significantly related to responses to the question "Did you keep your appointment on the scheduled day?" ($p < .01$). These results indicate that self-rating of appointment-keeping behavior is a valid measure for this sample.

RESULTS

Scales were developed from individual items. A multiple regression procedure was used with the following measures as predictor variables: social support; health locus of control; perception of susceptibility; perception of interference of disease; symptom checklist; feelings about the treatment environment; self-esteem; and perception of disease severity. The criterion variable was rating of appointment-keeping behavior. An adjusted R^2 of .21 was obtained, indicating that about one fifth of the variance in ratings of appointment-keeping behavior could be explained if these measures were used ($p < .05$.) Social support, health locus of control, feelings about the treatment environment, and self-esteem were the largest relative contributors in explaining appointment-keeping behavior. Social support was the strongest predictor in this study. Social support was also found to be significantly related to adherence to health behaviors such as watching diet, exercising, having regular blood pressure tests, and taking medication as prescribed ($r = .70, p < .01$).

The results of this study are limited to Black patients with sickle cell disease. However, the study findings can be used as a springboard for examining adherence issues in other minority populations with chronic illness. Because of the scarcity of research and clinical efforts related to adherence within minority populations, further investigation is needed.

GUIDELINES FOR ADHERENCE RESEARCH
IN MINORITY POPULATIONS

The following guidelines are recommended for developing adherence efforts in minority populations based on work performed at the Howard facility:

1. Development of a multidisciplinary, comprehensive approach that includes familial, community, social, historical, and cultural factors relevant to the individual.
2. Awareness of patient history that specifically focuses on the individual and family dynamics.

3. Utilization of the family to improve adherence behavior.
4. Utilization of community resources to improve adherence behavior.
5. Assessment of whether the treatment environment is positive for patients (e.g., monitoring clinic waiting time, obstacles in physician–patient relationships).
6. Encouraging patients to maintain as much control of their health care as possible.
7. Involvement of minority role models in health care experiences (e.g., physicians, social workers, psychologists, other successful patients).

SUMMARY

The purpose of this chapter has been to present factors related to health care adherence of minorities. The investigators discuss four factors—psychological, family, community, and societal or institutional.

Adherence behaviors are often shaped by the interaction of these factors in past and present experiences of the minority patient and his or her family. Perhaps most key to the conceptualization of this chapter has been the notion of cultural relativity in understanding health care utilization.

A research and clinical project at the Howard University Center for Sickle Cell Disease was presented as an illustration of one approach used for understanding and improving adherence in a Black chronically ill population. In a study of 70 patients with sickle cell disease, results illustrated that social support, health locus of control, feelings about the treatment environment, and self-esteem were contributing factors in explaining appointment-keeping behavior. A compliance clinic was then established as a treatment intervention for improving compliance. The major focus of the clinic was counseling and education, taking into account aspects of patients' family and community environments to address adherence issues.

It is clear from the review of the literature and the clinical and research efforts reported in this chapter that there is a need for further investigation. The findings at HUCSCD are limited to one minority group and one chronic illness. Studies of other minority populations and of other chronic illnesses are needed.

REFERENCES

Allen, W. (1978). The search for applicable theories of Black family life. *Journal of Marriage and Family, 40,* 117–129.

Anderson, P., & Hildreth, C. (1982). *Family ties of older blacks in diversity.* In B. Baptiste & L. Johnson (Eds.). Sweden: Uppsala International Library Press.

Aschenbrenner, J. (1975). *Lifelines: Black families in changes.* New York: Holt, Rinehart & Winston.

Becker, M. H., & Maiman, L. A. (1975). Sociobehavioral determinants of compliance with health and medical care recommendations. *Medical Care, 13*, 10-24.

Billingsley, A. (1968). *Black families in white America.* Englewood Cliffs, NJ: Prentice-Hall.

Caplan, G. (1974). *Support systems and community mental health.* New York: Behavioral Publications.

Charney, E. (1972). Patient-doctor communication. *Pediatrics Clinic of North America, 19*, 263-279.

Cobb, S. (1976). Social support as a moderator of life stress. *Psychosomatic Medicine, 38*(5), 300-314.

Dilworth-Anderson, P., & Slaughter, D. (1985). *Sickle cell anemia children and the Black extended family.* Paper presented at conference on Clinical and Research Directions in Sickle Cell Disease, Chicago, Illinois.

Franklin, J. H. (1974). *From slavery to freedom: A history of the Negro American* (4th ed.). New York: Alfred A. Knopf.

Gary, L. (1974). The sickle cell controversy. *Social Work, 19*(3), 263-271.

Harwood, A. (1981). *Ethnicity and medical care.* Cambridge: Harvard University Press.

Haynes, R. B. (1976). A critical review of the "determinants" of patient compliance with therapeutic regimens. In D. L. Sackett & R. B. Haynes (Eds.), *Compliance with therapeutic regimens.* Baltimore: Johns Hopkins University Press.

Hill, R. (1972). *The strengths of black families.* New York: Emerson Hall.

Levy, R. L. (1980). Social support and compliance: A selective review. In R. B. Haynes, M. E. Mattson, & T. O. Engebretsm (Eds.), *Patient compliance prescribed antihypertensive medical regimens* (NIH Publication 81-2102). Washington, DC: U.S. Government Printing Office.

Lewis, D. & Belgrave, F. Z. (1984). *The assessment of compliance patterns in patients with sickle cell disease: Pilot project summary.* Washington, DC: Howard University Center for Sickle Cell Disease.

Long, S. H. (1987). Public versus employment-related health insurance: Experience and implications for Black and Nonblack Americans. *Millbank Quarterly, 65*, 200-210.

Martin, E., & Martin, J. (1978). *The black extended family.* Chicago: University of Chicago Press.

McAdoo, H. (1983). Factors related to stability in upwardly mobile Black families. *Journal of Marriage and Family, 40*, 761-778.

McGoldrick, M. (1982). Ethnicity and family therapy: An overview. In M. McGoldrick, J. Pearce, & J. Giordano (Eds.), *Ethnicity and family therapy* (p. 5). New York: Guilford.

McQueen, A. J. (1977). The adaptations of urban Black families: Trends, problems and issues. Oberlin, OH: Oberlin College Public Service Studies.

Rakel, R. E. (1977). *Principles of family medicine.* Philadelphia, PA: Saunders.

Rosenberg, M. (1965). *Society and adolescents self-image.* Princeton, NJ: Princeton University Press.

Shontz, F., & Fink, S. (1961). A method for evaluating psychosocial adjustment of the chronically ill. *American Journal of Physical Medicine, 40*, 63-69.

Singer, B. P. (1967). Some implications of different psychiatric treatment of Negro and White patients. *Social Science and Medicine, 1*, 77-83.

Slaughter, P. J., & Anderson, P. D. (1983). Impact of sickle cell anemic children upon Black extended family functioning. Chicago, IL: Northwestern University.

Staples, R. (1971). Towards a sociology of the Black family: A theoretical and methodological assessment. 33(1), *Journal of Marriage and Family*, 119-135.

Travis, G. (1976). *Chronic illness in children*. Palo Alto, CA: Stanford University Press.

Tseng, W. G., & McDermott, J. F. (1981). *Culture, mind and therapy: An introduction to cultural psychiatry*. New York: Brunner/Mazel.

U.S. Department of Health and Human Services. (1985a). *Black and minority health*. Washington, DC: U.S. Government Printing Office.

U.S. Department of Health and Human Services. (1985b). *Health status of minorities and low-income groups*. Washington, DC: U.S. Government Printing Office.

Wallston, B. S., Wallston, K. A., Forsberg, P. R., & King, J. E. (1984). Measuring desire for control of health processes. *Journal of Personality and Social Psychology, 47*, 415-426.

Wilcox, B. (1981). Social support, life stress and psychological adjustment: A test of the buffering hypothesis. *American Journal of Communicy Psychology, 9*, 371-386.

Yamamoto, J., James, E., & Palley, N. (1968). Cultural problems in psychiatric therapy. *Archives of General Psychiatry, 19*(1), 44-49.

Zola, I. K. (1966). Culture and symptoms: An analysis of peoples presenting complaints. *American Sociological Review, 5*, 141-155.

15

Life-Style Interventions in the Young

Louis M. Aledort, Howard Weiss, Christine T. Parker, Judith R. Levi, Robert Simon

REVIEW OF THE LITERATURE

Life-style interventions in the young are a particularly difficult area of adherence research. Children and adolescents are not yet fully physically, cognitively, or emotionally developed and therefore may lack coordination, may lack ability to understand their diseases, and may be uncooperative or rebellious. In addition, the young are legally dependent for health care on parents or guardians, which necessitates parental understanding of disease and treatment regimen, ability to recognize symptoms, and motivation to adhere to the recommended therapies.

In an attempt to define some of the areas of particular difficulty with adherence in the young, Friedman and Litt (1986) described some of the obstacles facing adolescents. An example given was that adolescents have less privacy and mobility than adults (e.g., hiding contraceptives from parents may lead to forgetfulness; inability to travel to distant clinics). In addition, the young are hemmed in by school regulations and financial constraints, may lack experience in dealing with the health system, and are faced with family and social pressures that add obstacles to their path.

A controversy concerning patient adherence in the young is beginning to surface in the medical community. Although it has become almost a truism that adolescents are considerably less adherent to medical regimens than children or adults, little research (other than caregiver reports) exists to support this position. In order to determine if children and adolescents indeed have unusual problems with adherence, a literature review was performed to discover predictors of and life-style interventions for improved adherence to medical regimens in these populations.

Review Characteristics

Two search strategies were used for this review: (1) adherence in adolescents and children with chronic diseases; and, more generally, (2) adherence in adolescents and children. Inclusion criteria were that: (1) the majority of subjects within each study must have been under 20 years of age; (2) articles must be original research published since 1978; and (3) no reviews, letters, or book chapters were to be included.

The search found 211 articles; 58 met the inclusion criteria, although a review, one article by Bruhn (1983), reported preliminary results from 11 asthma studies, bringing the total number of studies meeting the inclusion criteria to 68.

Because of the wide range of diseases of the young, this review has been structured first, to describe correlates of adherence; second, to relate general statistics concerning rates of adherence; third, to describe the diversity of subjective measures of adherence; and fourth, to relate the type of interventions for improving adherence. After this review, original research on a population of young patients will be described.

Correlates of Adherence

Several correlates of adherence and nonadherence in the young were identified in the literature: (1) demographics; (2) perceptions of self and health; (3) role of the family; (4) disease characteristics; and (5) structure of care.

Demographics

Demographic predictors of adherence consistently included marital status and educational level (Becker et al., 1978; Becker, Maiman, Kirscht, Haefner, & Drachman, 1977; Korsch, Fine, & Negrete, 1978; Simonds, 1977). As would be expected, two-parent families and higher parental levels of education were predictive of adherence, while fatherless households and family instability were factors associated with nonadherence. Race (Buchanan, Siegel, Smith, & DePasse, 1982) and years since diagnosis (Passero, Remor, & Salomon, 1981) were not associated with adherence in the young.

What was not expected, however, was the total lack of consistent results regarding any other demographics. Younger patients were found to be better adherers in studies of patients with cystic fibrosis (Meyer, Dolan, & Mueller, 1975), cancer (Dolgin, Katz, Doctors, & Siegel, 1986; Jamison, Lewis, & Burish, 1986), renal transplants (Beck et al., 1980), and in appointment keeping (Irwin, Millstein, & Shafer, 1981; Pearce, O'Shea, & Wesson, 1979). Other studies showed that older patients with cystic fibrosis (Passero et al., 1981), asthma (Spector et al., 1986), and obesity (Becker et al., 1977) exhibited better levels of adherence. Another study found age to be a nonsignificant factor in cystic fibrosis (Finkelstein, Budd, Warwick, Kujawa, & Wienlinski, 1986).

Males were found to be less adherent to medical regimens in some studies (Clemmer & Hayes, 1979; Litt & Cuskey, 1984; Spector et al., 1986), while females exhibited less adherence in others (Beck et al., 1980, Irwin et al., 1981). No significant differences were found between males and females in studies on asthma (Cluss, Epstein, Galvis, Fireman, & Friday, 1984), cystic fibrosis (Finkelstein et al., 1986; Passero et al., 1981), and leukemia (Lansky, Smith, Cairns, & Cairns, 1983).

As mentioned earlier, much discussion on adherence in the young has centered around their lack of adherence to medical regimens, particularly in the case of adolescent males; research, as summarized above, does not support this contention. Replies that variety in the diseases studied may be an underlying cofactor creating differences between the sexes fail when it is noticed that in one particular disease, cystic fibrosis, age and sex were inconsistent factors in determining different rates of adherence.

Lower income has also been a favored rationale for failure of some patients to adhere to medical regimens. Discussions have centered on lack of money to support expensive treatments as a reasoned argument for lowered adherence to regimens. However, although spotty, the literature does not support this premise. Lower income was identified as a factor in adherence to immunosuppressive therapy in renal transplant patients (Korsch et al., 1978), but it was not a factor in asplenic, bone marrow transplant, or sickle cell disease patients (Buchanan et al., 1982); all four diseases demand expensive and continuing treatment.

Perceptions of Self and Health

Self-perceptions and perceptions relating to health status have long been a mainstay of paradigms of patient adherence (e.g., the Health Belief Model). The literature supports this contention to the extent that these types of perceptions appear to be consistent predictors of adherence or nonadherence in the young. Worry about future health (Bobrow, Ruskin, & Siller, 1985; Durant, Jay, Linder, Shoffitt, & Litt, 1984), low evaluation of personal health (Durant et al., 1984), and less belief that adherence will avoid or delay disease complications (Bobrow et al., 1985) have all been consistent factors in nonadherence to medical regimens.

Self-perceptions and psychosocial factors also have been consistent predictors of adherence in the young. If children exhibit higher self-esteem and autonomy (Denver [cited in Bruhn, 1983]; Litt & Cuskey, 1984; Litt, Cuskey & Rosenberg, 1982; Litt, Cuskey, & Rudd, 1980; Neel, Jay, & Litt, 1985), greater adaptiveness (Deaton, 1985), positive self or body image (Jamison et al., 1986; Litt & Cuskey, 1984; Stanford [cited in Bruhn, 1983]), and an internal locus of control (Jamison et al., 1986; Korsch et al., 1978), then there is a higher probability that they will adhere to medical regimens. This appears to hold true no matter the severity of disease or complexity of treatment. For example, self-esteem has been found to be a predictor in adherence to treatment for renal failure (Korsch et al., 1978), asthma (Denver [cited in Bruhn, 1983]), juvenile diabetes (Litt & Cuskey 1981), epilepsy (Friedman, Litt, & King, 1986), and contraceptive use (Neel et al., 1985).

Children also appear to adhere better when the social environment is positive. Children who have more interpersonal conflicts (Simonds, 1977), difficulty in discussing feelings, or are unable to share illness concerns with friends (Bobrow et al., 1985) have more trouble adhering to medical regimens.

Role of the Family

As one would expect, the family plays a major role in the adherence of children and adolescents to treatment regimens. As mentioned earlier, the young are dependent upon the family for payment of medical costs, and most need parental guidance in following their medical regimens. This dependency, particularly in terms of disease treatment, places enormous burdens on the family. Parental hostility, anxiety, or compulsive behavior (Lansky et al., 1983) and communication difficulties with the child-patient (Korsch et al., 1978) have profoundly negative effects on adherence. It is unclear from the literature whether these problems originate with the parent, the child, or interaction of the dyad; more research is necessary to determine the underlying processes.

More socially acceptable behavior by parents has been found to assist in adherence of the young to treatment regimens. The mother, not surprisingly, plays an integral part in adherence of her child. Adherence is increased if the mother is married, the family stable, and family problems few (Beck et al., 1980;

Bobrow et al., 1985; Korsch et al., 1978; Simonds, 1977). Increased concern of the mother for the ill child over other children, concern about other children's health, perceived vulnerability of the child to illness in general and this illness in particular, concern about general health, and the presence of a prevention orientation all improve the probability of adherence to the regimen (Becker et al., 1977, 1978).

Parental encouragement and increased supervision (Beck et al., 1980; Weinstein & Cuskey, 1985) also tends to increase adherence. What is interesting, however, is that parental accompaniment on clinic visits has not been a predictor (Passero et al., 1981). Parental scheduling of appointments has also been equivocal in its effects on adherence. In one study, it was a predictor of adherence (Irwin et al., 1981) in adolescents and children, while no significant differences were found in another study of adolescent girls (Durant et al., 1984). This may be an indicator that more research needs to be performed on what types of and to what degree parental involvement increases adherence. As the study of adolescent girls related to oral contraceptive use, perhaps medical condition—such as non-illness-related appointments—may be a cofactor in adherence with these populations.

One other finding of the literature must be noted. Patient or parent knowledge of the disease was an inconsistent predictor of adherence to regimen. It has been a truism in the study of patient adherence that knowledge alone is insufficient to change behavior; the results found in this review only confirm this assertion (Beck et al., 1980; Kaplan, Chadwick, & Schimmel, 1985).

Disease Characteristics

Several characteristics of diseases under study were found to be correlates of adherence. Duration of disease or illness (Litt et al., 1982; Litt & Cuskey, 1981) and time in specialist care (Becker et al., 1977; Radius et al., 1978), both components of disease chronicity, were found to affect adherence in the young. The longer the duration of disease and time in specialist care, the lower the probability of adherence to the regimen. However, there appears to be a contradiction of this assertion: one study (Allen, Tennen, McGrade, Affleck, & Ratzan, 1983) found that earlier onset of disease increased levels of adherence. A potential reason for this apparent contradiction is that onset of disease may be a cofactor in adherence. It may be that earlier onset allows for better habit formation for adhering to treatment regimens, particularly if that regimen does not change.

It is interesting to note that, contrary to most discussions by researchers in the field, disease severity is inconsistent as a predictor of adherence. In five studies, more severe diseases were found to increase adherence (Becker et al., 1977,

1978; Clemmer & Hayes, 1979; El-Mangoury, 1981; Jamison et al., 1986), while two other studies reported no significant differences (Finkelstein et al., 1986; Passero et al., 1981). This, again, may be due to the varying diseases under study. Increased severity of disease increased adherence in diseases as disparate as asthma (Becker et al., 1978), cancer (Jamison et al., 1986), orthodontia wear (Clemmer & Hayes, 1979), and obesity (Becker et al., 1977); however, it was not a predictor in cystic fibrosis (Passero et al., 1981).

This apparent inconsistency may be due less to the severity of disease than to its chronicity or to perception of benefits of the regimen. Asthma, orthodontia, and obesity usually show observable changes in a short time if patients adhere to their regimens; improvements in cancer treatment have extended life spans considerably or, in many instances, provided cures. Cystic fibrosis is a genetic disease that is universally fatal within the first three decades of life. It may be that, knowing the relative futility of treatment, patients may decide that adherence to a stringent regimen may not be worth the effort. More research in the area of treatment efficacy may be valuable in determining potential cofactors of adherence in this population.

A side note: increased numbers and severity of side effects of treatment were found to decrease adherence to treatment regimens (Lansky, Vats, & Cairns, 1979; Litt et al., 1982; Sleator, Ullman, & von Neumann, 1982). It is unknown at this time if there is a relationship between the number and severity of side effects and the severity of disease. This is another area where future research could be of much value.

As mentioned earlier, the development of strong behavioral habits may be a cofactor in patient adherence to medical regimens. Chronic diseases, by their nature, allow more time for the formation of habit in following a regimen; acute diseases, although potentially very serious, have a limited time frame in which adherence is necessary. This premise receives a small amount of support in one study (Glanz, Fiel, Swartz, & Francis, 1984), which found that number of attacks did not affect the level of adherence of asthma patients. Although asthma is a chronic disease, it tends to be episodic in nature, with treatment occurring during attacks rather than a complex daily treatment regimen.

Structure of Care

There were some interesting results concerning the structure of care. Although physician attitudes did not affect adherence (Pearce et al., 1979), increased patient and parent satisfaction with the physician, health care received, and prescribed regimen significantly increased adherence (Litt & Cuskey, 1984; Smith, Seale, Ley, Shaw, & Bracks, 1986). In addition, positive attitudes of the young toward self-care improved adherence to medical regimens (Kaplan et al., 1985).

Factors that decreased adherence included disruption of normal activities (Becker et al., 1978; Lansky et al., 1979) and complaints about the taste, scheduling, and relative inaccessibility for filling of prescriptions (Becker et al., 1978). Most surprisingly, perceived benefits of the regimen was a nonpredictor (Becker et al., 1977). Perhaps the constant problems associated with following the regimen causes its benefits to rank lower in importance. It also may be related to treatment efficacy, as mentioned earlier.

Summary

Inconsistent factors far outweigh those correlates of adherence found in the literature; this highlights the need for more research on adherence in the young. One of the most surprising results of this review was the lack of consistent support for some of the apparent truisms concerning adherence in this population. Data on lack of adherence in adolescent males when compared to children or to female adolescents were ambiguous. Disease severity, long thought to be a significant and consistent factor in adherence, was a nonpredictor in several studies.

Another surprising result was the lack of correlation between adherence and clinical outcome (Deaton, 1985; Finney, Friman, Rapoff, & Christophersen, 1985). This may be due to a variety of factors, not least of which could be the measures used for adherence or lack of strong treatment for the diseases under study.

All in all, few factors were discovered that were consistent predictors of adherence. It is clear, however, that many preconceptions concerning adherence in young populations must be tested, retested, and set aside where appropriate as data became available. In addition, it is clear that much more research must be performed before clear guidelines for interventions can be specified.

Rates of Adherence

In the present review, adherence in the young ranged from 10% to 94.8%, with a mean adherence rate across studies of 56.3%. These statistics conform to historical estimates of adherence (Haynes, Taylor, & Sackett, 1979). Only 26 of the 68 studies identified either full or partial adherence rates. Over 40 studies did not identify any rates; the others stated changes in rates of adherence but did not specify either baseline or final rates.

Measures of Adherence

Measures of adherence in the literature ranged from serum or urine assays to self-reports and appointment keeping. The diversity of measures leads to some problems with comparative analysis of results. Few of the studies used objective measures of adherence (e.g., assays, metered prescription instruments, pill counts). Many of the studies using nonobjective methods (e.g., self-report, caregiver reports) reported no data concerning the reliability or validity of the instruments used.

It is unwise to denigrate the use of nonobjective or objective measures of adherence: Proponents of both sides have a tendency to exhibit alarming behaviors—to the dismay of the denigrator. Measures such as the Guttman scale may obviate the need for partisan tactics (Jay, DuRant, Shoffitt, Linder, & Lift). A Guttman scale usually includes four measures of adherence: (1) avoidance of a behavior; (2) measurement of remaining medication; (3) appointment adherence; and (4) an assay. The first measure, avoidance of a behavior, can be measured nonobjectively, while the remaining three are objective in nature.

Similar measures to Guttman scales need to be developed, as reliance on one type of measure over another leads to problems in generalization of results. It is our contention that research on adherence must use not only the traditional objective and nonobjective measures but also measures such as case reports and interviews, to more accurately identify problems associated with adherence.

Objective methods, such as assays, provide information on the degree of adherence exhibited by a number of people. Nonobjective methods, such as questionnaires, assist in determining, although on a relatively superficial level, if a number of people share the same perceptions on health, disease, and treatment. Case reports and open-ended interviews allow in-depth measurement of motivations and explanations for behavior, although generalization to others may be in question. By the use of two or more types of measurement—objective measures, questionnaire, interview, case report—both superficial but generalizable and in-depth but nongeneralizable data may be used to develop a rich understanding of the motivations, perceptions, and behaviors that affect adherence, and the improvements in or restrictions to quality of life that adherence can bring.

Interventions

Over half the articles describe nonintervention studies (37 of 68); nonetheless, much useful information was garnered on potentially fruitful interventions to improve adherence. Interventions described in the literature ranged from educational to contractual to behavioral in nature. Unfortunately, few studies have used similar interventions, so little may be said concerning the effectiveness or generalizability to other populations of each type of intervention. Therefore, no attempt has been made here to describe the interventions in depth; only the relative effectiveness of each type has been presented.

Educational

Sixteen studies related experience with educational interventions. Twelve studies described educational interventions combined with methods as diverse as behavioral strategies, group seminars, recreational activities, counseling, and home visits. In several instances, no statistics were given as to the effectiveness of the interventions.

General educational interventions in asthma were found to increase knowledge (Buffalo, Denver, Pittsburgh, & Stanford [cited in Bruhn, 1983]; Smith et al., 1986), with improvements in school attendance, self-esteem, coping both by patient and family, and self-help skills. Interventions found to decrease emergency room visits and number of hospital stays involved recreational activities, group education, relaxation techniques, self-help skills, and general education (Buffalo, Columbia, Pittsburgh, Stanford, & UCLA [cited in Bruhn, 1983]).

Improvements in self-management through education were garnered through use of relaxation techniques (Columbia [cited in Bruhn, 1983]). The data on behavioral modification were more ambiguous. Two studies (Los Angeles, Palo Alto [cited in Bruhn, 1983]) indicated only that parents responded favorably, with no statistics given, while another found a 25% increase in adherence (Smith et al., 1986). The problem of no statistics or results being reported (other than description of the program) occurred in several instances. This may be because of the preliminary nature of the reports on these studies.

Other educational interventions were implemented with diabetic patients and general populations of adolescents. In diabetes, one educational program increased adherence as measured by negative urine samples (Epstein et al., 1981), while in another there was improved ability in problem-solving and social skills (Kaplan et al., 1985). Two studies found no significant correlation between knowledge and adherence (Beck et al., 1980; Kaplan et al., 1985), although parental involvement was a predictor (Beck et al., 1980) when counseling techniques were used.

One of the problems with reviewing educational interventions is the vast array of techniques used. As shown above, education alone was seldom used, appropriately, as the adherence literature has demonstrated that knowledge alone does not lead to adherence on measures of medical importance. When education is teamed with other approaches, changes in behavior are more apt to occur. However, few of the studies indicated baseline, interim, or follow-up adherence levels, making it difficult to assess the magnitude of effect of the interventions on behavior; in some instances, only descriptions of the interventions were reported.

Telephone Reminders

Telephone reminders were used in only two studies. In one study with a general pediatric population, reminders increased appointment keeping (Casey, Rosen, Glowasky, & Ludwig, 1985). In the other study, of asthma patients, no statistics were given as to the effectiveness of telephone reminders when coupled with parental encouragement (Weinstein & Cuskey, 1985).

This intervention highlights some of the difficulties with the literature. One problem is the lack of adequate documentation as to the effectiveness of the intervention in changing adherence patterns. Another relates to the behavior being measured. Appointment-keeping is a very minimal type of adherence behavior. Little, if any, literature exists that indicates that appointment-keeping is a predictor of either medical outcome or patients adhering to medical regimens outside the confines of medical clinics. Although many times difficult to determine, more direct, richer, and (if necessary) more intricate measures of adherence must be developed if meaningful progress is to be made in determining predictors of adherence.

Contracts

Only one study intervened by using contracts: research on adolescents with acne (Flanders & McNamara, 1985). Contingency and noncontingency contracts in addition to traditional self-management techniques were the three interventions. There were no significant differences found between the two types of contracts or between contract interventions and self-management; however, all were found to be significantly better at improving adherence than the control group receiving standard care. This study was interesting because it focused on comparing three interventions against a control group.

Such studies provide considerably more information to other researchers, as comparative analysis of different types of interventions, particularly well-defined ones, allows researchers to do more than throw the kitchen sink at their patient populations. They allow the development, albeit slow, of each component of a complement of interventions that will improve adherence in the young.

Self-Management

Eight studies used self-management techniques to modify adherence behavior. Although self-management was not found as a predictor in a study of asthma patients (Baum & Creer, 1986), it was a significant factor with diabetics (Daneman et al., 1982; Schafer, Glasgow, & McCaul, 1982), adolescent patients in general and those with acne or who were using contraceptives (Flanders & McNamara, 1985; Jay, DuRant, Shoffitt, Linder, & Litt, 1984), and pediatric patients who suffered from otitis media (Finney et al., 1985) and obesity (Becker et al., 1977).

Summary

The literature in self-management highlights the need to study specific life-style interventions in a variety of patient populations. Self-management has been studied in populations as diverse as asthmatics and acne sufferers in addition to healthy individuals using contraceptives. This diversity documents how a single type of intervention can be effective with a variety of populations. If too many types of interventions are implemented and tried on only one patient population, there is no evidence that these interventions can be of use with others; it may be of interest only to point at possibly fruitful avenues of research. It is too early in the evolution of research on adherence in the young to determine if interventions are population-specific; however, a cautious approach must be maintained so that interventions that are developed have a solid grounding in theory and past research in behavior. The following research on improving adherence to regimens for hemophiliacs through a family therapy intervention is an example of such work.

FAMILY THERAPY IN HEMOPHILIA: A CHRONIC DISEASE MODEL

Hemophilia affects approximately 15,000 American males. It is a chronic disease where a coagulation factor is not functioning. It leads to repeated, painful episodes of bleeding that are spontaneous and therefore unpredictable. Bleeding is usually into joints and leads to significant arthropathy, which impairs movement. Few, if any, intervention studies in chronic diseases, and particularly in genetic disorders, have demonstrated methods to alter outcomes.

Comprehensive Care in Hemophilia

For more than a decade, hemophilia care has been delivered in a comprehensive fashion for almost half the nation's patients. Multidisciplinary teams at satellite centers cover large portions of the country. Teams are prepared to care for the medical, dental, and psychosocial problems that this disease presents to the clinician. Members of teams are also ready to deal with the complex financial issues chronic disease entails. In addition, much effort is placed on educating schools, physicians, employers, and other community agencies as to the "do's and don'ts" of hemophilia.

Regional centers are actively engaged in outreach so that treatment plans can be easily translated for primary care physicians who may live far from any center and have little or no experience with hemophilia. A key element that has altered the life-style and makes possible early intervention for bleeding episodes was the introduction of home care. Home care meant that the human blood derivatives, which are required to stop bleeding, could be administered by the patient, his spouse, or a family member. Such care allowed early treatment to be performed with more rapid alleviation of pain, as well as abbreviation of long periods of waiting in emergency rooms. With this therapeutic modality in a setting of comprehensive care, patients live longer, miss school and work less, are employable, have better insurance underwriting of health care, and decrease health care costs. Table 15.1 demonstrates the dramatic advances made by this mode of care.

Adherence at the Mount Sinai Hemophilia Center

As in many chronic disorders, adherence by hemophiliacs is a major problem. Most adherence studies have dealt with the patient as the primary and essentially only focus for behavioral change; this is a linear approach that has not proven very successful. There is an emerging field of family approaches to chronic disease. There are more systemic approaches that look at multiple factors, including "well" members of the family unit. These approaches are an attempt to define those multiple factors that might affect the patient's behavior. In a case report, a noncompliant hemophiliac child (not using his factor appropriately) became compliant following an intervention with the patient and his family (Hanford, 1980).

The Mount Sinai Hemophilia Center has had a longstanding interest and commitment to family issues in its hemophilia population. Three years ago the center embarked on a National Heart, Lung, and Blood Institute-supported randomized prospective clinical trial using family intervention as one arm of the study of adherence in hemophilia patients.

Sample

One hundred and sixty-six patients at the Mount Sinai Medical Center were studied. Only 25.9% of the patient population was ineligible for participation in the trial. The distribution of the adherence issues of those who entered mirrored the distribution of adherence problems in the center as a whole; problems associated with a nonrepresentative, skewed population did not arise.

TABLE 15.1 Outcome Data from 31 Division of Maternal and Child Health-Funded Comprehensive Hemophilia Centers and Their Affiliates

Outcome data	Year before program (1975)	10th year of program (1985)	% increased or % decreased (+/−)
No. patients seen at primary centers	1,783	5,606	+214%
No. patients seen at affiliate centers	329	1,641	+399%
No. patients receiving regular comprehensive care	1,333	5,683	+326%
No. patients on self-infusion ("home care")	514	2,517	+390%
Average days/year lost from work or school	14.5	3.9	− 73%
Average hospital admissions/year	1.9	0.22	− 88%
Average days/year spent as inpatient	9.4	1.6	− 83%
Percent patients with third-party coverage	74	93	+ 26%
Out-of-pocket expenses/patient/year	$1,700*	$396	− 77%
Overall costs of care/patient/year	$31,600*	$8,127	− 74%
Percent unemployed adults	36	9.4	− 74%

*adjusted for 1985 dollars.
Data provided by the National Hemophilia Foundation.

Methods

Categories of Nonadherence

Patients were evaluated for three categories of nonadherence: medical management problems, social–behavioral problems, and substance abuse (see the appendix operational definitions).

Medical Management Indicators of Nonadherence. This category included: (1) number of bleeding episodes; (2) inappropriate factor use (overuse and underuse); and (3) failure to keep bleeding logs in accordance with program requirements (see Table 15.2). Other issues included inappropriate use of the treatment center (i.e., poor attendance at clinic or overuse of the clinic, missed appointments, or inappropriate use of the emergency room) and inability to be eligible for home care or to remain on home care because of poor management

TABLE 15.2 Operational Definitions of Nonadherence

I. Medical Management Indicators of Nonadherence
   A. Number of Bleeds
      1. Number of bleeds in the last 6 months at least double that of the previous 6 months. Doubling the number of bleeds in the more recent 6-month period compared to the previous half-year was presumed to be an indirect measure of chronic psychosocial forces on biological events.
      2. The maximum number of bleeds in any month in the last 6-month period was greater than the maximum number of bleeds in the previous 6-month period. Doubling the maximum number of bleeds in any *one* month in the more recent 6-month period compared to the previous half-year was presumed to be an indirect measure of acute psychosocial forces on biological events.
   B. Inappropriate Use of Blood Products
      1. Underuse of blood products: total number of times underused greater than one.
      2. Overuse of blood products: total number of times overused greater than one.
      3. The total number of bleeds and the amount of blood products actually used is consistently higher than would be expected (given the level of severity of the disease) AND there is clinical evidence of a pattern of inappropriate prophylactic use.
      4. There is a medically significant discrepancy between the total amount of blood products dispensed during the last 6 months and the reported amount of factor/cryoprecipitate actually used.
      5. Patient has reported to a clinical staff member not infusing for a bleed for which infusion was appropriate any time in the last 6 months (or delaying treatments).
   C. Nonsubmission of Bleeding Logs
      The patient has failed to submit self-report bleeding logs according to home care instructions more than once in the last 6 months.
   D. Inappropriate Treatment Center Utilization
      1. *Number of Clinic Visits:* The patient has at least two times the number of clinic visits in the last 6 months as he had the previous 6 months.
      2. *Number of Missed Appointments:* The patient has missed at least two times the number of appointments in the last 6 months as he missed in the previous 6 months.
      3. *Number of Emergency Room Visits:* The patient has gone to the emergency room at least two times the number of times in the last 6 months as in the previous 6 months.
   E. Inability to be Placed on Home Therapy
      The treatment team has determined that the patient should not be placed on home care because of disease-management issues.
   F. Inability to Remain on Home Therapy
      The patient has been taken off home care in the last 6 months because of inappropriate management.
II. Social–Behavioral Problems
   A. Days Lost from School
      The patient has missed at least two times as many days from school due to bleeding episodes (including his own or other's fears related to hemophilia) in the last year as in the previous year.

(continued)

TABLE 15.2 (*continued*)

B. Days Lost from Work
The patient has missed at least two times as many days from work within the last year due to bleeding-related factors or episodes (including his own or other's fears related to hemophilia).

C. Enmeshment with Physician or Other Team Member
The patient or a family member has an emotionally overinvolved or overdependent relationship with a physician or other team member (e.g., frequent unnecessary phone calls, acting as if the provider can read his or her mind, coalition with provider that excludes parent or spouse).

D. Identifiable Family Problem
The patient has reported family problems to a member of the treatment team that were sufficiently frequent or intense to threaten the unity of the family or to interfere with the effective management of the disease.

III. Substance Abuse

A. Drug Abuse
The patient has been identified as a drug abuser, with either a pattern of pathological use or impairment in social or occupational functioning due to drug use (DSM-III 304.9).

B. Alcohol Abuse
The patient has been identified as an alcohol abuser, with either a pattern of pathological use or impairment in social or occupational functioning due to drug use (DSM-III 305.0).

behavior. A total of 54.3% of the patients had medical management problems. Approximately 26% of the patients had medical management problems only. Another 28.3% of the patients had medical management problems in combination with social–behavioral or substance abuse problems.

Social–Behavioral Problems. This category included patients: (1) with excessive loss of time from work or school; (2) abnormally enmeshed with a clinic team member; or (3) with family problems that had a negative impact on disease management or threatened the unity of the family as a whole. A total of 42.8% of the patients had social–behavioral problems. Only 15.7% of the population had social–behavioral problems only; another 27.1% had social–behavioral problems in combination with medical management or substance abuse problems.

Substance Abuse. This category included patients with alcohol or drug abuse problems. They represented 12.6% of the clinic population; only 0.6% (one patient) had a substance abuse problem without exhibiting any problems from the other categories. Only 25.9% of the patient population was ineligible in all three categories.

Intervention

The family intervention was compared of a maximum of 10 sessions of family therapy performed by members of the Ackerman Institute of Family Therapy. Patients also continued with their traditional comprehensive care during the course of the trial. Sessions at the Institute were held, where the "cutting edge" issue—that is, entry adherence problem—was the focal point.

Procedures

A multidisciplinary team, similar to that described earlier, identified patients who were eligible for study. With appropriate informed consent, patients and their families were entered into the study. Each patient and his family were then interviewed, given questionnaires regarding demographics and attitudes, and baseline data on adherence problems gathered. The patient and his family were randomized into either the family intervention group or into traditional comprehensive care.

At the end of the intervention period, patients and families were reassessed (in both arms of the study) regarding any changes in adherence and attitudes about the adherence problem. The comprehensive team treating the patient also was assessed regarding these issues. A nontreating comprehensive hemophilia team was presented the case and asked their assessment of change in adherence given the initial problems, patient, and team and family observation after intervention.

Data now are being analyzed. The ultimate goal is to define whether family intervention should be an additional resource to comprehensive centers in dealing with the very high proportion of adherence problems in this disease.

Issues Affecting the Hemophilia Trial

Recruitment Issues.   Recruitment for biopsychosocial research is extraordinarily difficult. It is quite different from classic prevention clinical trials. It is particularly difficult in studies dealing with nonadherence. The population, by definition, is not following recommended treatment regimens. In the trial on hemophilia, it was observed that recruiting family members was an additional problem.

The approach taken by the study team to solve this problem was to choose, as recruiter for the trial, a social worker who was a longstanding member of the Mount Sinai program. Patients were contacted at their 6-month regular visits. Literature in English and Spanish was sent to all patients. The directors of the program sent letters to all their patients to explain the nature of the project, its relevance to their care, and value to the rest of the hemophilia population. All members of the team were educated about the study as well as its perceived value for hemophilia treatment. Recruitment into the study was 32% of eligible contactable patients.

Reasons for Nonparticipation.   The reasons for nonparticipation are of interest. Patients and families felt that the burden of the disease, especially with AIDS added to their worries, was a major issue. The commitment of time was another. Overparticipation in scientific studies was a significant issue. These patients, representing the most heavily transfused group in the world, have been asked repeatedly to enter many major longitudinal studies of transfusion-transmitted diseases. Distance from the treatment center was another issue. Lastly, but by no means minor, is that many patients felt they had built substantial defenses and were not prepared to disassemble them.

Impact of AIDS on the Hemophilia Population.   While carrying out the study, the threat of increasing numbers of AIDS cases occurring in hemophiliacs (first case, 1982) has added a major new dimension to adherence issues in hemophilia. Fear of getting the AIDS virsus from concentrate has increased the number of patients frightened to infuse. Recognition that the virus can be sexually transmitted had enhanced anxiety and wrought serious problems for this patient group. All patients who are constantly being exposed to the virus are educated concerning safer sexual practices. However, in a recent survey of the Mount Sinai population, 30% do not tell sexual partners that they are HIV-positive, and 51% do not practice safer sex. Of note: 98% exhibit appropriate levels of knowledge of sexual transmission of HIV infection. This represents another example of failure of traditional educational techniques in improving adherence behavior.

OBSTACLES TO ADHERENCE RESEARCH IN THE YOUNG

Access to patients is another important consideration in adherence research with the young. Many times parental involvement is necessary but, because of many conflicting responsibilities, cannot be assured. The use of children in research is especially a problem in areas concerning confidentiality.

Assessment of comprehension is a constant obstacle in adherence research with the young. Language and cultural barriers are additional factors. One study mentioned a cultural factor as affecting adherence (Kellaway & Brown, 1983) and suggested that nonadherence was due to language difficulties. These factors warrant further investigation.

SUMMARY

Compliance issues in chronic diseases are common. Little is known about the effectiveness of interventions for this group of diseases. Biopsychosocial research in this complex area is very difficult to carry out. The very nature of the population makes the "nonadherent" patient hard to reach—no less to change behavior. Recruitment of individuals, and especially families, to enter prospective controlled clinical trials is a monumental task. Review committees of federal research funding agencies such as NHLBI are not very sympathetic to this type of research agenda or design. We strongly encourage more research and financial support for this perplexing and critical area of health care delivery.

REFERENCES

Allen, D. A., Tennen, H., McGrade, B. J., Affleck, G., & Ratzan, S. (1983). Parent and child perceptions of the management of juvenile diabetes. *Journal of Pediatric Psychology,* 8(2), 129–141.

Baum, D., & Creer, T. L. (1986). Medical compliance in children with asthma. *Journal of Asthma,* 23(2), 49–59.

Beck, D. E., Fennell, R. S., Yost, R. L., Rodinson, J. D., Geary, D., & Richards, G. A. (1980). Evaluation of an education program on compliance with medication regimens in pediatric patients with renal transplants. *Journal of Pediatrics,* 96(6), 1094–1097.

Becker, M. H., Maiman, L. A., Kirscht, J. P., Haefner, D. P., & Drachman, R. H. (1977). The Health Belief Model and prediction of dietary compliance: A field experiment. *Journal of Health and Social Behavior,* 18, 348–366.

Becker, M. H., Radius, S. M., Rosenstock, I. M., Drachman, R. H., Schubert, K. C., & Teets, K. C. (1978). Compliance with a medical regimen for asthma: A test of the Health Belief Model. *Public Health Reports,* 93(3), 268–277.

Bobrow, E. S., Ruskin, T. W., & Siller, J. (1985). Mother–daughter interaction and adherence to diabetes regimens. *Diabetes Care,* 8(2), 146–151.

Bruhn, J. G. (1983). The application of theory in childhood asthma self-help programs. *Journal of Allergy and Clinical Immunology,* 72(5, Part 2), 561–577.

Buchanan, G. R., Siegel, J. D., Smith, S. J., & DePasse, B. M. (1982). Oral penicillin prophylasix in children with impaired splenic function: A study of compliance. *Pediatrics,* 70(6), 926–930.

Casey, R., Rosen, B., Glowasky, A., & Ludwig, S. (1985). An intervention to improve follow-up of patients with otitis media. *Clinical Pediatrics,* 24(3), 149–152.

Clemmer, E. J., & Hayes, E. W. (1979). Patient cooperation in wearing orthodontic headgear. *American Journal of Dental Care,* 75(5), 517–524.

Cluss, P. A., Epstein, L. H., Galvis, S. A., Fireman, P., & Friday, G. (1984). Effect of compliance for chronic asthmatic children. *Journal of Consultant and Clinical Psychology, 52*(5), 909–910.

Daneman, D., Epstein, L. H., Siminerio, L., Beck, S., Farkas, G., Figueroa, J., Becker, D. J., & Drash, A. L. (1982). Effects of enhanced conventional therapy on metabolic control in children with insulin-dependent diabetes mellitus. *Diabetes Care, 5*(5), 472–478.

Deaton, A. V. (1985). Adaptive noncompliance in pediatric asthma: The parent as expert. *Journal of Pediatric Psychology, 10*(1), 1–14.

Dolgin, M. J., Katz, E. R., Doctors, S. R., & Siegel, S. E. (1986). Caregivers' perceptions of medical compliance in adolescents with cancer. *Journal of Adolescent Health Care, 7*, 22–27.

Durant, R. H., Jay, M. S., Linder, C. W., Shoffitt, T., & Litt, I. (1984). Influence of psychosocial factors on adolescent compliance with oral contraceptives. *Journal of Adolescent Health Care, 5*(1), 1–6.

El-Mangoury, N. H. (1981). Orthodontic cooperation. *American Journal of Orthodontia, 80*(6), 604–622.

Epstein, L. H., Beck, S., Figueroa, J., Farkas, G., Kazdin, A. E., Daneman, D., & Becker, D. (1981). The effects of targeting improvements in urine glucose on metabolic control in children with IDD. *Journal of Applied Behavioral Analysis, 14*, 365–375.

Finkelstein, S. M., Budd, J. R., Warwick, W. J., Kujawa, S. J., & Wienlinski, C. L. (1986). Feasibility and compliance studies of a home measurement monitoring program for cystic fibrosis. *Journal of Chronic Diseases, 39*(3), 195–205.

Finney, J. W., Friman, P. C., Rapoff, M. A., & Christophersen, E. R. (1985). Improving compliance with antibiotic regimens for otitis media: Randomized clinical trial in a pediatric clinic. *American Journal of Diseases of Children, 139*, 89–95.

Flanders, P. A., & McNamara, J. R. (1985). Enhancing acne medication compliance: A comparison of strategies. *Behavioral Research Therapy, 23*(2), 225–227.

Friedman, I. M., & Litt, I. F. (1986). Promoting adolescents' compliance with therapeutic regimens. *Pediatric Clinics of North America, 33*(4), 955–973.

Friedman, I. M., Litt, I. F., & King, D. R. (1986). Compliance with anticonvulsant therapy by epileptic youth: Relationships to psychosocial aspects of adolescent development. *Journal of Adolescent Health Care, 7*, 12–17.

Glanz, K., Fiel, S. B., Swartz, M. A., & Francis, M. E. (1984). Compliance with an experimental drug regimen for treatment of asthma: Its magnitude, importance and correlates. *Journal of Chronic Diseases, 37*(11), 815–824.

Hanford, A. (1980). Effect of psychiatric intervention on use of antihemophilic factor concentrate. *American Journal of Psychiatry, 132*, 1254.

Haynes, R. B., Taylor, D. W., & Sackett, D. L. (1979). *Compliance in health care*. Baltimore, MD: John Hopkins University Press.

Irwin, C. E., Millstein, S. G., & Shafer, M. B. (1981). Appointment-keeping behavior in adolescents. *Journal of Pediatrics, 99*(5), 799–802.

Jamison, R. N., Lewis, S., & Burish, T. G. (1986). Cooperation with treatment in adolescent cancer patients. *Journal of Adolescent Health Care, 7*, 162–167.

Jay, M. S., DuRant, R. H., Shoffitt, T., Linder, C. W., & Litt, I. F. (1984). Effect of peer counselors on adolescent compliance in use of oral contraceptives. *Pediatrics, 73*(2), 126–131.

Kaplan, R. M., Chadwick, M. W., & Schimmel, L. E. (1985). Social learning intervention to promote metabolic control in Type 1 diabetes mellitus: Pilot experimental results. *Diabetes Care, 8*(2), 152–155.

Kellaway, G. S.M., & Brown, S. A. (1983). Compliance failure and counseling in paediatric drug therapy. *New Zealand Medical Journal, 96*(728), 207–209.

Korsch, B. M., Fine, R. N., & Negrete, V. F. (1978). Noncompliance in children with renal transplants. *Pediatrics, 61*(6), 872–876.

Lansky, S. B., Smith, S. D., Cairns, N. U., & Cairns, G. F. (1983). Psychological correlates of compliance. *American Journal of Pediatric Hematology and Oncology, 5*(1), 87–92.

Lansky, S. B., Vats, T., & Cairns, N. U. (1979). Refusal of treatment: A new dilemma for oncologists. *American Journal of Pediatric Hematology and Oncology, 1*(3), 277–282.

Litt, I. F., & Cuskey, W. R. (1981). Compliance with salicylate therapy in adolescents with juvenile rheumatoid arthritis. *American Journal of Diseases of Children, 135*, 434–436.

Litt, I. F., & Cuskey, W. R. (1984). Satisfaction with health care: A predictor of adolescent appointment keeping. *Journal of Adolescent Health Care, 5*, 196–200.

Litt, I. F., Cuskey, W. R., & Rosenberg, A. (1982). Role of self-esteem and autonomy in determining medication compliance among adolescents with juvenile rheumatoid arthritis. *Pediatrics, 69*(1), 15–17.

Litt, I. F., Cuskey, W. R., & Rudd, S. (1980). Identifying adolescents at risk for noncompliance with contraceptive therapy. *Journal of Pediatrics, 96*(4), 742–745.

Meyer, A., Dolan, T. F., & Mueller, D. (1975). Compliance and self-medication in cystic fibrosis. *American Journal of Diseases of Children, 129*, 1011–1013.

Neel, E. U., Jay, S., & Litt, I. F. (1985). The relationship of self-concept and autonomy to oral contraceptive compliance among adolescent females. *Journal of Adolescent Health Care, 6*, 445–447.

Passero, A. M., Remor, B., & Salomon, J. (1981). Patient-reported compliance with cystic fibrosis therapy. *Clinical Pediatrics, 20*(4), 264–268.

Pearce, T., O'Shea, J. S., & Wesson, A. F. (1979). Correlations between appointment keeping and reorganization of hospital ambulatory pediatric services. *Pediatrics, 64*(1), 81–87.

Radius, S., Becker, M. H., Rosenstock, I. M., Drachman, R. H., Schubert, K. C., & Teets, K. C. (1978). Factors influencing mothers' compliance with a medical regimen for asthmatic children. *Journal of Asthma Research, 15*(3), 133–149.

Schafer, L. C., Glasgow, R. E., & McCaul, K. D. (1982). Increasing the adherence of diabetic adolescents. *Journal of Behavioral Medicine, 5*(3), 353–357.

Simonds, J. F. (1977). Psychiatric status of diabetic youth matched with a control group. *Diabetes, 26*(10), 921–925.

Sleator, E. K., Ullmann, R. K., & von Neumann, A. (1982). How do hyperactive children feel about taking stimulants and will they tell the doctor? *Clinical Pediatrics, 21*(8), 474–479.

Smith, N. A., Seale, J. P., Ley, P., Shaw, J., & Bracks, P. U. (1986). Effects of intervention or medication compliance in children with asthma. *Medical Journal of Australia, 144,* 119–122.

Spector, S. L., Kinsman, R., Mawhinney, H., Siegel, S. C., Rachelefsky, G. S., Katz, R. M., & Rohr, A. S. (1986). Compliance of patients with asthma with an experimental aerosolized medication: Implications for controlled clinical trials. *Journal of Allergy and Clinical Immunology, 77*(1, Part 1), 65–70.

Weinstein, A. G., & Cuskey, W. (1985). Theophylline compliance in asthmatic children. *Annals of Allergy, 54,* 19–24.

BIBLIOGRAPHY

Babiker, M. A. (1986). Compliance with penicillin prophylasix by children with impaired splenic function. *Tropical Geographic Medicine, 38,* 119–122.

Chryssanthropoulous, C., Laufer, P., & Torphy, D. E. (1983). Assessment of acute asthma in the emergency room: Evaluation of compliance and combined drug therapy. *Journal of Asthma, 20*(1), 35–38.

de Wet, B., & Hollingshead, J. (1980). Medication compliance in paediatric outpatients. *South African Medical Journal, 58,* 846–848.

Gross, A. M., Stern, R. M., Levin, R. B., Dale, J., & Wojnilower, D. A. (1983). The effect of mother–child separation on the behavior of children experiencing a diagnostic medical process. *Journal of Consultant & Clinical Psychology, 51*(5), 783–785.

Kaufman, R. E., Smith-Wright, D., Reese, C. A., Simpson, R., & Jones, F. (1981). Medication compliance in hyperactive children. *Pediatric Pharmacology, 1,* 231–237.

Kleiger, J. H., & Dirks, J. F. (1979). Medication compliance in chronic asthmatic patients. *Journal of Asthma Research, 16*(3), 93–97.

Litt, I. F. (1985). Know thyself—Adolescents' self-assessment of compliance behavior. *Pediatrics, 75*(4), 693–695.

McCormick, M. C., Shapiro, S., & Starfield, B. H. (1981). The association of patient-held records and completion of immunizations. *Clinical Pediatrics (Philadelphia), 20*(4), 270–274.

Miller, K. A. (1982). Theophylline compliance in adolescent patients with chronic asthma. *Journal of Adolescent Health Care, 3,* 177–179.

Polowich, C., & Elliott, M. R. (1977). The juvenile diabetic: In or out of control? *Canadian Nurse, 73*(9), 24–27.

Schmitt, B. D. (1984). Preschoolers who refuse to be examined. *American Journal of Dental Care, 138,* 443–446.

Smith, N. A., Seale, J. P., & Shaw, J. (1984). Medication compliance in children with asthma. *Australian Paediatric Journal, 20,* 47–51.

Spector, S. L. (1985). Is your asthmatic patient really complying? *Annals of Allergy, 55,* 552–556.

Sublett, J. L., Pollard, S. J., Kadlec, G. J., & Karibo, J. M. (1979). Non-compliance in asthmatic children: A study of theophylline levels in a pediatric emergency room population. *Annals of Allergy, 43*, 95–97.

Tinkelman, D. G., Vanderpool, G. E., Carroll, M. S., Page, E. G., & Spanger, O. L. (1980). Compliance differences following administration of theophylline at 6 and 12 hour intervals. *Annals of Allergy, 44*, 283–286.

16

Problems with Adherence in the Elderly

Harold P. Roth

Problems with adherence to medical regimens are common among the elderly. One factor that contributes to the number of problems is the frequency with which the elderly take medications (Klein, German, & Levine, 1981). The likelihood of developing one or more chronic diseases increases with age. Furthermore, effective treatment for many of these diseases requires a prolonged or continuous therapeutic regimen, including potent drugs. Often the regimen must be followed meticulously if it is to prove effective, and side effects or even dangerous toxicity are to be avoided. Physiological effects of aging may increase the possibility of adverse effects; in addition, functional limitations that patients suffer with aging may make it more difficult for them to follow their regimens. Information on some of these issues and problems and possible ways of avoiding or dealing with them are presented in the material that follows.

DRUG USE IN THE ELDERLY

About 76% of individuals over 65 years of age were found to be taking at least one drug when a study was done at Dundein on a series of elderly from a large retirement area located near St. Petersburg and Clearwater, Florida (Hale, Marks, & Stewart, 1979). The individuals examined had come to Dundein to participate in a program to screen elderly patients for hypertension and other disorders. In preparation for this examination, patients were asked to list all medications that they were currently taking, whether prescription or nonprescription, and the intended therapeutic indications of each. The results showed that, on the average, men 65 to 69 years of age took 1.2 prescription drugs and women 1.7. For men in the 85 to 90 age group, the number of prescription drugs was 1.7; for women, it was over 2.2. Nonprescription drugs taken by elderly men averaged about 1, and elderly women averaged about 1.5; but both sexes showed a slight drop in the number of nonprescription drugs as subjects entered their late eighties.

Findings were only slightly different in household interviews conducted on 3,467 individuals in rural Iowa (Helling et al., 1987). Drug users in the 65 to 70 age group totaled 65.6%, with the average number of prescription drugs used being 1.4. The mean number of prescription and nonprescription drugs reported was 2.99 for women and 2.69 for men. Fifty percent of the prescription drugs taken were cardiovascular agents. A third of the nonprescription drugs could be classified as acting on the musculoskeletal system.

Medication intake was found to be larger in a study of 184 low-income elderly and disabled persons living in two federally supported high-rises in Seattle. The mean number of prescription drugs taken per person was 2.3, and for nonprescription drugs it was 2.1 (Ostrom, Hammarlund, Christensen, Plein, & Kethley, 1985).

Intake of drugs was even larger among residents in a high-rise subsidized housing unit in Indianapolis who agreed to participate in interviews in their apartments (Darnell, Murray, Martz, & Weinberger, 1986). The mean age of the 155 respondents was 71.6 years; 90% took prescribed drugs, with an average number of 4.5 per person. Ninety-six percent used over-the-counter drugs; the average number of these was 3.4. In London, use of medication was found to be similar. In a random sample of patients 65 and older from an inner-city family practice, 97% were taking medications (Kiernan & Isaacs, 1981).

Number of Drugs Taken by Those Not Healthy and Active

Elderly who are not as healthy or active as members of some of the populations described above usually take more drugs. Upon discharge from the Johns Hopkins Hospital 25% of those over 65 years of age received six or more drugs (Smith, 1979). However, several medications may have been given for a single disorder such as diabetes or heart disease (Hulka, Cassell, Kupper, & Eferd, 1976). Among 740 patients seen in an ambulatory clinic at Johns Hopkins, the average number of medications taken in the preceding month was 6.1, of which 4.9 were prescribed by a clinician and 1.2 were obtained over-the-counter (German & Klein, 1986).

A further indication of the use of medications among those who are not active and ambulatory is provided by the medications given to patients in nursing homes (Hale et al., 1979). The percentages of patients who received each of the following type of medications were: laxatives, 58.1%; analgesics, 51.3%; tranquilizers, 46.9%; vitamins, 34.1%; sedative-hypnotics, 34.7%; and cardiac drugs, 29.1% (Department of Health and Human Services, 1976).

A major concern in the use of medication by the elderly is that there is evidence that as the number of drugs prescribed is increased, patients' compliance with instructions for use decreases (Williamson & Chopin, 1980). Such problems with compliance are more commonly described with patients over 65 years of age, particularly when four or more drugs are prescribed (Klein et al., 1981). There are also more likely to be problems with compliance or misuse of drugs in older patients who have two or more physicians or pharmacists (Raffoul, 1986).

Review of the most common therapeutic indications and the actual names of the drugs most commonly prescribed shows that many of these medications require precise adjustment of dosages in order to attain the desired effect and avoid toxic effects. Thus, for many medications, the patient can have problems if precisely the right amount is not prescribed by the physician or taken by the patient.

DIFFICULTIES WITH DOSAGES IN THE ELDERLY

Doctors may find determination of precise doses of medication for aged patients difficult for a number of reasons (Halaris, 1986). Changes in metabolism and physiology can occur with aging. An aged patient (1) may not metabolize a given drug at the same rate and in the same way as a younger individual; (2) may not excrete the drug or its metabolites in urine at the usual rate, since renal functional impairment is not uncommon in the aged; (3) may have a low proportion of body water, causing distribution of the drug in the body to be altered; (4) may not respond to a drug in the usual way, as there may be alterations in physiologic receptors with age (Ouslander, 1981); or (5) may find that one drug may interact in an unusual way with another already being taken.

Even if the physician determines the dose carefully, he can be frustrated in his effort to provide effective and safe care when patients deviate from their prescribed regimens. These deviations can include (1) failure to take the prescribed amount; (2) overdoses of the prescribed drugs; or (3) taking, along with prescriptions, unknown to their physicians, over-the-counter drugs or medication given by another physician.

Certain over-the-counter drugs (Lundin, Eros, Melloh, & Sands, 1980) are taken commonly. These include vitamins, laxatives, and stomach preparations.

Among the latter are antacids that may interfere with absorption of other medications prescribed for the patient, including antibiotics. It is also not uncommon for patients to take over-the-counter drugs for specific problems such as "muscular aches," "colds," and "insomnia." These drugs may cause symptoms of their own (May, Stewart, Hale, & Marks, 1982) and may interact with medications given by prescription.

Thus, even though the physician has carefully selected a regimen that he or she believes should be effective and will not produce side effects or adverse reactions, if the desired effect is not obtained it can be important for the physician to carefully evaluate compliance. In a difficult, confusing case it may be useful to determine the level of the drug in the blood. If the level is low, inadequate intake may be considered; if the level is high, an overdose is a potential consideration. It may also be important to determine whether the patient is taking any drugs other than those prescribed.

EXAMPLES OF PROBLEMS WITH ADHERENCE IN COMMON DISORDERS

Some examples are given here of the problems that may occur in aged patients when they are given prescribed medications for some common diseases or disorders and deviate from their regimens.

Mental Illness

Mental illness, anxiety, insomnia, and depression are common among the aged (Luke et al., 1982). Hypnotics, tranquilizers, sedatives, and antidepressants are commonly prescribed. If the patient fails to take the medicine, effects expected of the drug may not be observed. However, if he or she takes too much, be it only a tranquilizer prescribed with the goal of treating anxiety, the patient may become confused, obtunded (less acute mentally), or depressed. This may also occur if the patient is taking a sedative drug purchased over-the-counter about which the current physician has not been informed, or if he or she is using a sedative given by another physician (Patrick, Peach, & Gregg, 1982).

Cardiovascular Disorders

Drugs acting on the cardiovascular system are among those most commonly given to the elderly. Most of these drugs require precise management to obtain and maintain the desired blood levels in the patient and yet avoid a level that is too high, which can cause serious or even dangerous side effects (Cusack et al., 1978). Digitoxin is such a drug: If the patient does not take the full, correct dose, cardiac failure may not be prevented; if he or she takes too much, there may be toxic effects such as arrhythmias. If a diuretic is also a part of the patient's regimen, the possibility of problems may be increased because of unanticipated or unrecognized changes in fluid volume or electrolyte levels.

Recommendations for fluid and electrolyte intake must be followed carefully by the patient in order to help adjust for the effects of diuretics. The elderly may have low fluid volume to begin with, and with fluid loss from a diuretic, they may suffer dehydration unless fluid intake is appropriately increased. Electrolyte balance may also be difficult to manage. Maintaining the correct level of potassium can create difficult problems in management for the physician with a patient who is taking digitoxin, since this patient then can be unusually sensitive to the level of that electrolyte. The problem of handling potassium levels is aggravated if the patient also has some impairment of kidney function, as occurs often in the elderly (Papper, 1973). Thus, when the patient is asked to take a potassium supplement along with diuretic therapy, there can be serious problems if the patient does not take the medication precisely as prescribed (Henschke, Spence, & Cape, 1981).

Hypertension

Hypertension is a disorder for which a drug regimen is often prescribed. A common problem in hypertension management is failure of the patient to take all or part of the medication, causing unsatisfactory control of blood pressure. However, occasionally, if the patient does have a lowering of blood pressure with antihypertensive drugs, there can be hypotensive episodes with weakness and falls (Fedder, 1984). Such episodes may occur if the patient is taking diuretics and there has been unrecognized and uncorrected major fluid loss. This problem can happen more readily in the elderly than in other patients because the elderly may have a low proportion of body water before any treatment is given (Forbes & Reina, 1970).

ADVERSE DRUG REACTIONS IN THE ELDERLY

Adverse drug effects among the elderly are common. The Royal College of Physicians estimates that 20% to 25% of all elderly admitted to acute-care hospitals present with adverse drug reactions. Comparable U.S. data show 12 to 17% of the elderly population present with adverse drug reactions; this is three to four times the rate for all adults. In one study, the incidence steadily increased with age, from 9.9% among patients in the 21 to 30 age group to 24.0% among patients 81 years old and older (Seidl, Thornton, Smith, & Cluff, 1966). Canadian data indicate that 30% of all elderly admitted to acute-care hospitals from nursing homes suffer from adverse drug reactions, and British data estimate that 40% of community-living elderly are probably affected by adverse reactions.

The single factor reported as contributing to or accounting for 80.9% of acute drug reactions among the elderly was misuse or abuse of drugs; that is, usually poor compliance with a prescribed drug regimen (Peterson & Thomas, 1975). Over-the-counter drugs were implicated in 186 drug-related admissions (Caranasos, Stewart, & Cluff, 1974).

REASONS FOR NONADHERENCE IN THE ELDERLY

As indicated earlier, poor compliance with a drug regimen is common. Evans and Spelman (1983) estimated that one half of patients do not take their medicine or do not take it as prescribed. Failure to adhere to a medical regimen may take many forms, and many different reasons may be given for it.

Reasons for patient failure to adhere to regimens were examined by Cooper, Love, and Raffoul (1982), who visited elderly in their homes in Lexington, Kentucky. Subjects were asked to provide medications in their containers and were asked about each medication. They found that 10% of reported nonadherence could be characterized as overuse. Patients decided that more of a drug was needed and so took more than 125% of the prescribed dosage for over a month. On the other hand, usually the breach reported was in taking less than the prescribed amount. The reason that patients gave most frequently for not taking the full dose was the decision that the dosage prescribed by the physician was too large. Side effects were also a reason given for diminishing the dose, but this reason was not commonly given. Some patients stated that they had forgotten or did not understand the prescription. Another reason that patients gave in this and other studies was that they simply could not afford the drug. The latter reason was also given for not taking the full dose; patients saved some medications for following days.

It should also be noted that many elderly patients live alone. Once such patients make mistakes in time or amount of drugs to be taken, they are likely to continue with the errors as there is no one to indicate the correct schedule or dosage.

Comprehension of Instructions

A factor that may contribute to elderly patients' failure to follow accurately their instructions for medication usage is the limited information that they receive and remember about their prescriptions. Often they have poor understanding of the nature of their regimens and the purpose of their medications (Cartwright & Anderson, 1981). Furthermore, instructions about the how and when to take their medicine may have been inadequate or confusing (Lundin, 1978). For example, directions such as "take as needed" can leave patients uncertain as to when the medicine is needed. Even commonly used instructions such as "take after each meal" can be confusing to a patient who is not consistently consuming three meals a day; the prescribing physician may have presumed that this was the case.

Problems with Containers and Labels

When 178 attendees at the General Medical Clinic of the New York Hospital were interviewed, 105 were committing some type of "medication error" (Schwartz, Wang, Zeitz, & Goss, 1962). A number of possible causes for patient confusion about their drug regimens were found by pharmacy and nursing students who visited patients in their homes and studied prescriptions in their containers. Discrepancies between prescribed regimens and labels on containers were common. Often a change in the dosage schedule had been made by the prescriber after the medication was dispensed that had not been entered on the label. The labels on some bottles were difficult for the patient to read; in some elderly it may be difficult to read the usual label because of impaired vision, and large type may be needed.

Some patients had difficulty dealing with childproof caps or were too weak or too poorly coordinated to remove them easily. This may have caused patients to transfer medications to other containers or to leave off the caps. Removing the medication from the original bottle can be risky—patients may try to recognize medicines in the new bottles by the color of the tablets, but it has been found that some patients cannot distinguish the colors of different medications (Murray, Darnell, Weinberger, & Martz, 1986).

Murray and his team (1986) also found that patients tended to keep medicines that were commonly used handy, for example, on the kitchen table. However, sometimes medications were stored in a place that was too warm or too moist. Some medications had been removed from their original bottles and labels on the new containers were wrong for that medication. It was also common for patients to store prescribed medications that were no longer in use.

Continued Use of Old Prescriptions

Patients also had a tendency not only to keep bottles of medication but to continue to take them without discussion with their physician (Cartwright & Anderson, 1981). In several studies, when physicians examined the drugs that patients were taking, they found that some of the drugs were unnecessary; this was true even for potent drugs like digitoxin (Gryfe & Gryfe, 1984).

322 Adherence Issues within Specific Populations

SUGGESTIONS FOR IMPROVING ADHERENCE IN THE ELDERLY

Written Instructions

Several suggestions for improving compliance have grown out of the studies of factors associated with poor compliance (Davidson, 1973). First, instructions should be written, as elderly patients may not fully hear instructions on prescriptions or remember them. Second, the use of large type for labels and instructions may be helpful, as imparied vision is common with this population. Third, labels can be a valuable source of information for patients, but they are usually not used to their full potential; with the elderly, it is particularly important to provide as much information as possible on the labels of medications (Wade & Bowling, 1986). Guidelines for labels have been developed by the American Pharmaceutical Association and the American Society of Internal Medicine and should be used by both physicians and pharmacists. Fourth, bottles containing tablets or pills should be easy to open. Physicians should indicate to the pharmacist those patients for whom childproof containers may present a problem or for whom childproof containers are unnecessary or undesired. Lastly, avoid tablets or capsules that may be too big for patients who could have trouble in chewing or swallowing them.

Some investigators have found no evidence that teaching patients about why the medicine works improves compliance (German, Klein, McPhee, & Smith, 1982). Others have stated that understanding the manner of action of a medication and why it is taken according to a schedule has proven helpful to patients. Understanding the way medication acts may provide an explanation for the times it should be taken.

Teaching and Counseling

There is little disagreement about the value of instructing patients about regimens. A leaflet containing information about a medication and its use has been described as a useful element in a program for instruction; however, it has been repeatedly suggested that the physician arrange time for discussion of prescriptions with patients. This time can provide opportunities to raise and discuss such questions as (1) why the medication is important to take; (2) why patients should take the medication at the times, in the amounts, and for the periods identified; (3) when is a regular, convenient, and consistent time for patients to take medicine—for example, in relation to meals or another of the patient's consistent daily activities (Zifferblatt, 1975); and (4) what is the manner of action of the medication, if the physician considers it appropriate.

Because of the declining memory of some aged patients, calendars and other memory aids have been found helpful (Macdonald, Macdonald, & Phoenix,

1977; Wandless & Davie, 1977). During or after discussions with patients, physicians may wish to provide written or printed descriptions of regimens.

A brief period of counseling proved helpful to one group of elderly patients (Edwards & Pathy, 1984). They were advised at the time of discharge from the hospital on dosage, frequency of administration, and mode of action of drugs that were prescribed for them. This counseling was associated with significantly better compliance to regimens as measured by pill counts. Counseling by physicians was associated with a slightly, but significantly, greater effect than counseling by nurses or pharmacists.

Role of the Pharmacist

A number of studies have shown the potential value of the pharmacist in answering questions of patients. Furthermore, pharmacists can maintain records of all medications and thus identify possible interactions that might occur among the drugs that patients are taking and notify their physicians. Pharmacists can improve compliance by talking to patients, and they can simplify medication schedules or supply memory aids ((Bayne, Caulfied, Kendrick, & Slack, 1983). The pharmacist may have a unique opportunity to help (Smith & Sharpe, 1984), particularly if patients use the same pharmacy for all prescriptions, as did 93% of the interviewees in a study in Seattle (Ostrom et al., 1985).

SUMMARY

Most individuals over 65 years of age are taking at least one drug; when they grow older and develop one or more of the chronic diseases that are common in the elderly, they begin to take several drugs. With an increase in the number of disorders, and in drugs taken to treat them, comes problems for the physician and the patient. Often these problems are due to poor compliance by the patient.

Serious problems in the elderly center around the large number of adverse drug reactions seen in the elderly. These may be due to the patient taking too large a dose or interactions of drugs taken for different conditions or drugs taken without the knowledge of the primary physician. In the latter case, primary physicians may be unaware of drugs in use by their patients because the drugs were prescribed by other physicians, obtained over the counter, or were previously prescribed and continued to be taken by patients without informing their physicians. Contributing to adverse reactions may be alterations in physiologic processes in the elderly such as distribution of fluids.

Another type of common problem can be an apparently poor response to ordinarily effective therapy that is actually due to failure of the patient to take any of or the full dose of the drug prescribed. The patient may forget to take the drug, think a full dose is not needed, or cannot afford the cost of the medication.

Both the adverse reactions and the failure to take an adequate dose may result from patients' lack of correct knowledge about their regimens. For the elderly who often may not hear or see normally and may have poor memories, it may be wise for their physicians to provide written instructions in large type and to discuss their regimens and problems with them in a brief counseling session.

REFERENCES

Bayne, J. R., Caulfield, P., Kendrick, R., & Slack, R. (1983). Pharmacists and their relationship with elderly patients. *Canadian Medical Association Journal, 129,* 35–37.

Caranasos, G. J., Stewart, R. B., & Cluff, L. E. (1974). Drug-induced illness leading to hospitalization. *Journal of the American Medical Association, 228,* 713.

Cartwright, A., & Anderson, R. (1981). *General practice revisited.* London: Tavistock.

Cooper, K., Love, W., & Raffoul, R. (1982). Intentional prescription nonadherence (non-compliance) by the elderly. *Journal of the American Geriatric Society, 30,* 329–334.

Cusack, B., Horgan, J., Kelly, J. G., LaVan, J., Noel, J., & O'Malley, K. (1978). Pharmacokinetics of digoxin in the elderly. *British Journal of Clinical Pharmacology 6,* 439.

Darnell, J. C., Murray, D., Martz, L., & Weinberger, M. (1986). Medication use by ambulatory elderly. An in-home survey. *Journal of the American Geriatric Society, 34,* 1–4.

Davidson, J. R. (1973). Presentation and packaging of drugs for the elderly. *Journal of Hospital Pharmacy, 31,* 180–184.

Edwards, M., & Pathy, J. S. J. (1984). Drug counselling in the elderly and predicting compliance. *The Practitioner, 228,* 291–300.

Evans, L., & Spelman, M. (1983). The problem of non-compliance with drug therapy. *Drugs, 25,* 63–76.

Fedder, O. (1984). Drug use in the elderly: Issues of noncompliance. *Drug Intelligence and Clinical Pharmacy, 18,* 158–162.

Forbes, G. B., & Reina, J. C. (1970). Adult lean body mass declines with age: Some longitudinal observations. *Metabolism, 19,* 653.

German, P. S., & Klein, L. E. (1986). Adverse drug experience among the elderly. In paper presented at *New research and new concerns: Pharmaceuticals for the elderly.* (pp. 40–48). Pharmaceutical Manufacturers Association and Hill and Knowlton, Washington, DC.

German, P. S., Klein, L., McPhee, S. J., & Smith, C. R. (1982). Knowledge of and compliance with drug regimens in the elderly. *Journal of the American Geriatrics Society, 30,* 568, 571.

Gryfe, C. I., & Gryfe, B. M. (1984). Drug therapy of the aged: The problem of compliance and the roles of physicians and pharmacists. *Journal of the American Geriatrics Society, 32*(4), 301–307.

Halaris, A. (1986). Antidepressant drug therapy in the elderly: Enhancing safety and compliance. *International Journal of Psychology in Medicine, 16*(1), 1–19.

Hale, E., Marks, G., & Stewart, B. (1979). Drug use in a geriatric population. *Journal of the American Geriatrics Society, 26,* 374–377.

Helling, K., Lemke, H., Semla, P., Wallace, B., Lipson, P., & Cornoni-Huntley, J. (1987). Medication use characteristics in the elderly: The Iowa 65+ rural health study. *Journal of the American Geriatrics Society*, 35(1), 4-12.

Henschke, P. J., Spence, J. D., & Cape, R. D. T. (1981). Diuretics and the institutional elderly: A case against routine potassium prescribing. *Journal of the American Geriatrics Society*, 29, 123-125.

Hulka, B. S., Cassell, J. C., Kupper, L. L., & Burdette, J. A. (1976). Communication, compliance, and concordance between physicians and patients with prescribed medications. *American Journal of Public Health*, 66, 847.

Kiernan, P. J., & Isaacs, J. B. (1981). Use of drugs by the elderly. *Journal of Research in Social Medicine*, 74, 196.

Klein, E., German, S., & Levine, M. (1981). Adverse drug reactions among the elderly: A reassessment. *Journal of the American Geriatrics Society*, 24(11), 525-530.

Luke, E. N., Norton, W., & Denbigh, K. (1982). Prevalence of psychologic impairment in an advanced-age population. *Journal of the American Geriatrics Society*, 30, 114-117.

Lundin, V., Eros, P., Melloh, J., & Sands, J. E. (1980). Education of independent elderly in the responsible use of prescription medication. *Drug Intelligence and Clinical Pharmacy*, 14, 335-342.

Macdonald, E. T., Macdonald, J. B., & Phoenix, M. (1977). Improving drug compliance after hospital discharge. *British Medical Journal*, 2, 618-621.

May, E., Stewart, B., Hale, E., & Marks, G. (1982). Prescribed and nonprescribed drug use in an ambulatory elderly population. *Southern Medical Journal*, 75(5), 522-528.

Murray, M. D., Darnell, J., Weinberger, M., & Martz, B. L. (1986). Factors contributing to medication noncompliance in elderly public housing tenants. *Drug Intelligence and Clinical Pharmacy*, 20, 146-151.

Ostrom, J. R., Hammarlund, E. R., Christensen, D. B., Plein, J. B., & Kethley, A. J. (1985). Medication usage in an elderly population. *Medical Care*, 23(2), 157-164.

Ouslander, J. G. (1981). Drug therapy in the elderly. *Annals of Internal Medicine*, 95, 711-722.

Papper, S. (1973). The effects of age in reducing renal function. *Geriatrics*, 28, 83.

Patrick, D. L., Peach, H., & Gregg, I. (1982). Disablement and care: A comparison of patient views and general practitioners knowledge. *Journal of the Royal College of General Practitioners*, 32, 429-434.

Raffoul, P. R. (1986). Drug misuse among older people: Focus for interdisciplinary efforts. *Health and Social Work*, 197-203.

Schwartz, D., Wang, M., Zeitz, L., & Goss, M. E. W. (1962). Medication errors made by elderly, chronically ill patients. *American Journal of Public Health*, 52, 2018.

Seidl, L. G., Thornton, G. F., Smith, J. W., & Cluff, L. E. (1966). Studies on the epidemiology of adverse drug reactions III. Reactions in patients on a general medical service. *Bulletin of the Johns Hopkins Hospital*, 119, 299.

Smith, C. R. (1979). Use of drugs in the aged. *Johns Hopkins Medical Journal*, 145, 61.

Smith, C., & Sharpe, T. R. (1984). A study of pharmacists' involvement in drug use by the elderly. *Drug Intelligence and Clinical Pharmacy*, 18, 525-530.

U.S. Department of Health, Education and Welfare (HEW) Office on Long-term Care. (1976). *Physicians' drug prescribing patterns in skilled nursing facilities* (DHHS Publication No. 76-50050), Washington, DC: U.S. Government Printing Office.

Wade, B., & Bowling, A. (1986). Appropriate use of drugs by elderly people. *Journal of Advanced Nursing, 11*, 47–55.

Wandless, I., & Davie, J. W. (1977). Can drug compliance in the elderly be improved? *British Medical Journal, 1*, 359–361.

Williamson, J., & Chopin, J. M. (1980). Adverse reactions to prescribed drugs in the elderly: A multicenter investigation. *Age and Aging, 9*, 73–80.

Zifferblatt, S. M. (1975). Increasing patient compliance through the applied analysis of behavior. *Preventive Medicine, 4*, 173–182.

Commentary: Adherence in Specific Populations

Merwyn R. Greenlick

The inclusion in this text of a section on adherence in specific populations implies that patient adherence issues in three populations are sufficiently different to require individual treatment. One wonders about this assumed conceptual difference, as it seems equally likely that the problems of achieving patient adherence are essentially the same in all populations.

In taking this view, one could assume that people comply with recommendations of health professionals when they are convinced that it is in their own interest to do so, and, further, that when adherence becomes a problem, something is blocking patients' acceptance of adherence as in their best interests. That blockage might be perceptual, it might be cognitive, or it might be attitudinal. Or, in fact, there might be no blockage at all: Individuals from whom adherence is sought could have weighed the demands or requests of their physicians and decided, on the basis of clear understanding and insight, that it is in their interests not to adhere to treatment recommendations.

If this latter perspective is the correct one, the only apparent reason for including specific populations in discussions of adherence is that health professionals continue, inappropriately, to ask members of these populations to adhere to protocols or treatments on the basis of incomplete understanding of patient situations or circumstances. Note, for example, the statement in Chapter 15 on life-style interventions with young hemophiliacs that describes the difficulty in recruiting families into hemophilia intervention studies. The authors report that "many patients felt they had built substantial defenses and were not prepared to disassemble them." This perspective of patients is presented as an obstacle to be overcome in order to recruit participants into studies. That is, the authors apparently assume that this perspective of patients is inappropriate, even though the next paragraph points out that "little is known about the effectiveness of interventions for this group of diseases [i.e., chronic diseases]." Given the uncertain effectiveness of the intervention, patient resistance might very well reflect an inherent wisdom.

It is possible to argue that adherence takes place when subjects perceive adherence to the protocol as appropriate or at least sensible. The premise for this section of the text is that differences exist between special populations and the investigators who study them that are so great that investigators will have difficulty in designing interventions, protocols, strategies, or treatments that make sense to members of these populations. For example, Roth posits a variety of hypothetical reasons for adherence difficulties in the elderly in Chapter 16; yet, some studies find little difficulty in achieving high levels of adherence in this population.

A specific example of high adherence in the elderly can be found in a report of the SHEP (Systolic Hypertension in the Elderly Program) pilot study. Data suggested that elderly patients can achieve high levels of adherence to antihypertensive medications (Black, Brand, Greenlick, Hughes, & Smith, 1987). In this study of 551 men and women over the age of 60 with a mean age of 72 years, three measures of adherence to the treatment protocol—pill counts, self-reports, and urine chlorthalidone assays—all indicated high levels of adherence in 80 to 90% of participants. These results were consistent at both 3 months and 1 year after randomization into arms of the study.

The high levels of adherence found in the SHEP study were not accidental. A standardized set of clinical procedures was designed to maximize adherence, and these procedures were applied at each of the five clinical sites. During the baseline phase of the study, participants were given good materials explaining the study and detailed and clear instructions about participation. At the final randomization visit, each participant was engaged in a standardized interview regarding adherence. The interview assessed the participant's knowledge of the study and the required medication schedule. It reinforced instructions regarding study procedures and identified any barriers to good adherence. A frequent schedule of visits for treatment, a large amount of clinical contact at each visit, availability of referrals for other medical problems, and a self-report form on adherence that was administered at each visit were all reported to increase the enthusiasm and adherence of participants.

An interesting finding of the SHEP pilot study was the strong relationship between high levels of adherence and achievement of goal levels for blood pressures in both the active *and* the placebo groups. This finding was similar to that reported by the Coronary Drug Project Research Group (1980), which identified a relationship between adherence to clofibrate or its placebo and 5-year mortality rates. While both studies concluded that analyses of treatment efficacy in groups determined by postrandomization responses (such as adherence to therapy) were problematic and should be avoided, the similar findings do make one wonder whether patients really do have some finely tuned ability to decide when and whether adherence makes sense.

In dealing with any specific population, a major problem is to ensure that participants understand why they must adhere to the recommendations of the investigator or clinician. To do this, it is extremely important to understand the mind of any given participant. In Chapter 14, Lewis, Belgrave, and Scott assert that "individuals with an internal orientation are expected to exhibit more positive health behaviors, including adherence, since these individuals feel they make a difference in health outcomes." This statement, if true, would seem to be equally true in a Black sickle cell disease patient, an elderly hypertension patient, a young hemophiliac, or anyone else. The problem is not that the trait—internal locus of control in this case—is differentially distributed in populations. The problem in design of research projects and treatment protocols is that researchers and theorists do not know with much certainty what really does make a difference in specific individuals. And this, in turn, could be the result of an even broader problem—namely, that researchers and clinicians do not have sufficient empathy with the ideas, needs, and desires of their patients to request adherence with recommendations that make sense to patients on their terms.

REFERENCES

Black, D. M., Brand, R. J., Greenlick, M. R., Hughes, G., & Smith, J. (1987). Compliance to treatment for hypertension in elderly patients: The SHEP pilot study. *Journal of Gerontology, 42*(5), 552–557.

The Coronary Drug Project Research Group. (1980). Influence of adherence to treatment and response of cholesterol on mortality in the Coronary Drug Project. *New England Journal of Medicine, 303*(18), 1038–1041.

SECTION V

Adherence Issues in Clinical Trials

Jeffrey L. Probstfield, Editor

The adherence of study participants is a critical component in the conduct of clinical trials. Indeed, the integrity of the results of a trial can be undermined if participants are not able to follow through with protocol requirements. If the effect of a treatment is to be evaluated, such as the efficacy of a drug, the drug has to be taken. Well-designed and well-managed trials do not automatically guarantee optimal adherence from participants. An adherence perspective must be an integral part of each phase of a trial from its planning and design through its conduct and interpretation, as discussed in the chapters in this section.

A legacy of the large clinical trials of the 1970s and 1980s has seen increased attention to the management of participant adherence, and much that has been learned from this clinical research offers the promise for broader application in routine clinical practice. For example, the concept of an adherence counselor, as developed in the Lipid Research Clinics Coronary Primary Prevention Trial (LRC-CPPT), suggests a feasible approach for the management of patients with high blood cholesterol. Such a model is important in light of the results of the LRC-CPPT that reducing high levels of blood cholesterol reduced the incidence of coronary heart disease and that benefit was directly proportional to the amount of cholesterol lowering achieved (Lipid Research Clinics Program: I and II, 1984). In response to these results, new treatment guidelines were developed, and these have immediate implications for primary care (Cholesterol Adult Treatment Panel Report, 1988). According to the guidelines, relatively large numbers of people will have to be brought into care; all will require diet intervention, and those patients whose cholesterol response to diet change is insufficient will also require drug intervention.

For the most part, cholesterol therapy will be lifelong, and the ability of patients to make and maintain life-style changes will determine the outcome of these preventive efforts. Although physicians believe that such care is warranted, they are concerned about the practicalities of administering extensive, long-term therapy, especially diet therapy (Schucker, Wittes, Cutler, et al., 1987). Alternative care models that can provide clinical and adherence management within the constraints of practice are needed. The emergence of the adherence counselor as the mainstay of the allied health care model of the LRC-CPPT is described by Hunninghake in Chapter 17, and he suggests a practical solution. He argues for a slight modification in the way practices are organized so that physicians can continue to provide overall supervision of therapy while other office personnel assume responsibility for adherence counseling. In fact, variations on this model, especially instances of nurses playing an expanded role in the management of high blood cholesterol, have already been shown to be successful in a variety of practice settings (Blair, Bryant, & Bocuzzi, 1988; Jones, Davies, Dove, Collinson, & Brown, 1988).

The following chapters address different aspects of adherence; some are unique to the conduct of clinical trials while others relate to the needs of clinical practice as well as clinical research. Hunninghake, in Chapter 17, "The Interaction of the Recruitment Process, with Adherence," describes the complex relationship between recruitment and adherence by showing how the philosophies and practices of staff during the recruitment phase can influence, often adversely, subsequent participant adherence. Because the goals of recruitment are short-term and adherence goals long-term, investigators have to be careful that these different goals do not conflict. Hunninghake shows how an easy solution to a recruitment problem could have devastating consequences on the maintenance of adherence.

Because of the importance of adherence to the outcome of a trial, it is very tempting to consider enrolling into a study only those individuals who will guarantee perfect or near-perfect adherence. But this raises questions of whether such selection is possible and, if it is, whether or not such preselection could have any untoward consequences. In Chapter 18, "Prerandomization Compliance Screening: A Statistician's View," Davis shows how the statistical power of a trial can be increased by excluding those who will not follow a treatment regimen. He then examines the tradeoff between increased study power and loss of generalizability of study results.

Addressing the question of whether or not early detection of poor adherence is possible, Dunbar reviews the literature on compliance for evidence relating personal behaviors and characteristics such as psychological, motivational, and somatic factors to adherence outcomes. In Chapter 19, "Predictors of Patient Adherence," she also presents 7-year follow-up data from the LRC-CPPT. The finding that the initial adherence performance of those participants was strongly associated with their long-term adherence efforts is worthy of note. It suggests that researchers and clinicians early on should preferentially allocate time and resources for the management of the initial adherence problems that people encounter as they attempt to adopt a new regimen rather than emphasize remedial efforts during the course of treatment.

In Chapter 20, "Strategies for Enhancing Adherence in Clinical Trials," Gorkin and colleagues set the stage for a discussion of adherence strategies with a comprehensive overview of clinical trial methodology. They point out the unique demands that methodology places on study participants as well as the implications these demands have for participant adherence and, in turn, the ramifications of poor adherence on trial outcome and interpretation. Gorkin et al. present a wide range of interventions that can be used in an effort to increase adherence. The strategies are targeted at problems emanating from different sources, including the treatment regimen, participant characteristics, the research team, the health care system, and finally the family and community.

One category of poor adherence is the dropout. This is a double-barreled problem in which participants are lost both to care and to follow-up. In Chapter 21, "Dropouts from a Clinical Trial, Their Recovery and Characterization," Probst-field and colleagues, describe a dropout recovery program that was developed in one of the Lipid Research Clinics. He characterizes dropouts in terms of "who, why and when." This leads to practical lessons in how to prevent participants from falling into the dropout category.

There are several underlying messages for managers of clinical trials in these chapters. One, already mentioned, is that an adherence perspective must dominate each phase of a trial. A corollary message relates to the issue of who has responsibility for adherence. Obviously participants are ultimately responsible for their own adherence behaivors, and designated staff will have specific responsibilities. But in a collaborative trial, everyone involved, no matter what their function, can potentially influence adherence, and thus responsibility for successful adherence should be thought of as a collaborative responsibility.

BETH SCHUCKER

REFERENCES

Blair, T. P., Bryant, F. J., Bocuzzi, S. (1988). Treatment of hypercholesterolemia by a clinical nurse using a stepped-care protocol in a nonvolunteer population. *Archives of Internal Medicine*, 148 (May), 1046-1048.

Cholesterol Adult Treatment Panel Report. (1988). Report of the National Cholesterol Education Program Expert Panel on Detection, Evaluation, and Treatment of High Blood Cholesterol in Adults. *Archives of Internal Medicine*, 148 (Jan.), 36-39.

Jones, A., Davies, D. H., Dove, J. R., Collinson, M. A., Brown, M. R. (1988). Identification and treatment of risk factors for coronary heart disease in general practice: A possible screening model. *British Medical Journal*, 296 (June), 1711-1714.

Lipid Research Clinics Program. (1984a). The Lipid Research Clinics Coronary Primary Prevention Trial Results: I. Reduction in Incidence of Coronary Heart Disease. *Journal of the American Medical Association*, 251(3), 351-364.

Lipid Research Clinics Program. (1984b). The Lipid Research Clinics Coronary Primary Prevention Trial Results: II. The Relationship of Reduction in Incidence of Coronary Heart Disease to Cholesterol Lowering. *Journal of the American Medical Association*, 251(3), 365-374.

Schucker, B. H., Wittes, J. T., Cutler, J. A., Bailey, K., MacKintosh, D. R., Gordon, D. J., Haines, C. M., Mattson, M. E., Goor, R.S., & Rifkind, B. M. et al. (1987). Change in physician perspective on cholesterol and heart disease. *Journal of the American Medical Association*, 258(24), 3521-3526.

The Interaction of the Recruitment Process with Adherence

Donald B. Hunninghake

There is a gradually expanding number of publications that deal with predictors of adherence or compliance. (The term *adherence* is used throughout this chapter. However, there is limited information on the predictors of adherence in clinical trials, especially in multicenter trials. A preliminary report on the predictors of adherence in the Lipid Research Clinics Coronary Primary Prevention Trial (LRC-CPPT) was presented at a workshop of the Society of Clinical Trials (Lipid Research Clinics Coronary Primary Prevention Trial, 1986; also, see Chapter 19).

There are no definitive studies of the impact of recruitment procedures on adherence. Hence, the information contained in this chapter is based upon experiences derived either from my own clinical center, which has been involved in numerous clinical trials and unpublished observations of other clinical trial centers in a variety of clinical trials.

This chapter addresses two general areas where adherence and recruitment activities have the potential for significant interaction:

- The first area relates to those adherence activities that either must be implemented prior to initiation of the recruitment process or implemented simultaneously with the recruitment process. In many clinical centers, staff members will be actively involved in both recruitment and adherence activities.
- The second major area relates to those recruitment activities that can either directly or indirectly affect adherence, with more emphasis on recruitment activities that negatively affect adherence.

INITIATION OF RECRUITMENT

The following must be implemented either prior to initiation of recruitment or during the recruitment process:

1. *Planning and Study Design*: It is essential that consideration of adherence issues be incorporated into the study design. Reduced adherence can decrease the likelihood of success in all clinical trials, but adherence issues are especially important if the trial is multicenter, involves a prolonged period of treatment, or the treatment is especially difficult. For multicenter trials, adherence planning by the sponsor is essential to assure that all participating centers possess the fundamentals for achieving good adherence. This may require centralized training in the fundamentals of adherence and strategies for achieving and maintaining adherence. Inclusion of expert consultants in the original planning phase or for monitoring adherence during the course of a trial may be advisable. Both centralized as well as local monitoring of adherence during the entire trial is essential.

Provisions must also be made for feedback on adherence data. Protocols that involve a prerandomization test period of adherence to either study medication or placebo may eliminate many poor adherers (Davis, this volume; Probstfield, Russell, Insull, & Yusuf, this volume). Initiating therapy with small dosages of drugs with a gradual increase in dosage may also be desirable in certain studies. Studywide goals for adherence must be used in the power calculations to determine sample size. The crucial point is that adherence must be considered both in study design and from the very beginning of the implementation of recruitment in large multicenter trials as well as in smaller trials.

2. *Responsible Person*: In all large studies, it is important to designate a person who is in charge of coordinating the adherence effort (Adherence Coordinator). An Adherence Coordinator is necessary for each clinical center participating in the study, and there should also be a central coordinator in a multicenter trial. Ideally, the Adherence Coordinator will have had prior experience in clinical trials. If not, this person must be creative but also use common sense and possess

a caring and sensitive attitude. The principal investigator should be cognizant of the difficulties of achieving good adherence and must be supportive of the role of the coordinator and provide status for this position.

3. *Staff Selection*: The Adherence Coordinator should have significant input in the hiring of other personnel who will be involved in adherence activities. Consideration of the type of health professional that will be used for adherence counseling must be considered. The principal investigator and other physicians participating in the trial can make invaluable contributions to the adherence effort. However, physicians are usually not effective adherence counselors, either because they do not have the time or because they are unwilling to pay adequate attention to essential details of adherence. Efforts should be made to utilize other health professionals such as nurses, dietitians, or physician assistants.

4. *Prerandomization Evaluation of Participants by Adherence Staff.* It is essential that adequate personnel time be devoted to adherence during the recruitment process. It is easy to focus on other study details and ignore the implementation of effective adherence procedures or monitoring adherence. It is helpful to have individuals who are responsible for maintaining adherence in the postrandomization phase see the participants during the prerandomization phase. This may not be possible due to the design of certain studies. The adherence counselors should feel reasonably comfortable with the participants who will be randomized and have an expectation that adherence can be maintained.

Although there have not been conclusive data to document the characteristics of good adherence to study protocols, the subjective impression is that certain poor adherers to study protocols can be identified. The LRC-CPPT is currently developing an extensive monograph on predictors of adherence in that trial. In addition to the adherence counselor seeing the participant, regular staff meetings must be held to review each person being considered for randomization. If there is strong sentiment among the staff that a given individual poses a high risk for poor adherence, that person will not be randomized. Some of the major considerations for exclusion include serious concerns about study design such as placebo, blinding, or fear of taking medication. Other factors include alcoholism, erratic life-style or behavior, frequent missed appointments, multiple somatic complaints, extensive travel if frequent visits are required, and an inability of staff members to effectively communicate with the participant. The degree of discomfort with excluding participants for subjective reasons only will vary among clinical centers.

In some trials there is a separate screening staff that is responsible for the initial contact with prospective participants. If this is the case, the Adherence Counselor must work carefully with the screening staff to make them aware of participant traits that may be predictors of poor adherence. There may be tremendous pressures to randomize all potentially eligible participants, and the principal investigator must formally establish a policy that excludes potentially poor adherers. Although adherence cannot be accurately predicted in some participants, there is no doubt that certain participants (traits mentioned above) are at high risk for poor adherence. Adherence means adherence to all aspects of the study protocol. This may include taking study medication, changing multiple behaviors, and adhering to the details of each scheduled visit. The staff must understand that the study will be more powerful with a smaller total number of participants who are good adherers than with a larger total number of participants, many of whom are poor adherers.

5. *Constant Caretaker Model*: It is advantageous to have the same individual or a limited number of individuals on the staff see the participant in the prerandomization phase and continue the adherence maintenance program during the postrandomization follow-up. A counselor who has developed an effective relationship with the participant can be especially useful if difficulties arise in the immediate postrandomization period to various aspects of the study protocol, including study medication. The participants' early experience can determine adherence for the entire trial. It is highly desirable that adherence personnel develop an effective relationship with the participants prior to randomization.

6. *Patient and Staff Education*: It is important that the participant be given an adequate and realistic description of the entire study. If a medication is being used, it is essential that they know the characteristics of the medication, the potential side effects, and that mechanisms for dealing with side effects are available. In the LRC-CPPT, staff members demonstrated the proper method for mixing and administering cholestyramine. The participant is more likely to be willing to work on problem solving if given adequate information beforehand.

Staff members must receive adequate education and training regarding all aspects of the study protocol. An informed staff member is more likely to be able to deal with participant problems and instill confidence. Uninformed or poorly trained staff members may also unknowingly transfer to study participants their own concerns about issues, which could be minimized by proper education. There should also be periodic meetings of Adherence Counselors, both local and central, for identifying and solving adherence issues.

7. *Patient Selection*: The success of any trial is not only dependent upon the number of participants who are randomized, but also upon the adherence of the participants to the study protocol. A large number of poor adherers in the active treatment group could significantly decrease the power of the study. It is therefore imperative that individuals who are potentially poor adherers not be randomized. As described previously, there are high-risk situations for poor adherence, but there are no absolute criteria for predicting adherence. However, certain commonsense rules appear to apply. If the person has a preexisting disease or condition that will be aggravated by the study medication, poor adherence is more likely. For example, an individual with a symptomatic hiatal hernia or severe constipation is unlikely to tolerate large doses of drugs such as cholestryramine. Menopausal or postmenopausal women may not tolerate drugs

such as nicotinic acid that produce significant flushing. A low success rate is common with the high-risk individuals identified above.

8. *Recruitment Sources*: This is an area where more definitive work is needed. Obviously, if one were able to implement recruitment strategies that are likely to generate better adherers this would be desirable. The experience in the LRC-CPPT suggests that individuals recruited from specific sources such as blood banks, community screens, or from prior participation in clinical studies adhere better to the drug, cholestyramine, than individuals recruited from physician or clinical laboratories (unpublished data, 1984).

9. *Clinic Organization*: There was considerable variation in the adherence to the drug, cholestyramine, among the various clinical centers in the LRC-CPPT (unpublished data, 1984). The reason for the variability in adherence among clinical centers in various trials has not been clearly defined. Unpublished experience supports the general experience that clinical centers that have principal investigators or project directors who are very actively involved in the clinical trial and that have organizatonal structures that pay careful attention to the details of a smoothly functioning clinic have better adherence. For example, waiting time in the clinic has been inversely correlated with adherence in medical care settings (Finnerty, Shaw, & Himmelsbach, 1973; Rockart & Hofman, 1969). It is easy for clinic functions to be seriously disrupted because of the volume of participants seen during the recruitment phase. This creates a bad image for the clinic. Participants are expected to be precise in terms of adhering to study protocols. The participants should then have the right to expect careful attention to their needs, which may include minimal waiting time; pleasant, courteous and informed staff; and adequate parking.

RECRUITMENT AND ADHERENCE

There are a number of ways in which recruitment efforts can either directly or indirectly influence adherence.

An efficient recruitment effort that is randomizing participants at the scheduled rate can have positive effects on adherence. There is a general sense of optimism, and morale is high. These feelings are transmitted throughout all phases of the study to both staff and participants. In contrast, if recruitment is seriously lagging or in danger of collapse, serious repercussions may occur. Staff resources and energy may be diverted from adherence to recruitment efforts. There may be a sense of panic and a lack of optimism. Staff and participant morale may be low, and this could translate into lack of enthusiasm for the entire study, including adherence. The study could be terminated or prolonged. In the latter case, participants my object to continuing the study beyond their original commitment. Even if recruitment is eventually successful, there may be a late surge of activity, creating an uneven workload for the entire duration of the study.

1. *Effective Recruitment*: It is beyond the scope of this chapter to extensively review approaches to recruitment. A comprehensive monograph describing the recruitment experience in a variety of clinical trials is available (*Recruitment experience in NHLBI-sponsored clinical trials*, 1987). This monograph includes a brief review of the available literature on recruitment (Hunninghake, Darby, & Probstfield, 1987).

Recruitment for large multicenter trials has frequently been either unsuccessful or required much longer periods of time than anticipated. Lack of recruitment experience by investigators, lack of published data on recruitment, and lack of appreciation for the multiple problems that can be encountered in recruitment are among the potential reasons for this problem. Recruitment is almost always more difficult than originally anticipated. There is no good correlation between the number of eligible participants and eventual recruitment success. The efficiency of various recruitment strategies is quite variable. Contingency plans are frequently not available if the original recruitment strategies fail.

The elements of a successful recruitment effort include adequate planning at both the national and local level for multicenter trials. Adequate planning necessitates an understanding of various recruitment strategies, their probable yield over time, and adequate contingency plans.

There must be effective management. This includes a strong administrative component, appropriate allocation of resources, provisions for monitoring the recruitment effort, and implementation of contingency plans when necessary. Consideration of physician and participant attitudes and characteristics is also important for recruitment success. These characteristics and attitudes have only been partially developed for recruitment. There is also a need for definition of physician and participant attitudes and characteristics that are important for achieving good adherence.

2. *Consequences of Recruitment Delays or Failures*: Failure to recruit enough participants could result in termination of a trial and total loss of expended funds or energy. The trial could be completed with inconclusive results.

Delays in recruitment generally result in increased costs, which may mean fewer resources for adherence. The diversion of resources from adherence and the potential negative effect on both participant or staff morale has been previously discussed.

A major problem related to recruitment delays is that there is frequently a late surge of recruitment activity with markedly uneven rates of entry for participants. Many study protocols are designed so that a much more extensive evaluation is required at certain visits such as the annual visit, and the available staff are frequently reduced in the postrandomization phase. The uneven workload may necessitate diversion of staff activities at critical times from adherence to other needs of the study.

If recruitment is delayed and the duration of follow-up of participants is increased, study participants may be unwilling to extend their participation beyond the time originally specified in the consent form. It may be difficult to maintain adherence during the extension of the study.

SUMMARY

There are a number of significant interactions that can occur between the recruitment and adherence efforts in clinical trials, although much of the information is subjective rather than objective. Adherence issues must be included in the original study design, and appropriate measures for achieving good adherence must be implemented throughout the entire recruitment phase. Appropriate personnel and adequate personnel time for adherence efforts must be available throughout the entire recruitment period. Recruitment is frequently more difficult than anticipated, and the temptation to divert resources from adherence to recruitment should be avoided. A uniform accrual rate of participants into the study will ensure an even workload for the duration of the trial. Provisions must be made for adequate training or education of both staff and participants in all phases of the study protocol, including adherence. Special attention must be devoted to clinic function during recruitment because a disorganized clinic may negatively influence adherence. The criteria for defining good and poor adherence are poorly developed, but certain individuals are unlikely to be good adherers and should not be randomized. If adherence issues are considered in the planning process and throughout the recruitment process, the chances of achieving good adherence are enhanced.

REFERENCES

Finnerty, F. A., Shaw, L. W., & Himmelsbach, C. K. (1973). Hypertension in the inner city. *Circulation, 47,* 76-78.

Hunninghake, D. B., Darby, C. A., & Probstfield, J. L. (1987). Recruitment experience in clinical trials: Literature summary and annotated bibliography. *Controlled Clinical Trials, 8*(Suppl.), 6S-30S.

Lipid Research Clinics Coronary Primary Prevention Trial. (1986). Risk factors for adherence: Experience of the Lipid Research Clinics Coronary Primary Prevention Trial (LRC-CPPT). *Controlled Clinical Trials, 8*(Suppl.), 223.

Lipid Research Clinics Coronary Primary Prevention Trial. Unpublished data, 1984.

Recruitment experience in NHLBI-sponsored clinical trials. (1987). *Proceedings of a Workshop. Controlled Clinical Trials, 8*(Suppl.), 1S-149S.

Rockart, J. R., & Hofman, P. B. (1969). Physician and patient behaviour under different scheduling systems in a hospital outpatient department. *Medical Care, 7,* 463-470.

18

Prerandomization Compliance Screening: A Statistician's View

C. Edward Davis

In the conduct of clinical trials, the "intent to treat" rule is used as a standard data analysis procedure. The intent to treat rule states that the data from a participant entered into a clinical trial should be analyzed with the group to which he or she was assigned regardless of whether the intended treatment was applied. For example, in a clinical trial of medicine versus surgery in the treatment of severe coronary disease, patients assigned to medical treatment who subsequently have surgery would be treated as though they were only treated by medical means. This rule is used in order to ensure that the comparison of the two (or more) treatment groups is unbiased. If the more severely ill patients among those assigned to medical treatment were to have surgery, counting subsequent deaths among these patients as attributable to surgical treatment would make the medically treated group appear to fare better than it actually did.

The use of the intent to treat rule in data analysis leads to another similar issue related to patient adherence to the behavior regimen assigned within a particular treatment. For example, if participants assigned to a diet or drug therapy do not adhere to the regimen, their data will be analyzed as though they had in fact followed the prescription. This concept has led to the proposal that prospective participants in a clinical trial should be excluded if they are unable or unwilling to follow the procedures that will be used in the trial. Such issues as reporting to the clinic as requested or keeping a dietary record may be used as possible tests to see if the *potential* participant is likely to cooperate during the trial. An additional possibility is to ask the participant to take medication, usually placebo, single-blinded, to determine capability to adhere to the required medication schedule (the reader is referred to the chapter by Probstfield, Russell, Insull, and Yusuf in this volume for further details). The participant, if unable to follow the prescribed behavioral pattern well, is not entered into the full study. In this brief presentation, I review some of the pros and cons of this latter procedure and briefly describe the interim results of an NIH-sponsored trial that is using the method.

SHOULD A PRERANDOMIZATION ADHERENCE SCREEN BE USED?

The major reason for using a prerandomization adherence screen is to protect the statistical power of the clinical trial. Suppose we are to conduct a clinical trial using a response variable that is normally distributed with means μ_1 (control group) and μ_2 (treated group), and common variance δ^2. If the proportion of participants in the treated group who do not adhere to the assigned regimen is p, it follows that the expected treatment difference is $(1 - p)(\mu_1 - \mu_2)$, rather than $\mu_1 - \mu_2$. With perfect adherence, the sample size for significance level α and power $1-\beta$ is

$$2n = \delta^2 (z_\alpha + z_\beta)^2/(\mu_1 - \mu_2)^2.$$

However, with the proportion of participants in the treated group not adhering equal to p, the sample size is:

$$2n = \delta^2 (z_\alpha + z_\beta)^2/(\mu_1 - \mu_2)^2 (1 - p)^2$$

Thus the size of the study is increased by a factor of $(1 - p)^{-2}$. The following short table gives values for the increase in sample size for a given level of adherence.

Increase in Sample Size for Adherence p

p	k
.01	1.02
.05	1.11
.10	1.23
.20	1.56
.50	4.00

To use the table, one can compute the sample size assuming all participants adhere and then multiply that sample size by k (a constant) to account for poor adherence. For example, if we computed an estimated sample size of 100 for a trial, then assuming that 10% of the participants would not adhere to the treatment implies that we should have a sample of $100 \times 1.23 = 123$ participants; that is, a 10% poor adherence proportion leads to a need for 23% more participants in order to maintain the same statistical power.

In the above sample computation, we assume that poor adherence to placebo will not effect the study. Of course, if participants who are assigned to the placebo group begin to receive the active treatment, the power will be further diminished. Clearly, the cost of poor adherence is great, and thus we should try our best to minimize poor adherence. This has led to the proposal for a prerandomization adherence screen (run-in).

This proposal is based on the assumption that those participants identified as poor adherers in the prerandomization screen will be the same as those who would subsequently be poor adherers in the main study. There is some evidence to support this idea from observational data. In Chapter 19 of this volume, Dunbar presents data from the LRC-CPPT indicating that participants who took their medication regularly during the early portion of the study tended to take their medication regularly throughout the study. While this observation certainly supports the idea that we should be able to predict persons who will be poor adherers, it would be preferable to have a well-designed randomized study to investigate this assumption in more detail. For example, one might have a study with a prerandomization screen but enter all patients regardless of whether they passed the screen. It would then be possible to directly measure the effect of the prerandomization screen and in particular to determine if the assumption concerning the ability to predict future adherence is correct. Obviously this would add a cost to the main study but potentially could save costs on future studies and would give us a better scientific basis from which to argue the mertis or demerits of prerandomization adherence screening.

The major criticism of the prerandomization adherence screen is that the removal of a subset of potential participants restricts the generalizability of the results. If we ask the question "Does drug A reduce the mortality in patients with disease X?", we are asking what will happen if we apply drug A to the entire population of patients with disease X. However, if we remove from consideration those patients who do not follow instructions during the prerandomization phase, we are answering the question "Does drug A reduce mortality in patients with disease X who behave as we request?" This criticism will be valid in some settings and not in others.

For example, if I want to design a trial to answer the question "Will the introduction of a low-fat diet reduce the *incidence* of coronary disease in the population?", it would not be proper to have a prerandomization adherence screen, since the question is clearly asking what will happen in the entire population. However, if we design a trial to answer the question "Will a low-fat diet reduce the *risk* of coronary disease?", we may choose to eliminate from the study those persons who do not pass a prerandomization screen, since the question concerns whether the diet has any effect at all on coronary disease. In demonstration and prevention research where the acceptability of an intervention may play a role we should rarely use prerandomization screening, but in research designed primarily to look at the efficacy of treatment, such a screen may be warranted and in fact appears necessary. Clearly, we should think carefully about these issues before making such a decision.

There are, of course, logistical problems associated with a prerandomization screen, particularly in double-blind studies. If a participant takes a placebo for a few days and then at randomization is given the active treatment, the side effects or symptomatic relief may lead them to conclude that they are on the active treatment and thus threaten the blind. The degree to which this might effect the validity of the study will no doubt be dependent on the type of treatment and its side effects. Nonetheless, the possibility of damaging the study through breaking the blind should be considered before one embarks on a run-in.

Two other potential problems associated with a run-in period should be noted. First, to the extent that nonadherers are misidentified, the gain in statistical power may be reduced. Second, the addition of a run-in period will almost certainly make recruitment more difficult.

PRERANDOMIZATION SCREENING IN SOLVD

The National Heart, Lung, and Blood Institute is currently sponsoring a clinical trial in patients with low ejection fractions (reduced emptying of the ventricular chamber associated with normal beating of the heart), the Studies of Left Ventricular Dysfunction (SOLVD). In this study, potential participants with ejection fractions less than or equal to 35 are randomly assigned to an angiotensin-converting enzyme inhibitor (enalapril) or a placebo. The endpoint of interest is total mortality, and follow-up will be for a minimum of 2 years.

In this study there are in fact two types of prerandomization screenings. Since it has been reported that in a small number of persons the first exposure to enalapril may lead to severe hypotension, it was decided to give each potential participant a small test dose of the active drug so that participants in whom the drug was contraindicated could be excluded. Thus at the first clinic visit each patient is put on a 2.5 mg bid dose of the active drug for a period of from 2 to 7 days. Although the intent of this "test dosing" is to protect the safety of the participants, it was decided to exclude participants who took less than 75% of the prescribed medication during this period. A participant judged to be eligible

TABLE 18.1 Participants Excluded from SOLVD, March, 1987—Preliminary Data

			Excluded			
Visit	Included	Percentage	Poor adherence	Percentage	Other	Percentage
Test dose	1390	97.0	30	2.1	13	0.1
Placebo dose	1230	96.2	26	2.0	22	1.7

following this "test dosing" is then prescribed 2 weeks of placebo. Participants who do not take at least 80% of the medication during this 2-week period are excluded from the trial.

SOLVD began recruitment in July 1986 and as of the data presented here, 1342 participants have been entered toward a goal of 7100. Table 18.1 gives a summary of the results of the prerandomization screening to date. Clearly, a small proportion (approximately 4%) of the potential participants are being excluded for lack of adherence. Nevertheless, if we use the rough rule outlined above, correcting for a 4% reduction in adherence, we would need 8.5% more participants to make up for this loss in power. Thus, although the percentage of potential participants excluded is small, the potential gain in the power of the study is not negligible.

It is interesting to consider the question of the effect of the prerandomization adherence screen on the generalizability of the study. Table 18.2 compares some of the characteristics of the participants excluded for poor adherence with those of the participants who were not excluded. Since these data are very preliminary and subject to change over the continued recruitment, I have chosen not to report any tests of statistical significance. After the recruitment is complete, the

TABLE 18.2 Characteristics of Participants Excluded in SOLVD Compared to Those Not Excluded, March, 1987—Preliminary Data

	Not Excluded		Excluded poor adherence	
Characteristic	E dose[a]	P dose[b]	E dose[a]	P dose[b]
Mean age (yrs.)	59	59	63	61
Percentage male	85	86	73	77
Percentage white	82	83	73	62
Percent NYHA > 2	24	23	50	35
Taking vasodilators (%)	29	27	36	36
Mean EF (%)	25	26	23	25

[a]enalapril; [b]placebo.

SOLVD investigators will prepare a detailed report concerning the prerandomization screening.

In Table 18.2 it is noticeable that characteristics that seem to be associated with poor adherence are older age, female sex, nonwhite race, more severe disease (as noted by the NYHA classification but not by ejection fraction), and taking vasodilators. This latter characteristic is probably not a surprise, since it seems well recognized that the more behaviors we ask of a person, the less likely they are to be able to carry out all of them. It appears from these preliminary data that SOLVD is slightly changing the characteristics of its sample by requiring adherence to be good during the prerandomization phase. The effects of this on the generalizability of the study are debatable.

SUMMARY

The exclusion of potential participants who will not follow a treatment regimen likely increases the statistical power of the clinical trial. However, this increase in power may be purchased by reducing the generalizability of the results of the study, possibly interfering with the double-blinding and possibly making recruitment more difficult. Thus one should consider the relative merits of these issues in deciding whether or not to have a prerandomization adherence screen in any particular study. It would be of great interest to see if we can confirm the basic underlying assumption that persons who adhere poorly prior to randomization are more likely to adhere poorly after the study begins.

19

Predictors of Patient Adherence: Patient Characteristics

Jacqueline Dunbar

With nonadherence rates ranging from 20% to 80% in practice and research settings, considerable health care resources are utilized in either remediating nonadherence or in treating the consequences of inadequately treated disease or risk factors. In the clinical research arena further resources may be expended in the recruitment and management of additional subjects to compensate for the loss of power due to dropouts or poor adherers. Resources might be better utilized at the outset of treatment or subject recruitment if those individuals likely to have difficulty adhering could be identified. And, indeed, investigations have been undertaken directed toward the prediction of adherence.

A number of studies have examined factors under the control of the provider that are likely to lead to nonadherence, such as prescribing multiple and/or complex regimens, a lack of consistency in care providers, care provider behavior toward patients, adequacy of instructions, and convenience. Another set of predictors are those that are more specific to the person than to the regimen, provider, or clinical setting. It is this latter set of factors that is addressed in this review. That is, what characteristics of the individual are likely to influence subsequent adherence to a health care regimen? A number of areas have been examined, including (1) psychological characteristics, (2) cognitive–motivational factors, (3) behavior itself, and (4) somatic factors.

PSYCHOLOGICAL CHARACTERISTICS AS PREDICTORS OF ADHERENCE

Overall, the literature shows little support for personality traits as predictors of patient adherence. On the other hand, certain psychological states may influence adherence. Depression and anxiety in particular have been found to be associated with poor adherence (Blumenthal, Williams, Wallace, Williams & Needles, 1982; Heiby, Onorato & Sato 1985; Nelson, Stason, Neutra, Solomon, & McArdle, 1978; O'Leary, Rohsenow, and Chaney, 1979). Higher scores on the MMPI depression scale have been associated with dropouts from cardiac rehabilitation exercise programs and from alcohol treatment (Blumenthal et al., 1982; O'Leary et al., 1979), while high anxiety has been associated with poor medication adherence among hypertensives (Nelson et al., 1978). At the opposite end of the mood spectrum, feelings of euphoria after training runs have predicted completion of a marathon (Heiby, Onorato, & Sato, 1985).

In a study undertaken in the Lipid Research Clinics–Coronary Primary Prevention Trial[1] (LRC-CPPT), psychological distress, which included the self-reported presence or history of tranquilizer use, excessive fatigue, difficulty sleeping, moodiness, and irritability, as well as depression, was assessed during prerandomization screening. A multiple regression analysis showed statistical significance ($p < .001$) between tranquilizer use and excessive fatigue and reduced adherence at year 1. Further, these two factors and difficulty sleeping were associated with reduced adherence over 7 years. However, such a small proportion of the variance was accounted for ($r = .012$, $r = .022$ respectively) that one could conclude that psychological distress did not predict adherence (Dunbar & Knoke, 1986). The pattern of the relationship between psychological distress and adherence, however, was toward lower adherence given the presence of psychological distress during the prerandomization period or ever in the past (see Table 19.1).

The question arises as to why psychological states might predict adherence. A study examining a cognitive–behavioral model of adherence to health-related

[1]The Lipid Research Clinics–Coronary Primary Prevention Trial (LRC-CPPT) was a multicenter, randomized, double-blind, controlled clinical trial testing the cholesterol hypothesis among healthy, hyperlipidemic males aged 35 to 59 at entry. Participants were on a cholesterol-lowering medication or placebo dispensed in packets for at least 7 years. All volunteers completed a medical history and examination during the screening phase of the recruitment effort, prior to randomization into the study. Three months after this assessment was completed, the volunteers were randomized to either active medication or placebo and followed at bimonthly clinic visits for the 7 to 10 years of participation. Adherence was assessed at each clinic visit by means of an unobtrusive packet count. The predicted behavior was adherence over the first year of the trial and over 7 years of the trial.

TABLE 19.1 History of Tranquilizer Use and Medication Adherence at Year 1 and Over 7 Years in the LRC–CPPT: Cumulative Adherence as Measured at Two-Time Intervals in a Study

	1 year	7 years
Never used	81%	66%
Used in past	77%	59%
Used during screening	71%	48%

exercise by Heiby and colleagues (1985) suggests that depression and anxiety may be components of motivation. In a factor analysis, these investigators found that trait anxiety, depression, self-reinforcement, and self-motivation loaded on the same factor such that low trait anxiety and low depression scores were associated with the high self-reinforcement and high self-motivation. It may be speculated that the pessimistic and self-deprecating cognitions typically found in depression contribute to lowered self-reinforcement and self-motivation. This would be an interesting avenue for further exploration.

COGNITIVE-MOTIVATIONAL PREDICTORS OF ADHERENCE

Beliefs and other cognitions have also been examined as potential predictors of patient adherence. It is in this area that much of the research on the characteristics of the patient as an influence on adherence has taken place. The principle models include health beliefs, intentions, and self-efficacy.

Most commonly cited is the Health Belief Model, a cognitive-motivational model described by Rosenstock in 1966 and further refined by Becker and others (e.g., Becker, Drachman, & Kirsch, 1974; Rosenstock 1974; Janz & Becker, 1984). The model essentially states that recommended health actions will be taken if an individual believes: (1) himself susceptible to the illness; (2) the consequences of the illness or of noncompliance are serious; (3) the recommended action is beneficial or efficacious in reducing risk or severity; and (4) the barriers or costs of action do not exceed the benefits. In addition to these beliefs, general health motivation is, at times, included in the model. General health motivation consists of both positive factors, for example, engagement in healthy behaviors, as well as negative factors, for example, worry or concern over health.

Most investigations of the utility of the health belief model have been concurrent or retrospective studies. Behavior of interest and health beliefs were assessed at the same time. These studies have shown modest relationships between beliefs and behavior.

Fifteen prospective studies have been reported in the literature that have undertaken an examination of the influence of health beliefs on subsequent behavior. Two of these studies were intervention studies designed to change health beliefs through educational procedures and measured postintervention adherence (Inui, Yourtee, & Williamson, 1976) and contraceptive practices of adolescents (Eisen, Zallman, & McAlister, 1985). The postintervention assessment was carried out on a group of patients largely different from those assessed pretreatment in the Inui et al. (1976) study. Further, the inclusion of an intervention targeted to the modification of health beliefs confounded the utility of initial beliefs as predictors of adherence in the absence of a control group in the Eisen et al. (1985) study. These two studies will not be included in this discussion. Thus, 13 prospective prediction studies remain.

The types of behaviors and the period between assessment of health beliefs and subsequent adherence varied among these 13 prospective prediction studies. For example, these studies variously examined health care utilizataion (3), attendance at screening programs (3), the acquisition of immunizations (1), self-report of drinking and driving (1), smoking cessation (1), weight loss (1), breast self-examination practices (1), and medication adherence (2). The period between assessment of health beliefs and subsequent behavior ranged from 1 week (screening attendance) to 8 years (smoking cessation). Susceptibility, severity, benefits, and health motivation were typically assessed. In general, barriers were not examined in these studies.

Eight of the prospective studies examined perceived susceptibility to disease. Variations were found in the populations and the health behaviors that were associated with this patient characteristic. Perceived susceptibility was associated with medical care utilization among medical facility populations (Berkanovic, Telesky, & Reeder, 1981) and HMO populations (Leavitt, 1979), but not in a population-based random sample (Berkanovic et al., 1981). Perceived susceptibility predicted well-child visits but not illness or accident visits in a pediatric clinic (Becker, Nathanson, Drachman, Kirscht, 1977b). Further, it predicted medication adherence and appointment-keeping for children with otitis media (Becker, et al., 1974) and children's weight loss in an obesity program (Becker, Maiman, Kirscht, Haefner, & Drachman, 1977a). It did not predict adherence to antihypertensive medications among adults (Taylor, 1979). Lastly, perceived susceptibility predicted participation in a breast-screening program (Calnan, 1984; Calnan & Moss, 1984), but not the actual practice of breast self-examination (Calnan & Moss, 1984). Even when perceived susceptibility was successful as a predictive variable, power was low with gamma coefficients[2] ranging from .3 to .5 and correlation coefficients ranging from .01 to −.03.

[2]Gamma is an index of rank-order association. In the special case of the 2×2 table, gamma is a function of the odds ratio. A simple way to test its significance is to compute and test the contingency chi-square value. Numerically gamma is larger than the corresponding phi coefficient, which is equal

Personal susceptibility was examined in the LRC–CPPT program in a somewhat different manner (Dunbar & Knoke, 1986). In this case, personal susceptibility was dichotomously operationalized as the presence or absence of known risk factors for cardiovascular disease during the screening period. This type of definition is similar to that utilized by Croog and Richards (1977) in assessing health beliefs and smoking cessation. That is, symptoms or risk factors are seen as associated with a threat to individual susceptibility. Croog and Richards (1977) used such indicators as occurrences of chest pain, heart palpitations, breathlessness, and other symptoms as well as rehospitalization, use of physician services, and disability days. In the LRC–CPPT the risk factors included: (1) systolic blood pressure greater than 104 mmHg and/or diastolic blood pressure above 90mmHg; (2) greater than 120% of ideal weight using the 1979 Metropolitan Life tables; (3) current smoker; (4) lack of exercise; (5) over age 47; (6) previously advised by a physician to follow a cholesterol-lowering diet; and (7) a family history, in a first-degree relative, of cardiovascular disease or stroke. These particular risk factors were all those that were in the subject's awareness.

Family history of cardiovascular disease, age, and smoking were statistically significant predictors of adherence both during the first year of the trial and over the 7-year duration of the study; however, the proportion of variance accounted for was low. The multiple regression equation yielded an R^2 of .024 ($p = .0001$) for year 1 and an R^2 of .039 ($p = .001$) over the 7 years of the trial. However, with the exception of smoking, the trend across all of the risk factors was for higher susceptibility to be associated with higher adherence.

The results of these studies suggest that the utility of perceived susceptibility as a predictor of adherence may vary with the timing of assessment, the population sampled, and the health behavior of interest. Susceptibility appears to be associated with attendance at screening or prevention visits as well as with mothers' adherence to pediatric regimens and childhood weight loss, at least when assessed after diagnosis is made. It does not appear to be predictive of health practice or medication adherence when assessment is prior to diagnosis, at least for adult populations. While some interesting and consistent trends were noted in an adult clinical trial population with the above definition for susceptibility, the proportion of variance accounted for by this patient characteristic had little if any predictive power.

Perceived severity is the second component of the Health Belief Model. It has been shown to predict well-child and illness visits in a well-child clinic popula-

---

to the Pearson Product Moment Correlation between 0–1 indicator variables. In the case of the 2 × 2 table, for crude test purposes, or for comparing it with results stated as correlations, dividing the gamma by two is not too misleading for gammas up to .60. A computational formula can be found in the SPSS Statistical Algorithms manual, and a more detailed discussion in Goodman and Kruskal (1954). (Richard Ulrich, MS, Research Assistant Professor of Psychiatry, University of Pittsburgh, Pittsburgh, PA personal communication.)

tion (Becker et al., 1977b) weight loss among obese children (Becker et al., 1977a), and treatment adherence among children with otitis media (Becker et al., 1974). The gamma coefficients range from .16 for well-child visits to .5 for weight loss. The proportion of variance accounted for is again low. Perceived severity did not, however, predict visits in an adult HMO (Leavitt, 1979) or in an adult community sample (Berkanovic et al., 1981). It is interesting to note that mothers' management of children's health care appears to be the population where severity is most likely to influence subsequent behavior. An examination of the interaction of populations and health behavior with beliefs about severity of the illness or its consequences and the effects on health behavior would be of interest.

Perceived benefits or efficacy of health behaviors as a modifier of disease, a third component in the Health Belief Model, were found to be predictive of screening attendance, but had little predictive power (Calnan, 1984; King, 1984). Modest correlations (r .25, .27 respectively) also were found with adolescent self-report of driving while drinking (Beck, 1981) and of mothers' adherence to medication regimen for children with otitis media (Becker et al., 1977b). It is interesting that little attention has been given to this factor in the prospective prediction studies, particularly in light of the recent work in the area of efficacy and health behavior.

With the exception of studies examining mothers' management of children's health regimens, there appears to be some inconsistency in the findings regarding the ability of health beliefs to predict subsequent behavior. Less favorable findings appear when adult health practices are examined, for example, studies on breast self-examination practices and adherence to antihypertensive drug regimens, than when screening practices are examined. The predictive ability of health beliefs may vary between populations, as noted in the examination of studies of perceived severity and medical care utilization. The number of studies in each of the abovementioned areas is small, but those that have been undertaken suggest than an important direction in the study of health beliefs is an examination of the interaction of specific beliefs with types of health behaviors prescribed, as well as with the population of patients and the setting in which patients are seen.

A complicating factor in evaluating the effect of health beliefs on adherence is the time at which the assessment of health beliefs was undertaken in relation to diagnosis. Health beliefs may be modified with experience with a particular regimen (Beck, 1981; Taylor, 1979). In the single study that assessed health beliefs prior to diagnosis and again 6 months and 12 months after diagnosis and initiation of treatment, prediagnostic beliefs did not predict subsequent adherence (Taylor, 1979). After 6 months of exposure to antihypertensive treatment, beliefs both corresponded to current adherence as well as offered some prediction of adherence at 12 months. It would appear from this study that the ability of health beliefs to predict behavior is related to whether or not the individual has experienced the behavior and adjusted his beliefs accordingly. This is consistent with much of the attitude/behavior research.

A number of studies found other cognitive-motivational factors to be more predictive than health beliefs. Six of the 13 studies reported that behavioral intentions were the most powerful predictor of behavior (Beck, 1981; Calnan, 1984; Calnan & Moss, 1984; Cummings, Jette, Brock, & Haefner, 1976; King, 1982, 1984). These findings are consistent with the cognitive-motivational model posed by Fishbein (1975), which postulated a major role of intention in predicting subsequent behavior. Interestingly, three of these studies found associations between selected health beliefs and intentions. Perceived severity was related to intentions, as was perceived efficacy (Cummings et al., 1976; King, 1982, 1984). The nature of these studies did not lend themselves to an examination of the direction of influence. However, a path model developed by Cummings et al., (1976) suggests that perceived severity effects perceived efficacy. This in turn effects behavioral intention both directly and in conjunction with other variables such as past experience and social influence. The findings of these studies suggest an interesting avenue for further exploration, that is, the role of behavioral intentions in predicting adherence and the influence, if any, of health beliefs on those intentions.

Following yet a third cognitive-motivational model, Bandura (1977) has postulated in his Self-Efficacy Theory of behavior that individuals will engage in or persist with a behavior to the extent that they believe themselves able to carry out that behavior and to the extent that they believe the behavior will lead to a desired outcome. Conversely, "people avoid activities that they believe exceed their coping cabilities" as well as those in which "they expect their efforts to give no results" (Bandura, 1982). Moreover, these expectations tend to be specific to the behavior in question rather than general expectations of outcomes or competence (Kaplan, Atkins, Reinsch, 1984). Interestingly, this specificity was also a finding in the Health Belief area (Becker et al., 1977b).

Recent research suggests that the self-efficacy model has utility in explaining why individuals adopt or sustain health behaviors. It also suggests interventions that may stimulate action (Bandura, 1977, 1982; O'Leary, 1985; Strecher, DeVillis, Becker, Rosenstock, 1986). Bandura (1982) proposes behavioral skills training and practice as a method of altering self-efficacy on the precept that authentic mastery experiences are the best mechanism for providing efficacy information. This has been demonstrated in the research on self-efficacy. For example, Kaplan et al., (1984) reported that patients with chronic obstructive pulmonary disease who were given training in compliance with a walking prescription significantly increased their exercise in contrast to a control group of patients who were just given the exercise prescription and attention. They found that efficacy expectations regarding walking mediated the gains in exercise. Expectations regarding gains in behaviors other than walking changed as a function of their similarity to walking. Similar findings were reported in a study of the effects of exercise testing on physical activity patterns among men postmyocardial infarction (Ewart, Taylor, Reese, DeBusk, 1987). Further, self-efficacy was found to be a factor in the adoption of new behaviors in a study of self-management among children with asthma (Evans, 1987).

Cognitive-motivational models, therefore, have contributions to make to the understanding of patient adherence to a health care regimen. Each proposes a slightly different schema for the understanding of the relationship between motivational cognitions and subsequent behavior. In most cases the proportion of the variance in adherence behavior accounted for is low. Further, studies in the health belief area suggest that the effect of beliefs on behavior may vary as a function of the population and setting studied as well as a function of the time at which assessment of beliefs is undertaken. Intentions and self-efficacy seem particularly promising as predictors of adherence. Aspects of health beliefs also appear to be promising in predicting mothers' adherence behaviors and more general screening behaviors. They may also have a mediational role with intentions. Both self-efficacy and health beliefs appear to be influenced by experience, suggesting that studies need to assess these dimensions prior to the onset of the regimen of interest, if interest is in initial adherence. This is not to diminish the role of altered cognitions of this sort as predictors of longer-term adherence once experience has been gained with the regimen. As self-efficacy and health beliefs, however, appear to change in the direction of the behavior change, one wonders if behavior itself would be predictive of future adherence.

HEALTH BEHAVIORS AS PREDICTORS OF SUBSEQUENT ADHERENCE

Health behavior as a predictor of subsequent adherence can be examined along two dimensions. The first is whether adherence to a specific behavior predicts adherence to that same behavior in the future. The second is whether adherence to a specific behavior or set of behaviors predicts adherence to another health behavior in the future.

It can be hypothesized that if an individual adheres to a health care regimen at one time he is likely to do so at a later time. Indeed, such a hypothesis is supported in studies that have examined the effect of adherence to a specific regimen on subsequent adherence to that same regimen. Becker et al., (1974) reported that mothers with prior experience with ear infections were more likely to have their children adhere to the medication regimen and follow-up appointment when the child had otitis media. Similarly, Calnan and Moss (1984) reported that the best predictor of breast self-examination (BSE) practice following the offering of a BSE class was previous practice.

Support for the value of adherence as a predictor of subsequent adherence was found in an examination of the LRC–CPPT participants (Dunbar & Knoke, 1986). Adherence to the study medication during the first month postrandomization was examined as a predictor of adherence during the first year of the study and over the entire 7 years of the study. Initial adherence accounted for 34.5% of the variance in adherence during the first year. This was the best predictor of those examined of adherence in the LRC–CPPT study. Indeed, the addition of the next three patient predictors of adherence, age, smoking status, and psychological distress, to a multiple regression equation only increased the R^2 to .36 ($p = .001$). The same set of factors predicted adherence over the 7 years of the study with an R^2 of .24 ($p = .001$). Initial adherence continued to make the major contribution. The ability of initial adherence to predict subsequent adherence over a 7-year duration suggests a certain stability to adherence within a specific regimen based upon a pattern established early. This suggests an interesting and valuable direction for continued study of adherence to health regimen.

Health behaviors other than early adherence performance to an intervention do not predict adherence to a specific regimen. For example, while prior experience with otitis media predicted mothers' adherence to follow-up appointments for otitis media care, it did not predict adherence to appointments for other reasons (Becker et al., 1974). In the LRC–CPPT study, visit attendance during the first month postrandomization was associated with subsequent medication adherence in the first year and over the 7 years of the study. However, the substitution of initial visit adherence for initial medication adherence in a multiple regression equation lowered substantially the proportion of variance accounted for in subsequent medication adherence ($R^2 = .095$ contrasted with $R^2 = .36$). Thus, a related but not identical health behavior reduced the ability to predict future adherence.

Other behaviors were examined among the LRC–CPPT participants to determine the predictive ability of health-oriented behaviors on subsequent adherence to the medication regimen. During screening the participants were interviewed regarding their current and past practices with regard to smoking, exercise, weight, alcohol intake, and multivitamin use. Univariate analyses showed no statistically significant association over 1 year or over 7 years for regularity of exercise, relative weight, alcohol consumption, or multivitamin usage. While smoking status during screening did predict medication adherence over 1 year and over 7 years, the proportion of variance accounted for was very small, 1.2% the first year and 2% over the 7 years. Smokers had lower adherence than nonsmokers.

These studies suggest that behavior can predict behavior. The more similar the initial behavior is to the behavior to be predicted, the greater the ability to predict. However, there does not appear to be a set of behaviors characterizing an individual that would allow prediction of adherence to a specific health regimen; that is, there is not an individual who is health-oriented, as defined by the practice of a set of healthy behaviors, whose adherence could be predicted on the basis of that practice alone. However, the studies suggest that a history of adherence to a specific regimen would predict subsequent adherence to that regimen. Further study of the ability of behavior to predict subsequent adherence would be of interest and would be most useful in the selection of subjects for clinical research efforts where maximal adherence to protocol regimen is desired.

Somatic Factors as Predictors of Adherence

A number of studies have examined the aversive effects as well as the relief of symptoms due to treatment as a predictor of adherence. For example, physical discomfort during running does predict dropping out of a marathon training program (Heiby et al., 1985). Indeed, the amount of running done by the dropouts was a function of the number of injuries experienced. Similarly, adherence to self-management procedures for adults with diabetes, hypertension, and/or pulmonary disease was negatively associated with symptoms (Nagy & Wolfe, 1984). Thus patients with more symptoms were less likely to follow self-management procedures.

Given, Given, and Coyle (1985) noted further that patients with hypertension participating in an intervention study who perceived themselves to have more severe symptoms were more likely to drop out. This investigation suggests that beliefs about symptoms may be important predictors of nonadherence. This notion is further supported by Meyer, Leventhal, & Gutmann, (1985) in a study of hypertensive patients' models of their illness. These investigators noted that a majority of patients believed they could monitor their own blood pressure changes through physiological symptoms. Indeed, 71% of new patients, 92% of continuing patients, and 94% of returning patients reported such an ability. Those patients who believed treatment relieved their symptoms reported adhering to treatment. Thus the notion of somatic factors predicting subsequent adherence may be confounded by the patient's perception of those symptoms and by the inclusion of somatic factors in their model of a disease and its treatment.

SUMMARY

A variety of factors specific to the patient have been reviewed that predict subsequent patient adherence. Included in these factors are psychological characteristics, particularly psychological distress; cognitive–motivational factors drawn from theories regarding health beliefs, intentions and behavior, and self-efficacy; and health behaviors and somatic complaints. While each of these areas has something to contribute to the prediction of patient adherence to a health care regimen, the predictive power tends to be modest at best for any single factor. The most promising of these seem to be self-efficacy, intentions, and adherence behavior itself. Not to be lost, however, is the role of psychological distress, perceived vulnerability or susceptibility to illness or its consequences, and the experience or perceived experience of somatic complaints. Many questions still arise in the area of prediction of patient adherence. Among these are such questions as how beliefs interact with populations, health care settings, and type of behavior to influence adherence. Also, how do these multiple factors interact, if at all, to lead to adherence or nonadherence? Further, how do each of these factors independently act to influence adherence, if at all? While more is becoming known about patient factors predictive of adherence, the relatively modest associations suggest that there is still much to be learned.

REFERENCES

Bandura, A. (1977). Self-efficacy: Toward a unifying theory of behavioral change. *Psychological Review, 84*(2), 191–215.

Bandura, A. (1982). Self-efficacy mechanism in human agency. *American Psychologist, 37*(2), 122–147.

Beck, K. H. (1981). Driving while under the influence of alcohol: Relationship to attitudes and beliefs in a college population. *American Journal of Drug and Alcohol Abuse, 8*(3), 377–386.

Becker, M. H., Drachman, R. H., & Kirscht, J. P. (1974). A new approach to explaining sick-role behavior in low-income populations. *American Journal of Public Health, 64*(3), 205–216.

Becker, M. H., Maiman, L. A., Kirscht, J. P., Haefner, D. P., & Drachman, R. H. (1977a). The health belief model and prediction of dietary compliance: A field experiment. *Journal of Health and Social Behavior, 18*(December), 348–366.

Becker, M. H., Nathanson, C. A., Drachman, R. H., & Kirscht, J. P. (1977b). Mothers' health beliefs and children's clinic visits: A prospective study. *Journal of Community Health, 3*(2), 125–135.

Berkanovic, E., Telesky, C., & Reeder, S. (1981). Structural and social psychological factors in the decision to seek medical care for symptoms. *Medical Care, 19*(7), 693–709.

Blumenthal, J. A., Williams, R. S., Wallace, A. G., Williams, R. B., & Needles, T. L. (1982). Physiological and psychological variables predict compliance to prescribed exercise therapy in patients recovering from myocardial infarction. *Psychosomatic Medicine, 44*(6), 519–527.

Calnan, M. (1984). The health belief model and participation in programmes for the early detection of breast cancer: A comparative analysis. *Social Science and Medicine, 19*(8), 823–830.

Calnan, M. W., & Moss, S. (1984). The health belief model and compliance with education given at a class in breast self-examination. *Journal of Health and Social Behavior*, 25(June), 198–210.

Croog, S. H., & Richards, N. P. (1977). Health beliefs and smoking patterns in heart patients and their wives: A longitudinal study. *American Journal of Public Health*, 67(10), 921–930.

Cummings, K. M., Jette, A. M., Brock, B. M., & Haefner, D. P. (1976). Psychosocial determinants of immunization behavior in a swine influenza campaign. *Medical Care*, 17(6), 639–649.

Dunbar, J., & Knoke, J. (1986). *Prediction of medication adherence at one year and seven years: Behavioral and psychological factors*. Paper presented at the Society for Clinical Trials Annual Conference, Montreal, Canada.

Eisen, M., Zellman, G. L., & McAlister, A. L. (1985). A health belief model approach to adolescents' fertility control: Some pilot program findings. *Health Education Quarterly*, 12(2), 185–210.

Evans, D. (1987). *School-based health education for children with asthma*. Paper presented at the NHLBI National Working Conference on the Adoption and Maintenance of Behaviors for Optimal Health, Bethesda, Maryland.

Ewart, C. K., Taylor, C. B., Reese, L., & DeBusk, R. F. (1987). *The effects of early exercise testing on physical activity patterns after myocradial infarction*. Paper presented at the NHLBI National Working Conference on the Adoption and Maintenance of Behaviors for Optimal Health, Bethesda, Maryland.

Fishbein, M. (1975). *Belief, attitude, intention, and behavior*. Reading, MA: Addison-Wesley.

Given, C. W., Given, B. A., & Coyle, B. W. (1985). Prediction of patient attrition from experimental behavioral interventions. *Nursing Research*, 34, 293–298.

Goodman, L. A., & Kruskal, w. H. (1954). Measures of association for cross classifications. *Journal of the American Statistical Association*, 49:732–764.

Heiby, E. M., Onorato, V. A., & Sato, R. A. (1985). *A cognitive–behavioral model of adherence to health-related exercise*. Poster session presented at the American Psychological Association Convention, Los Angeles, CA.

Inui, T. S., Yourtee, E. L., & Williamson, J. W. (1976). Improved outcomes in hypertension after physician tutorials: A controlled trial. *Annals of Internal Medicine*, 84(6):646–651.

Janz, N. K., & Becker, M. H. (1984). The Health Belief Model: a decade later. *Health Education Quarterly*, 11:1–47.

Kaplan, R. M., Atkins, D. J., & Reinsch, S. (1984). Specific efficacy expectations mediate exercise compliance in patients with COPD. *Health Psychology*, 3(3), 233–242.

King, J. B. (1982). The impact of patients' perceptions of high blood pressure on attendance at screening: An extension of the health belief model. *Social Science and Medicine*, 16, 1079–1091.

King, J. B. (1984). Illness attributions and the health belief model. *Health Education Quarterly*, 10(3/4), 287–312.

Leavitt, F. (1979). The health belief model and utilization of ambulatory care services. *Social Science and Medicine*, 13A, 105–112.

Meyer, D., Leventhal, H., & Gutmann, M. (1985). Common sense models of illness: The example of hypertension. *Health Psychology*, 4(2), 115–135.

Nagy, V. T., & Wolfe, G. R. (1984). Cognitive predictors of compliance in chronic disease patients. *Medical Care*, 22(10), 912–921.

Nelson, E. C., Stason, W. B., Neutra, R. R. Solomon, H. S., & McArdle, P. J. (1978). Impact of patient perceptions on compliance with treatment for hypertension. *Medical Care*, 16(11):893–906.

O'Leary, A. (1985). Self-efficacy and health. *Behavior Research and Therapy*, 23(4), 437–451.

O'Leary, M. R., Rohsenow, D. J., and Chaney, E. F. (1979). The use of multivariate personality strategies in predicting attrition from alcoholism treatment. *Journal of Clinical Psychiatry*, 40(4):190–193.

Rosenstock, I. M. (1974). The historical origins of the health belief model. Health Education. Monographs, 2:238.

Strecher, V. J., DeVillis, B. M., Becker, M. H., & Rosenstock, I. M. (1986). The role of self-efficacy in achieving health behavior change. *Health Education Quarterly*, 13(1), 73–91.

Taylor, D. W. (1979). A test of the health belief model in hypertension. In R. B. Haynes, D. W. Taylor, & D. L. Sackett (Eds.), *Compliance in health care* (pp. 103–109). Baltimore: Johns Hopkins University Press.

Ulrich, R. Personal Communication, 1988.

20

Strategies for Enhancing Adherence in Clinical Trials

Larry Gorkin, Michael G. Goldstein, Michael J. Follick, R. Craig Lefebvre

---

Enhancing adherence in clinical trials has received relatively little attention in the literature. We will describe why low adherence is a problem in the treatment of chronic disease, the particular concerns that make adherence even more important to the conduct of clinical trials, the complex and multivariate factors that predict low adherence rates, and possible strategies to increase adherence within trials.

Concerns regarding patient adherence are of particular importance in the context of clinical trials research—the vehicle by which basic science and applications to human disease merge. Clinical trials are designed to evaluate an experimental treatment relative to placebo or standard care, via the randomization of patients to the various treatment arms of the trial.

Clinical trials are designed to test the efficacy of interventions that prevent or treat disease. The subjects in these trials may be asymptomatic or symptomatic. In research with asymptomatic individuals (e.g., to achieve risk-factor reduction to lower the incidence of coronary artery disease), generating clinically meaningful outcomes is difficult because interventions are often not very powerful (Levy & Kannel, 1988). In trials that assess symptomatic patients, the endpoints of interest are often low-frequency events, such as mortality or sudden cardiac death. Thus large numbers of subjects are required for the successful conduct of both types of clinical trials.

One recent trend within clinical trials that is important to the present discussion is the movement toward addressing the "efficacy trials" rather than the "acceptability trials" research question. The former term refers to a trial designed to maximize adherence to the study protocol and, thereby, assess the validity of treatment efficacy under optimal conditions. Within this approach, one can proceed to an analysis of the physiologic substrates or other mechanisms that are hypothesized to mediate observed treatment effects. The cost of this approach is that the clinical efficacy of the treatment, once it has been approved for commercial use, may or may not mirror the results observed in the more contrived and standardized setting of the clinical trial. It is assumed that demonstration of efficacy will encourage adherence. In contrast, a trial designed to address the "dissemination to the public" question more accurately reflects conditions that will exist if and when the intervention is introduced to the public.

To maintain standardization of methods and to monitor protocol adherence, the trial often imposes strict management (1) of patients, including random and blinded assignment to experimental conditions; (2) of staff, prescribing and proscribing certain behaviors and activities that they may engage in with patients, as well as blinding them to patient assignment status; and (3) of data, including storage and analysis in a facility separate, in location and personnel, from sites of data collection.

Assuming that adequate enrollment and randomization of eligible patients is achieved, the success of the trial is then largely dependent upon patient adherence to the experimental protocol. Adherence in clinical trials takes two primary forms: (1) enactment of the assigned treatment regimen for the duration of the trial, be it surgical, pharmaceutical, utilizing a device, or behavioral, and (2) adherence to the scheduled assessment of outcome measures, be it laboratory workup, stress testing, or self-report.

Problems with patient adherence can threaten the validity of ongoing trials in several ways. Loss of patients can threaten internal validity, particularly if differential attrition occurs across treatment groups (Bhaskar, Reitman, Sacks, Smith, & Chalmers, 1986). Even when patient numbers are sufficient, external validity, or generalizability, of findings from a trial may be compromised by high rates of attrition of enrolled patients independent of treatment assignment, or by shifts in the type of patient who enrolls over time.

If patients who "drop out" for reasons not sanctioned by the trial protocol have to be replaced. This phenomenon can have far-reaching consequences on the power of the trial. Participating clinical centers may suffer financial cutbacks or termination of support. Such consequences pose further demands on the remaining centers to increase their productivity, may lead to changes in the protocol to bolster sagging subject numbers (Lipid Research Clinics Program, 1983), and increase total costs to the trial (Friedman, Furberg, & DeMets, 1985).

Once the trial is complete, it is unclear how to "treat" patients, statistically, who withdraw due to compliance difficulties, particularly if they are lost to follow-up. Does one ignore them, count them as treatment failures, or devise some other analytic strategy? The researcher must determine, notwithstanding random assignment of patients to conditions, whether rates of patient termination from the trial due to nonadherence are comparable across conditions and, more importantly, whether similar individuals, except for treatment assignment, remain in both experimental and control groups.

With this background, it is clear why clinical trials researchers are now motivated to analyze what factors are contributing to low adherence and then to design strategies to enhance patient adherence to research protocols. But this is a recent development in that clinical trial researchers in cardiovascular disease had previously shied away from active interventions to improve adherence. This policy had been based on the assumption that such active involvement would undermine the trial by confounding the generalizability of the findings. As enrollment and adherence issues become more critical to the success of trials, however, there has been greater willingness to challenge this a priori assumption. The argument presented herein is quite the opposite; when trial researchers integrate adherence-improving interventions conducted by individuals blind to treatment assignment, the design-confounding issue becomes a non sequitur. Accordingly, a successful trial with sufficient power to address the "mechanisms of action" question is more likely to be achieved.

To date there appears to be little in the literature on the assessment of factors contributing to patient nonadherence within clinical trials of cardiovascular disease, and even less on interventions to improve adherence. Using a methodology not designed to address this question directly, patients who participated for the duration of either the National Heart, Lung, and Blood Institute (NHLBI) clinical trial, Aspirin Myocardial Infarction Study (AMIS), or the Beta-Blocker Heart Attack Trial (BHAT) were asked what barriers to participation in the trial existed. Patient reports focused on frustration with clinic visits, such as transportation problems or scheduling inconvenience (Mattson, Curb, & McArdle, 1985). Unfortunately, patients who did not complete these research protocols were not queried regarding their decision to withdraw from participation. Because of the paucity of data on adherence in trials of cardiovascular disease, we have gathered evidence from a variety of research settings. Research on compliance with therapeutic regimens provides a wealth of data that may help us to understand adherence within clinical trials. However, it is noted that the populations within general medical practice may not extrapolate to the populations that agree to enroll in clinical trials.

There appear to be multiple factors within clinical trials that influence adherence by exerting both independent and interactive effects. These include: (1) aspects of the experimental protocol; (2) subject characteristics and behaviors; (3) interactions between subjects and health care providers (e.g., trial research team, personal physicians); (4) patient's relationship to family members; (5) organizational and environmental factors (e.g., use of community resources). These factors will be reviewed, in turn, in the following sections of this chapter.

ASPECTS OF THE EXPERIMENTAL PROTOCOL

The experimental regimen is itself a critical determinant of adherence. In general, adherence diminishes with greater complexity of the regimen, manifested by the frequency of dose or length of time for which treatment is prescribed (Cockburn, Gibberd, Reid, & Sanson-Fisher, 1987; Zifferblatt, 1975). In adapting to a more complex regimen, adherence is more likely to be maintained to the degree that the therapeutic regimen can be incorporated into the patients' life-style, for example, coincident trial medication administration with relatively reliable and easily demarcated daily events, such as mealtimes.

Given the lower rates of adherence to behavioral change regimens (Haynes & Dantes, 1987), integrative methods may be even more critical to achieving successful adherence to such regimens. A life-style exercise regimen (e.g., walking to and from school) was found to be a more effective, long-term strategy to produce weight loss in obese children than was a specific aerobic training regimen (Epstein, Wing, Koeske, & Valoski, 1985). Differences in this randomized trial were maintained at the 2-year follow-up, although training duration for both groups was limited to 8 weeks. Hence, it is incumbent upon investigators to adapt their protocol to patient life-styles to achieve high rates of adherence both during and following the trial.

When a behavioral change (e.g., dietary change, change in exercise pattern, smoking cessation) is a component of the treatment protocol in clinical trials, subject skill deficits may compromise both adherence and treatment outcome. Helping the subject to implement behavioral changes by providing specific behavioral skills training is likely to improve adherence more than information and instruction alone. For example, dietary treatment of hypertension is enhanced when patients receive skills training including self-monitoring, goal-setting, and changing antecedents and consequences for dietary behavior (Caggiula, Milas, & Wing, 1987; Schlundt, 1987). Also, patients who receive nicotine gum as a smoking cessation treatment are more successful if they also receive behavioral skills training, which includes relaxation training and training in the use of problem-solving and cognitive/behavioral strategies to deal with smoking cues as well as relapse situations (Goldstein, Niaura, Follick, & Abrams, 1989; Killen, Maccoby, & Taylor, 1984). Moreover, several studies that assess the effectiveness of nicotine gum provided by physicians without behavioral treatment show no significant effect (British Thoracic Society, 1983; Jamrozik, Fowler, Vessey, & Wald, 1984; Schneider, Jarvik, & Forsythe, 1983). Thus trial protocols that include behavioral skills training and evaluation will facilitate validity checks regarding the intervention and will be more likely to advance knowledge of the mechanisms responsible for the effective or ineffective behavior change or adaptation.

Although there has been much expected in terms of biologic markers of pharmacologic agents, to date such approaches have had little impact on clinical trials (Mattson & Friedman, 1984). Individual differences in the way that medications are absorbed and metabolized and subject voiding patterns have limited the reliability and validity of blood levels achieved for a given dose.

The mainstay for determining adherence in trials is by pill counts. This method provides information about medication availability, which is then interpreted relative to expected consumption rates. The information derived does not reflect actual amount or pattern of consumption, but of potential consumption. One amplification of the pill-counting approach has been to screen patients prior to randomization and thereby ensure randomization of only "good adherers" in the trial proper (see Davis and Probstfield chapters in this volume). Although the use of more sophisticated devices that record temporal pattern of dispensement has been discussed, cost and availability have hampered their integration into clinical trials (Mattson & Friedman, 1984).

PATIENT CHARACTERISTICS AND BEHAVIORS
Demographic Characteristics

Empirical research on adherence with therapeutic regimens has observed that patient characteristics such as age, gender, education, socioeconomic status, religion, and marital status have little association with adherence tests (see review by Haynes, 1976). For example, though it is often assumed that the elderly have poor rates of adherence to long-term treatment regimens due to factors such as cognitive deficits, multiple drug regimens, and greater social isolation (Lipton & Lee, 1988), this has not been found in clinical studies. Data from a clinical trial, the Systolic Hypertension in the Elderly Program (SHEP) (Black, Brand, Greenlick, Hughes, & Smith, 1987), suggested that adherence rates were high (80–90%) at both 3 and 12 months follow-up when assessed by either pill count, self-report, or by urine chlorthalidone assay.

Subject Knowledge and Beliefs

The subject's knowledge about the prescribed regimen, beliefs about personal vulnerability to disease, and efficacy of treatment have been found to influence adherence to therapeutic regimens (see reviews by DiMatteo & DiNicola, 1982; Haynes, 1976). For example, in a study of adherence to prescribed short-term antibiotics, knowledge regarding the name of the medication and greater perceived disease severity were associated with compliance (Cockburn et al., 1987). These variables can be altered by close attention to proper education of the patient about the nature of the study and requirements of the protocol, as described in the section below on patient–researcher interactions.

Increased knowledge of physical condition and education about the treatment of heart disease were consistently noted as reasons patients gave for participating in the BHAT or AMIS trials (Mattson et al., 1985). To address these concerns, some centers within recent trials (e.g., the Studies of Left Ventricular Dysfunction) have incorporated newsletters that are sent to patients periodically to convey information about cardiac disease and treatment and to keep adherence to the protocol salient.

Disease Status and Side Effects

The symptomatic status of subjects and, correctively, the side effects of other complications experienced by subjects are variables that predict adherence. For example, trials involving dietary modification to reduce cholesterol intake have been observed to produce greater adherence among patients with coronary heart disease (CHD) (Bierenbaum, Fleischman, Green, et al., 1970; Woodhill, Palmer, Leelarthaepin, et al., 1978) relative to normal populations or asymptomatic individuals at increased risk for CHD due to hypercholesterolemia (Mojonnier, Hall, Berkson, et al., 1980; Reeves, Foreyt, Scott, et al., 1983). This adherence difference may reflect the impact of beliefs regarding vulnerability to illness, as noted in the prior section.

An alternative explanation is that, by definition, asymptomatic individuals can only be made "worse" by the therapeutic intervention. For instance, in a randomized trial of antihypertensive medications (the angiotensin-converting enzyme captopril, the centrally acting sympathomimetic agent methyldopa, and the beta-blocker propranolol) among asymptomatic males, side effects predicted premature withdrawal from the trial (Croog, Levine, Testa, et al., 1986). Captopril was associated with significantly less withdrawal than methyldopa (8% vs. 20%), with propranolol between these two (13%). It was the more frequent reports of fatigue and blurred vision with methyldopa that led to greater patient attrition. Symptoms to the intervention related to the disease may be important and can be dealt with in the prerandomization period (Probstfield, Russell, Insull, & Yusuf, this volume). These results are of particular interest because there were no differences between medications in terms of blood pressure reduction.

Affective Status

Patients without a clinical disorder but who are somewhat anxious, fearful, or depressed may also be less willing or able to adhere to a therapeutic protocol (Richardson, Marks, Johnson, et al., 1987). Patient distress may interfere with comprehension of treatment instructions or motivation to follow the protocol. It is noted that psychological support as an adjunct to medical care produced a significant increase in cooperation with treatment after myocardial infarction (MI) or surgery (Mumford, Schlesinger, & Glass, 1982). A stress intervention trial on mortality among post-MI patients produced results that suggested that intervention increased adherence with cardiac medication (Frasure-Smith & Prince, 1987). This study will be described in more detail in the section on organizational and environmental factors.

PATIENT INTERACTIONS
Patient and Research Staff

Patient satisfaction with the health care provider is correlated with adherence to recommendations by such a provider (Haynes, 1976). It is likely that this relationship between satisfaction and adherence will generalize to clinical trials as well. Congruence between patient and researcher perceptions regarding the rationale for the trial is important to adherence. Results from a recent antiepileptic drug study (Cramer, Collins, & Mattson, 1988) may well have implications for trials other than those for epilepsy and for cardiovascular disease specifically. Factors assessed at baseline that predicted nonadherence to the protocol included the patient questioning the diagnosis or the need for medication, particularly focusing on the need for double-blinded research design. It is therefore important that all physicians and nurses who work on the trial be knowledgeable and comfortable with the research protocol and be skilled communicators or recruitment and adherence are likely to suffer (cf., Hall & Roter, 1988).

The research team is also charged with scheduling subjects for screening assessments and follow-up sessions. It is noted that a special referral clerk who helps to overcome barriers to appointment-keeping such as transportation and babysitting needs can increase attendance at referral appointments (Sackett, Haynes, & Tugwell, 1985). In a recent study of nonelective hospitalization rates among diabetic patients, an intervention package designed to increase office visits was evaluated relative to a usual-care control in a randomized trial (Smith,

Weinberger, & Katz, 1987). The intervention consisted of mailings of information, appointment reminders, and vigilant follow-up of patients who missed appointments. Results indicated that the intervention group averaged 9% more appointments than the control group over a 2-year period. In contrast, the groups did not differ in their rates of nonelective hospitalizations. In the context of clinical trials aimed at slowing the progression of cardiovascular disease, the Smith et al. (1987) results are, however, promising. Similar strategies might also increase adherence to appointments within clinical trials of cardiovascular disease.

There is also an accumulating literature assessing the influence of style, content, and "readability" of communications from physician to patient. This literature points to the need for simple, direct, and repetitive communications that convey the crucial points of the proposed treatment plan (Hunninghake, Darby, & Probstfield, 1987). Recall is enhanced if it is presented (1) in specific categories within a logical sequence (e.g., diagnosis, testing, treatment, patient responsibilities), rather than shifting between categories (Ley, Bradshaw, Eaves, & Walker, 1973), and (2) if presented in both verbal and visual form, rather than in just one modality (Boyd, Covington, Stanaszck, & Coussons, 1974). However, long-term adherence is not affected greatly by instruction or patient education alone (Daltroy, 1985; Sackett et al., 1985). Long-term adherence improves when more attention is focused directly on the behaviors required to follow the therapeutic regimen. Such interventions as self-monitoring, feedback, shaping, and reinforcement of the desired health behaviors and contingency contracting have been shown to be effective in clinical trials (Sackett et al., 1985). For example, behavioral training to foster adherence to a low-cholesterol diet involved modeling of shopping and cooking behaviors and monitoring of foods eaten (Meyer & Henderson, 1974).

It is clear that these points regarding communication need to be adopted by the research team at the time of enrollment, and as part of obtaining informed consent from patients. Although these strategies may lead to a slightly lower rate of enrollment among eligible patients (cf., Simes, Tattersall, Coates, et al., 1986), such strategies are likely to produce, among those who enroll, a much higher rate of patient adherence for the duration of the trial.

Patient and Personal Physicians

Patients enrolled in clinical trials are likely to have a primary care physician (e.g., internist, family physician) and/or a specialist (e.g., cardiologist) involved in their ongoing care. These personal physicians frequently develop strong relationships with their patients and have significant influence over their patients' choice of health behaviors. Because of these circumstances, involvement of patients' personal physicians in the research protocol may increase patient adherence. To achieve this result, it is important that personal physicians be fully informed about the study rationale, design, and methodology. The physician's concerns about the trial (e.g., drug safety, exacerbation of patient condition, loss of practice patients to the trial) should also be elicited and addressed by a research team representative, preferably another physician.

Providing personal physicians with feedback about patient status will help ensure the saliency of the trial for physicians and their patients. This may be accomplished by the assessment of risk factors for coronary disease that will provide a more developed clinical profile of patients. Feedback from fractionated lipid, cotinine, glucose intolerance, and/or ambulatory blood pressure monitoring could be provided to attending physicians with the encouragement to discuss results with their patients. This strategy would be a cost-effective and meaningful way to maintain physician and patient interest in the trial and thereby influence adherence.

PATIENT RELATIONSHIPS TO FAMILY MEMBERS

Most participants in clinical trials of cardiovascular disease are not isolated. For example, in the post-MI trial, the Cardiac Arrhythmia Pilot Study (CAPS), 74% reported being married, with an average of three persons living in the patient's household (CAPS Investigators, 1988). Similarly, 80% reported being married in a large hypertension trial (Croof et al., 1986). Accordingly, a logical source for improving adherence in trials is to involve the participant's social support system. In the absence of intervention, family members are likely to exert an influence, positive or negative, on adherence rates.

Participation of spouses in treatment and training in supportive behaviors appear to enhance initial outcomes and maintenance of gains for treatment of certain addictive disorders (cf., Brownell, Heckerman, Westlake, et al., 1978). It is reasonable to assume, for example, that spouses can be instrumental in achieving initial compliance and particularly in maintaining gains from dietary treatments of lipid disorders. Spouses are often involved in food selection and preparation. Moreover, studies have demonstrated that changes in blood lipids tend to covary among family members (Witschi, Singer, Wu-Lee, & Stare, 1978). Therefore, it is likely that training of spouses in dietary skills and behaviors supportive of dietary changes will increase the patient's dietary compliance and ultimately produce positive lipid changes over time.

It is also noted, however, that increased levels of perceived support do not necessarily translate into higher adherence rates. This can be seen in a study of social support on diabetic control among men and women with type II diabetic patients (Kaplan & Hartwell, 1987). Diabetic control was defined as glycosylated hemoglobin (HbA1C), providing an average reading over a 4- to 8-week period. Results indicated that although high levels of perceived support were associated with greater diabetic control in women, high levels of support were associated with less diabetic control for men. In contrast to the expected effect of support on women, support forms satisfactory to men may reinforce patterns of eating, drinking, and exercise that are incompatible with diabetic control.

From this perspective, cardiac rehabilitation is a social process that can be facilitated or impeded by the attitudes and behaviors of spouses and family members. One of the major problems experienced by the post-MI patient is that the family members often perceive the patient as incapacitated by the clinical event. This perception is particularly strengthened if the family members feel impotent to act in case of recurrence or exacerbation of clinical symptoms. Educating the supportive individual in terms of prognosis, expectations for recovery, and behaviors that will enhance the likelihood of positive outcomes is recommended. It is assumed that "significant others" are in a potentially critical position to shape the behavior of the patient. Significant others can monitor the patient's behavior and encourage direct adherence to the prescribed medical, dietary, and psychological regimens. Significant others may themselves engage in and thereby model the target behaviors that result in reductions in coronary heart disease risk. If a spouse changes his or her health habits simultaneously with the target patient, this mutual engagement and encouragement may decrease the perceived and actual difficulty of succeeding at and maintaining behavior change.

One of the most frequently expressed concerns of the wife of the MI patient involves her anxiety over her husband's level of activity (Sikorski, 1985). This concern would be salient if the patient was enrolled in a randomized clinical trial such as one involving early return to work versus usual care among men with uncomplicated MIs (Dennis, Houston-Miller, Schwartz, et al., 1988). In this context, an intervention that might influence the wives' behavior may produce beneficial results toward the conduct of the trial. A unique example would be to provide all spouses with the experience of performing exercise tolerance testing (ETT) (Taylor, Bandura, Ewart, et al., 1985). These authors found that wives who actually performed on the treadmill for 3 minutes at the level achieved by their husbands were more likely to view their husbands as capable of handling physical or cardiac stressors than wives assigned randomly to watch their husbands perform ETT (but not perform ETT themselves) or those wives who simply waited in the next room while their spouses performed ETT. Accordingly, an intervention that increases the confidence of a spouse regarding her partner's capabilities following an MI may produce enhanced adherence in trials aimed at cardiac rehabilitation.

ORGANIZATIONAL AND ENVIRONMENTAL FACTORS

Strategic use of environmental and organizational factors may also contribute to the success of trials by influencing adherence rates. This can include the use of specific health care or other organizations outside the research setting that are attended by trial patients or the use of environmental resources to intercede in the lives of patients to produce greater adherence.

Organizational Factors

Patients are more likely to view the trial protocol as integrated into their overall health care if the study intervention is provided at the site where they receive their usual health care rather than located at a tertiary care university center. For increasingly large numbers of patients, a Health Maintenance Organization (HMO) may be an ideal site for a trial center because virtually all of the outpatient care and health promotion activities are provided for patients and their families. Hence, involvement of a spouse or other family members in the trial may be facilitated if an HMO is utilized as a research site.

Another level to the organizational impact to clinical trials is the large number of resources available in the community that have been untapped by clinical investigators. In the context of dietary or pharmacologic treatment of hypercholesterolemia, nutritional information programs can be implemented in restaurants and grocery stores to encourage people to adopt and maintain healthy eating patterns (Lefebvre, 1987). The use of worksites or churches as enrollment, intervention, and follow-up sites has been employed in community-based trials aimed at reducing cardiovascular risk factor levels (e.g., Lasater, Wells, Carleton, & Elder, 1986; Nelson, Sennett, Lefebvre, et al., 1987; World Health Organization European Collaborative Group, 1986). In approaching such settings, it is important to gain the support of the "gatekeepers" (i.e., people who control access to a population group), who have both their own prestige and the welfare of their constituents to uphold. Through church leaders or factory foremen, for example, access to others who might help with adherence, such as company nurses, may be obtained. These individuals may provide additional dividends as health policy moves toward commercial availability of the intervention for the public.

Environmental Factors

The influence of an environmental system on patient adherence may be illustrated by the results of a clinical intervention involving crisis management. This project was conducted with male survivors of an uncomplicated MI (Frasure-Smith & Prince, 1985). No single theory or approach to stress reduction was tested; instead, nurses with a manageable caseload and access to referral and consultative services initiated and constituted the intervention. In this prospective, randomized design, 539 subjects were assigned to either the experimental intervention or standard hospital care. The experimental treatment consisted of monthly telephone calls involving a psychological distress interview. High stress scores resulted in home visits, and rehospitalization resulted in bedside visits. Control subjects were contacted by phone twice during the study, but these calls did not lead to nurse interventions.

Results revealed that control patients were twice as likely to die from ischemic heart disease as were experimental patients. After 4 months there was a clear divergence of the two groups with regard to patient mortality. Although the authors initially attributed the mortality reduction to stress reduction, a secondary finding suggested an alternative explanation relating to adherence. The mortality effect was most striking for patients prescribed beta-blockers at the time of hospital discharge (Frasure-Smith & Prince, 1987). It is therefore possible that the nursing intervention led to reduced mortality via increased adherence to the cardiac medication. It is this type of aggressive intervention, systematically built into a trial, that would allow for the optimal test of the "mechanisms of action" question.

CONCLUSION

We have argued that adherence is problematic in the treatment of chronic disease, and the concern is greater within clinical trials where decisions about treatment safety and efficacy regarding experimental interventions or applications are made. Given the size and cost of trials the need for high rates of adherence is of paramount importance.

We have seen that a number of creative avenues can be pursued in the attempt to increase adherence to health behaviors within clinical trials. These involve interventions at the level of patient characteristics and behaviors, research staff, attending physicians, and support-systems—both naturally occurring and those generated externally, via the health care system and community. A range of interventions has been offered that differ in scope and feasibility. Reasonable questions can be raised regarding the willingness of clinical trial researchers to incorporate these suggestions within their protocols. However, because trial investigators have made the decision to pursue "efficacy trials," active strategies to enhance adherence to trial protocols will be necessary to ensure the long-term success of such research.

REFERENCES

Bhaskar, R., Reitman, D., Sacks, H. S., Smith, H., Jr., & Chalmers, T. C. (1986). Loss of patients in clinical trials that measure long-term survival following myocardial infarction. *Controlled Clinical Trials, 7,* 134-148.

Bierenbaum, M. L., Fleischman, A. I., Green, D. P., Raichelson, R. I., Hayton, T., Watson, P. B., & Caldwell, A. B. (1970). The 5-year experience of modified fat diets on younger men with coronary heart disease. *Circulation, 42,* 943–952.

Black, D. M., Brand, R. J., Greenlick, M., Hughes, G. & Smith, J. for the SHEP Pilot Research Group (1987). Compliance to treatment for hypertension in elderly patients: The SHEP pilot study. *Journal of Gerontology, 42,* 552–557.

Boyd, J. R., Covington, T. R., Stanaszck, W. F., & Coussons, R. T. (1974). Drug defaulting—Part I: Determinants of compliance. *American Journal of Hospital Pharmacology, 31,* 362–364.

British Thoracic Society. (1983). Comparison of four methods of smoking withdrawal in patients with smoking related diseases. *British Medical Journal, 286,* 595–597.

Brownell, K. D., Heckerman, C. L., Westlake, R. J., Hayes, S. C., & Monti, P. M. (1978). The effect of couples training and partner cooperativeness in the behavioral treatment of obesity. *Behavior Research and Therapy, 16,* 323–333.

Caggiula, A., Milas, C. N., & Wing, R. R. (1987). Optimal nutritional therapy in the treatment of hypertension. In M. D. Blaufox & H. G. Langford (Eds.), *Non-pharmacologic therapy of hypertension* (pp. 6–21). Basel, Switzerland: Karger.

The Cardiac Arrhythmia Pilot Study (CAPS) Investigators. (1988). Recruitment and baseline description of patients in the CAPS. *American Journal of Cardiology, 61,* 704–713.

Cockburn, J., Gibberd, R. W., Reid, A. L., & Sanson-Fisher, R. W. (1987). Determinants of non-compliance with short-term antibiotic regimens. *British Heart Journal, 295,* 814–818.

Cramer, J. A., Collins, J. F., & Mattson, R. H. (1988). Can categorization of patient background problems be used to determine early termination in a clinical trial? *Controlled Clinical Trials, 9,* 47–63.

Croog, S. H., Levine, S., Testa, M. A., Brown, B., Bulpitt, C. J., Jenkins, C. D., Klerman, G. L., & Williams, G. H. (1986). The effects of antihypertensive therapy on the quality of life. *New England Journal of Medicine, 314,* 1657–1664.

Daltroy, L. H. (1985). Improving cardiac patient adherence to exercise regimens: A clinical trial of health education. *Journal of Cardiac Rehabilitation, 5,* 40–49.

Dennis, C., Houston-Miller, N., Schwartz, R. G., Ahn, D. K., Kraemer, H. C., Gossard, D., Junean, M., Taylor, C. B., & DeBusk, R. F. (1988). Early return to work after uncomplicated myocardial infarction. *Journal of the American Medical Association, 260,* 214–220.

DiMatteo, M. R., & DiNicola, D. D. (1982). ,Achieving patient compliance: The psychology of the medical practitioner's role. New York: Pergamon Press.

Epstein, L. H., Wing, R. R., Koeske, R., & Valoski, A. (1985). A comparison of lifestyle exercise, aerobic exercise, and calisthenics on weight loss in obese children. *Behavior Therapy, 16,* 345–356.

Frasure-Smith, N., & Prince, R. H. (1985). The Ischemic Heart Disease Life Stress Monitoring Program: Impact on mortality. *Psychosomatic Medicine, 47,* 431–445.

Frasure-Smith, N., & Prince, R. H. (1987). The Ischemic Heart Disease Life Stress Monitoring Program: Possible therapeutic mechanisms. *Psychology and Health, 1,* 273–285.

Friedman, L. M., Furberg, C. D., & DeMets, D. L. (1985). *Fundamentals of clinical trials* (2nd Ed.) (pp. 161–171). Littleton, Mass.: PSG.

Goldstein, M. G., Niaura, R. S., Follick, M. J., & Abrams, D. B. (1989). Effects of behavioral skills training and schedule of nicotine gum administration on smoking cessation. *American Journal of Psychiatry, 146*, 56–60.

Hall, J. A., & Roter, D. L. (1988). Physicians' knowledge and self-reported compliance promotion as predictors of performance with simulated lung disease patients. *Evaluation and The Health Professions, 11*, 306–317.

Haynes, R. B. (1976). A critical review of the "determinants" of patient compliance with therapeutic regimens. In D. L. Sackett & R. B. Haynes (Eds.), *Compliance with therapeutic regimens* (pp. 26–39). Baltimore: The Johns Hopkins University Press.

Haynes, R. B., & Dantes, R. (1987). Patient compliance and the conduct and interpretation of therapeutic trials. *Controlled Clinical Trials, 8*, 12–19.

Hunninghake, D. B., Darby, C. A., & Probstfield, J. L. (1987). Recruitment experience in clinical trials: Literature summary and annotated bibliography. *Controlled Clinical Trials, 8*, (Supplement), 6–30.

Jamrozik, K., Fowler, G., Vessey, M., & Wald, N. (1984). Placebo controlled trial of nicotine chewing gum in general practice. *British Medical Journal, 289*, 794–797.

Kaplan, R. N., & Hartwell, S. L. (1987). Differential effects of social support and social network on physiological and social outcomes in men and women with type II diabetes mellitus. *Health Psychology, 6*, 387–398.

Killen, J. D., Maccoby, N., & Taylor, C. B. (1984). Nicotine gum and self-regulation training in smoking relapse prevention. *Behavior Therapy, 15*, 234–248.

Lasater, T. M., Wells, B. L., Carleton, R. A., & Elder, J. P. (1986). The role of churches in disease prevention research studies. *Public Health Reports, 101*, 125–131.

Lefebvre, R. C. (1987). A case history of nutritional information on menus. *The Journal of Food Service Systems, 1*, 153–158.

Levy, D., & Kannel, W. B. (1988). Cardiovascular risks: New insights from Framingham. *American Heart Journal, 116*, 266–272.

Ley, P., Bradshaw, P. W., Eaves, D., & Walker, C. M. (1973). A method for increasing patients' recall of information presented by doctors. *Psychosomatic Medicine, 3*, 217–220.

Lipid Research Clinics Program. (1983). Participant recruitment to the Coronary Primary Prevention Trial. *Journal of Chronic Disease, 36*, 451–465.

Lipton, H. L., & Lee, P. H. (1988). *Drugs in the elderly: Clinical, social and policy perspectives.* Palo Alto, CA: Stanford University Press.

Mattson, M. E., Curb, J. D., McArdle, R., and the AMIS and BHAT Research Group (1985). Participation in a clinical trial: The patient's point of view. *Controlled Clinical Trials, 6*, 156–167.

Mattson, M. E., & Friedman, L. M. (1984). Issues in medication adherence assessment in clinical trials of the National Heart, Lung, and Blood Institute. *Controlled Clinical Trials, 5*, 488–496.

Meyer, A. T., & Henderson, J. B. (1974). Multiple risk factor reduction in the prevention of cardiovascular disease. *Preventive Medicine, 3*, 225–236.

Mojonnier, M. L., Hall, Y., Berkson, D. M., Robinson, E., Wethers, B., Pannbacker, B., Pardo, E., Stamler, J., Shekelle, R. B., & Raynor, W. (1980). Experience in changing food habits of hyperlipidemic men and women. *Journal of the American Dietetic Association, 77*, 140–148.

Mumford, E., Schlesinger, H. J., & Glass, G. V. (1982). The effects of psychological intervention on recovery from surgery and heart attacks: An analysis of the literature. *American Journal of Public Health, 72,* 141-151.

Nelson, D. J., Sennett, L., Lefebvre, R. C., Loiselle, L., McClements, L., & Carleton, R. A., (1987). A campaign strategy for weight loss at worksites. *Health Education Research: Theory and Practice, 2,* 27-31.

Reeves, R. S., Foreyt, J. P., Scott, L. W., Mitchell, R. E., Wohlleb, J., & Gotto, A. M. (1983). Effects of a low cholesterol eating plan on plasma lipids: Results of a three-year community study. *American Journal of Public Health, 78,* 873-877.

Richardson, J. L., Marks, G., Johnson, C. A., Graham, J. W., Chan, K. K., Selser, J. N., Kishbaugh, C., Barranday, Y., & Levin, A. M. (1987). Path model of multidimensional compliance with cancer therapy. *Health Psychology, 6,* 183-207.

Sackett, D. L., Haynes, R. B., & Tugwell, P. (1985). *Clinical epidemiology: A basic science for clinical medicine.* Boston: Little, Brown.

Schlundt, D. G. (1987). Compliance wth dietary changes. In M. D. Blaufox & H. G. Langford (Eds.), *Non-pharmacologic therapy of hypertension* (pp. 22-28). Basel, Switzerland: Karger.

Schneider, N. G., Jarvik, M. E., Forsythe, A. B., & Read, L. L. (1983). Nicotine gum in smoking cessation: A placebo-controlled, double-blind trial. *Addictive Behavior, 8,* 253-262.

Sikorski, J. M. (1985). Knowledge, concerns, and questions of wives of convalescent coronary artery bypass graft surgery patients. *Journal of Cardiac Rehabilitation, 5,* 74-85.

Simes, R. J., Tattersall, M. H. N., Coates, A. S., Raghaven, D., Solomon, H. J., & Smart, H. (1986). Randomized comparison of procedures for obtaining informed consent in clinical trials of treatment for cancer. *British Medical Journal, 293,* 1065-1068.

Smith, D. M., Weinberger, M., & Katz, B. P. (1987). A controlled trial to increase office visits and reduce hospitalizations of diabetic patients. *Journal of General Internal Medicine, 2,* 231-237.

Taylor, C. B., Bandura, A., Ewart, C. K., Miller, N. H., & DeBusk, R. F. (1985). Exercise testing to enhance wives' confidence in their husbands' cardiac capability soon after clinically uncomplicated acute myocardial infarction. *American Journal of Cardiology, 55,* 635-638.

Witschi, J. C., Singer, M., Wu-Lee, M., & Stare, F. J. (1978). Family cooperation and effectiveness in a cholesterol-lowering diet. *Journal of the American Dietetic Association, 72,* 384-389.

Woodhill, J. M., Palmer, A. J., Leelarthaepin, B., McGilchrist, C., & Blacket, R. B. (1978). Low fat, low cholesterol diet in secondary prevention of coronary heart disease. *Advances. Exp. Medical Biology, 109,* 317-330.

World Health Organization European Collaborative Group. (1986). European collaborative trial of multifactorial prevention of coronary heart disease: Final report on the 6-year results. *Lancet, I,* 869-872.

Zifferblatt, S. M. (1975). Increasing patient compliance through the applied analysis of behavior. *Preventive Medicine, 4,* 173-182.

21

Dropouts from a Clinical Trial, Their Recovery and Characterization: A Basis for Dropout Management and Prevention

Jeffrey L. Probstfield, Michael L. Russell,
William Insull, Jr., Salim Yusuf

> The remarkable increases in sample size because of dropouts and dropins strongly argue for major efforts to keep noncompliance to a minimum during trials.
>
> —Friedman, Furberg & Demets

Sackett and Snow (1979) have documented that adherence to the study protocol is a major problem in a wide variety of clinical trials. This is illustrated in a summary table adapted from their work (Table 21.1). Table 21.2 provides examples of adherence rates and attendance problems in some recent cardiovascular (CV) clinical trials of hypertension and myocardial infarction (*Cardiac Arrhythmia*

TABLE 21.1 Adherence Rates in Clinical Trials (Adapted from Sackett & Snow)

Activity	Type of trial	% Adherence*	Range (%)
Appointment keeping			
	Prevention (8)	39	10–65
	Management or cure (7)	78	55–84
Short-term medication (taking some study drug)			
	Prevention (2)	62	60–64
	Treatment (2)	78	77–78
Long-term medication (taking some study drug)			
	Prevention (4)	63	33–94
	Treatment (8)	59	41–69

*Weighted averages.

Pilot Study, unpublished data; *Five-year Findings of the Hypertension Detection and Follow-up Program*, 1979; Hulley et al., 1985; *A Randomized, Controlled Trial of Aspirin in Persons Recovered from Myocardial Infarction*, 1980; *A Randomized Trial of Propranolol in Patients with Acute Myocardial Infarction*, 1982).

A dropout is the extreme of poor adherence in a clinical trial and has been defined as a study participant who is unwilling or unable to return to the study clinic for regular follow-up visits (Meinert, 1986). Dropouts have been tradition-

TABLE 21.2 Examples of Adherence Rates in Cardiovascular Clinical Trials

	Withdrawn (%)	Adherence in remainder (%)	Average duration of follow-up (mos.)
Hypertension trials			
Pilot SHEP	17.0	89 (≥ 80%)[†]	12
HDFP	9.5	79 Rx Gp.	24
Post-MI trials			
AMIS	6.4	89	36
BHAT	15.0	NA*	36
CAPS	9.0	77 (> 80%)	12

† = the average of 3 methods of determination; * = no pill counts done.
AMIS = aspirin in myocardial infarction study; BHAT = beta-blocker heart attack trial; CAPS = cardiac arrhythmia pilot study.

ally considered an unavoidable and irremediable part of a clinical trial (Laskey, 1962; Sackett & Snow, 1979). Regardless, statements assuring the participant of the ability to withdraw at any time during the study are required in many consent forms and are made by the well-meaning investigator at the outset. However, all staff with more than a rudimentary knowledge of clinical trials methodology understand that dropouts must be kept to a minimum.

In several recent clinical trials major efforts have been devoted to improving adherence to medication or other forms of trial interventions. The most important reason for this concerted effort has been the realization that poor adherence has profound effects on the sensitivity of the study to demonstrate treatment effects. Poor adherence affects power to an extent that is related to the square of the proportion of participants complying with their original treatment assignment (Lachin, 1981). Those who are at the extremes of adherence have the most profound effect on the overall adherence in a study because they represent the two largest groups of participants. The plot of the distribution of adherence values by quartiles (Grodis, Markowtiz, & Lilienfeld, 1969) or deciles (Allport, 1934) clearly shows that outside the large number of participants who have excellent adherence, the next most prevalent group is that with no medication-taking, the dropouts and zero adherers (U- or J-shaped distribution). The optimal use of the "intention to treat" analysis and the potential for a worst-case analysis because of those not identifiable at trial closure make it imperative that all randomized participants be included in the potential for a worst-case analysis because of those not identifiable at trial closure make it imperative that all randomized participants be included in the primary analysis of trial results, including the dropouts (Freidman, Furberg, & Demets, 1985). This precept has not always been followed (*Dropouts from Clinical Trials*, 1987).

This chapter describes that group of poor adherers from clinical trials, the zero adherers and dropouts, and focuses primarily on the dropouts. Some aspects of five issues related to dropout participants will be described: who this group is, why they drop out, when they are likely to drop out, and how to manage them. Specific features and the results of a successful recovery program and long-term follow-up of recovered dropouts will be described. Based upon the experience of the authors with the first four issues, an outline for a preventive program is suggested.

A special group not dealt with in this chapter are those participants assigned to placebo who fail to adhere to their assigned study intervention and are knowingly prescribed the active intervention of the study. These participants are defined as dropins. Such participants are included in the zero adherers or dropouts when estimating adherence, but because they are taking the active drug this leds to an additional decrease in study power (Wu, Fisher, & Demets, 1980).

DROPOUTS IN CLINICAL TRIALS
Who Are They?

Little has been written about dropouts from clinical trials. Further, few descriptions have been made of their characteristics. Before 1978 there was no written description of whether or not dropouts are different from others who participate in a clinical trial. The following attempt to characterize dropouts was done in 1978 in the Lipid Research Clinic Coronary Primary Prevention Trial (LRC–CPPT). The design and results of the CPPT have been recorded in detail elsewhere (The Lipid Research Clinics program, 1979; 1983a, 1983b, 1984). Briefly, there were 12 North American clinics within this program involving a common protocol. The major hypothesis being tested in the CPPT was: Does plasma cholesterol lowering in primary hypercholesterolemic men who are clinically free of coronary heart disease and otherwise healthy lead to a reduction in definite myocardial infarction (both fatal and nonfatal) over a 7-year period of follow-up? Prerandomization visits (5) eliminated those who had secondary hypercholesterolemia and those who were relatively dietary sensitive. The trial consisted of 3,806 male volunteers between the ages of 35 and 59 who were continued on a moderate cholesterol-lowering diet throughout the trial. They were also randomly assigned in a double-blind fashion to one of two equal groups taking either cholestyramine, a bile acid sequestering agent, or its placebo, a biologically inert silica mixture, 24g daily in divided doses. The scheduled clinic visits were every 2 months with sufficient medication dispensed for the intervening period only.

The participants in the LRC–CPPT were men only, and therefore no information on potential gender effects could be collected. However, the information on age at entry, marital status, level of education, and type of employment were available for the entire LRC–CPPT, the Baylor-Methodist Clinic (B-MC) cohort, and the groups of nondropouts and dropouts at the B-MC (Table 21.3).

While the data in Table 21.3 show little difference in the demographic features of those who were in the dropout group as opposed to others who have adherence problems (described further below), additional analyses demonstrate a lower level of social support among dropouts (Dunbar, 1989). Cramer, Collins, and Mattson (1988) demonstrated the following reasons to be more frequently associated with those in seizure disorder trials who dropped out as opposed to others with adherence problems: alcohol or drug abuse, other neurological problems, and psychiatric disorders. The reasons for dropping out were not detected in about 10% of cases.

Differential mortality and morbidity within the randomized groups may theoretically lead to bias in analysis and either a Type 1 (concluding a treatment works when it actually doesn't) or Type 2 error (concluding a treatment doesn't work when it actually does). Examples with a possibility of the latter are from the

TABLE 21.3 Demography of Entire, Nondropout, and Dropout Cohorts at the Baylor-Methodist Clinic (B-MC) CPPT vs that of All Clinics, CPPT

	Entire B-MC cohort	Nondropout B-MC cohort	Dropout B-MC cohort	All clinics, CPPT
Age (years)	46.1	46.4	43.7	47.7
Marital status (% married)	92	92	90	92
Education (% college graduates)	58	59	47	37
Job classification (% white-collar)	83	84	77	76

Nottingham Studies of beta-blockade in those who had suspected myocardial infarction (Wilcox, Roland, Banks, Hampton & Mitchell, 1980; Wilcox et al., 1980). In both studies the early withdrawal rate among patients assigned to an active therapy was high, and a documented higher mortality rate occurred among the withdrawals. One study showed no significant benefit of treatment over placebo; the other was terminated prematurely because of early withdrawal in an active treatment group. Analysis of trial results by response to medication taken can lead to erroneous conclusions and misinformation related to a Type 1 error if great care is not exercised (The Coronary Drug Project Research Group, 1980). While potential for bias in analysis is the overriding problem in the two studies by Wilcox and coworkers, the unresolved problem remains of whether or not the group that withdrew early and had a differential morbidity or mortality had other differences as well.

Why Do Participants Drop Out of Clinical Trials?

In an attempt to discern why dropouts occur and what specific reasons the participants have for dropping out of a clinical trial, the 36 men who were dropouts on October 15, 1978 and who had been absent from the B-MC for varying lengths of time from 10 months to over 4 years were questioned about their reasons for dropping out at the initial telephone contact or at their initial clinical visit during the recovery program (described below) (Table 21.4).

Whether or not dropouts have special adherence problems was not known. In an attempt to determine whether or not the problems related to reduced adherence for those who do and those who do not drop out are similar, we identified a group of participants in the same trial, the LRC–CPPT, who had adherence problems but did not drop out and compared their reasons for reduced adherence with the reasons of those who had dropped out (Table 21.4). The following methodology was used:

In the spring of 1980 a cross-sectional chart review analysis revealed that within the B-MC cohort 202 of the 305 participants had adherence problems at some time during the trial but did not drop out (the 36 dropouts described above not included in the 202). They fulfilled the arbitrary definition of adherence problems by a 10% drop in medication adherence between two visits or a 10-day delay outside the "window" for a scheduled clinic visit at some point during the first 3½ years of the trial. Table 21.4 shows the distributions of reasons given by the dropouts and those given by others with adherence problems. While this is a relatively crude analysis, with the reasons for nonadherence obtained by strikingly disparate methods, the general distribution of reasons for nonadherence is similar in those with adherence problems and among the dropouts and is consistent with previously published data (Cramer, Collins, & Mattson, 1988; Haynes, 1979).

Recently, Cramer and colleagues reported a retrospective analysis of 622 participants in an antiepileptic drug study. Using previously established definitions for case quality (Cramer & Mattson, 1980) and entry criteria (Mattson, Cramer, & Collins, 1985), some differences in the characteristics of participants who dropped out were detected. Dropouts were usually younger, had a longer history of seizures, younger age of onset, were more frequently unemployed with less evidence of social support, and more frequently abused alcohol.

Further descriptive analyses of the large category of psychosocial reasons given for nonadherence to protocol among the dropouts and others with adherence problems in the CPPT suggested that relocation of residence, fear of drug toxicity (without symptoms or signs), concern about placebo, objections to protocol, and dissatisfaction with staff were reasons more commonly stated by dropouts. The overriding reasons among those with adherence problems were reduced motivation and, to a much lesser extent, domestic difficulties (Table 21.5). Lack of motivation for some is due to the occurrence of boredom and/or questioning the

TABLE 21.4 Distribution (%) of Reasons for Adherence Problems Encountered within the Group of Dropouts and Others with Adherence Problems in an RCT

Type of reason	Dropouts	Others
N	(36)	(202)
Adverse drug effects	19	22
Somatic problems	11	20
Psychosocial problems	69	58

TABLE 21.5 Distribution (%) of Psychosocial Problems: Comparison of Dropouts and Others with Adherence Problems in the Baylor-Methodist Clinic

Category of Reason	Dropouts (25)	Other (117)
Work-related	24	26
Relocation	24	0
Fear of drug toxicity	12	5
Concern about receiving placebo	8	1
Objections to protocol	8	0
Lack of motivation (vacation)	8	50* (5)
Dissatisfaction with staff	8	0
Domestic	4	11
Alcoholism	4	3
Anxiety	0	4
	100	100

*Includes vacation category.

importance of the investigation during the trial's follow-up or intervention maintenance phase.

In clinical trials that last several years a phenomenon occurs that we will call "study fatigue." Participants who experience this are usually very conscientious and have been excellent adherers to the protocol. They return to the clinic with a drastic and sudden decrease in adherence performance. Frequently the participant is unaware of the change. This situation must be met with much reassurance to the participant that occurrences of this nature are not uncommon and that good performance in the study almost always (over 90% of cases) returns. Continued participation in the clinic visits, especially the data collection portion of these visits, is to be encouraged and reinforced. Most of these participants will stay with the trial but experience the adherence problems as defined above. "Study fatigue," however, is a difficult situation to manage and may be associated with some who drop out if it is not handled judiciously (Probstfield & Russell, unpublished data 1983.)

When Do Dropouts Occur in the Course of a Clinical Trial?

With surprising consistency, a very large percentage, and in many cases the majority, of dropouts in a clinical trial occurs early, even within the period between randomization and the first scheduled postrandomization visit to the clinic. A review of five National Heart, Lung, and Blood Institute-funded trials and a trial in the United Kingdom reveals that between 16 and 60% of all participants who dropped out during the course of these trials either failed to return to or stopped medication consumption by the first follow-up visit (Table 21.6). Analyses of these and other data suggest that this can be determined as early as the first month of follow-up. As described more fully in another chapter, adherence performance with study medication during the first month in the LRC–CPPT was the most predictive variable in the description of a participant's medication-taking behavior for the remainder of the trial (Dunbar, 1989).

The Management of Dropouts from a Clinical Trial: The Recovery of Dropouts, A Specific Approach

A specific program for the recovery of dropouts to a clinical trial had not been published prior to 1986. Part of the description that follows has been published elsewhere (Probstfield, Russell, Henske, Reardon, & Insull, 1986). This chapter expands on the previous description and adds other points not previously reported.

Even if all the precautions during screening and recruitment are carefully observed and the staff members are sensitive and skillful in follow-up procedures, dropouts from clinical trials will still occur. The following are the key points of the recovery program, including generic aspects of negotiation with participants who are attempting to drop out of a clinical trial.

TABLE 21.6 Dropouts (%) at First and Last Visit Postrandomization in Long-Term Studies

Study	% dropouts	Time of Visits
BHAT	3.5, 15	1 mo., 36 mo.
AMIS	3, 6	1 mo., 36 mo.
U.K. Physicians	18, 30	6 mo., 72 mo.
CAPS	4, 9	3 mo., 12 mo.
LRC CPPT	1, 1.8, 6.1	2 wks, 4 wks, 7.4 yrs.
B-MC*	2, 4, 0.6	2 wks, 4 wks, 7.4 yrs.

*The 36 dropouts at the beginning of the recovery program.
wks = weeks
mo = months
yrs = years
AMIS = aspirin myocardial infarction study; BHAT = beta-blocker heart attack trial; CAPS = cardiac arrhythmia pilot study; LRC-CPPT = lipid research clinic's coronary primary prevention trial; UK Physicians = United Kingdom physicians trial of prophylactic aspirin for cardiovascular disease mortality.

Background

The specific dropout recovery program described here was conducted in the Baylor-Methodist Clinic cohort of the CPPT. The participants at that clinic consisted of 305 employed male volunteers from a pool of approximately 30,000 screenees. The most common reason (over 90%) for exclusion, as at other clinics, was a plasma LDL cholesterol level below protocol criteria at one of the prerandomization visits. No formal psychological tests were used as exclusion criteria in the trial, but those with evident psychosocial instability or evidence of substance abuse were excluded.

While dropouts were present at all clinics throughout the CPPT, the recovery program as described here was employed in its entirety originally at the B-MC. There were several reasons for this. First, the B-MC at the inception of the recovery program had more dropouts than any other clinic in the CPPT. Second, there had been no systematic approach previously to dropouts at the B-MC. A review of clinic information suggested that no unusual circumstances existed at the B-MC that would produce more dropouts there than at the other LRC clinics. Third, the B-MC had just initiated what was at the time a unique "fail-safe" computer-based surveillance system (described further below) that would allow careful tracking of activities in the recovery program.

Although dropouts have been considered to be unrecoverable, only limited previous reports have been published of attempts at doing so (Caldwell, Cobb, Dowling, & De Jongh, 1979; Gillum & Barsky, 1974). There had been some information published on prerandomization characteristics that would potentially identify who might drop out (Caldwell et al., 1970; Gordis et al., 1969; Lipman, Rickels, & Uhlenhuth, 1965). Further, there was a report in 1982 with only descriptive information identifying staff attitudes toward complaints, willingness to reduce participant medication requirements, and vigorous pursuit of those who fail to keep clinic appointments as key elements in reducing dropouts (Goldman, et al., 1982).

Despite these reports, which appeared both prior to and during the conduct of the dropout recovery program at the Baylor-Methodist Clinic, the issues that appeared critical remained largely untested. The questions that this specific dropout recovery program sought to address were as follows: (1) Can dropouts from a randomized controlled trial (RCT) be recovered? (2) If so, what method(s) is/are effective? (3) Once dropouts are recovered, can the trial protocol, including the study medication, be reinstituted and maintained by these participants?

Recovery Program: Design and Methods

The dropout recovery program was designed because of the need for intensive staff effort to have its maximal impact over a 6-month period and consisted of three key elements: (1) a computer-based surveillance system for monitoring all aspects of a participant's adherence in the trial, e.g., visit attendance, dietary and medication adherence; (2) six basic principles for counseling and corresponding goals specifically devised for the approach to dropout participants in an attempt to enhance protocol adherence; and (3) a 13-step operational sequence of activities and procedures for the reinstitution of the protocol during dropout recovery.

Principles and Goals for Participant Counseling

The six principles and corresponding goals used in the participant counseling procedures are summarized in Table 21.7. Since no successful methodology had been previously tested or published, these served as the foundation for the recovery program. Subsequently, anything new that was implemented for an individual dropout participant that represented a deviation from past procedures in the dropout recovery program was matched against this set of principles and goals for consistency. Since the trial director, a physician, saw most of the participants at each visit and conducted the majority of the retrieval program, these deviations from previous procedures were relatively easy to track. A diary of telephone conversations and all clinic visit activities was kept for each dropout so that review and continued planning for each individual's retrieval

TABLE 21.7 Principles and Goals for Participant Counseling of the Baylor-Methodist Coronary Primary Prevention Trial Dropout Recovery Program

Principles for counseling	Corresponding goals
1. To establish contact with participants.	1. To maintain contact with participants.
2. To undercut participant's resistance for reinstitution of some aspect of the trial protocol.	2. To complete as much of the trial protocol as possible.
3. To convey a caring attitude to the participant about his overall health status and the importance of health care to these participants.	3. To resolve any somatic, adverse drug effects, or behavioral problems preventing protocol adherence.
4. To maximize the participant's opportunities for success of protocol completion using standardized behavioral techniques.	4. To reinstate the protocol in small increments using informal contracts and shaping.
5. To give positive reinforcement for fulfillment of protocol activities.	5. To emphasize the positive contribution at any level of protocol adherence.
6. To resume study drug was given a low but definite priority for the participant.	6. To restore and maintain study power.

program was possible. Further, the individual retrieval programs were constructed with the addition of items consistent with the consecutive order as outlined in Table 21.7.

The first three principles from Table 21.7 were all used while scheduling for and during the initial contact with the dropout. Participant contact was imperative; virtually any rational approach that would allow for contact to occur and be maintained was used. Some dropout participants preferred a home or business face-to-face discussion about the study and perceived problems preventing protocol adherence rather than any substantive discussion of these issues by telephone or at the clinical trial center. If a face-to-face contact was not possible, then a minimum of regular telephone contact was expected with very specific guidelines on time and subjects to be discussed during each telephone contact. Before this minimum of contact was accepted, however, one face-to-face contact was requested to review issues of concern with the stated expectation that the issues might be resolved. Continued efforts to establish this face-to-face contact were attempted until a specific request for minimum contact was requested or face-to-face contact occurred.

Strict adherence was expected by trial staff to the guidelines for the regular phone calls allowed for maintenance of contact until the participant felt sufficiently comfortable to make the commitment for a face-to-face contact. Two dropouts allowed only phone contact after the initial phase of the recovery program and during the remainder of the follow-up phase of the trial. This form of communication was maintained until the end of the study. In one instance this made possible the attendance of the dropout participant for a closeout interview at his doctor's office and collection of an EKG and other crucial historical and physical information that would not have been otherwise available.

In the initial negotiations with all dropout participants, major emphasis was placed on the general health status and medical follow-up of the individual for his benefit as well as the value to study. Informal contracts were powerful tools used to gain the increasing acceptance and confidence of the dropout participants and also to secure increasing levels of participation. At every step the participant was urged to act in a collaborative fashion with the trial staff to set new goals or suggest how to maintain levels of performance (Haynes et al., 1976). Any contribution toward the fulfillment of the protocol was positively reinforced by trial staff (Cialdini & Schroeder, 1976). The participant's active agreement and cooperation in planning was necessary for the institution of any new protocol elements or any increase in study medication dosage.

Surveillance System for Adherence to the Protocol

The availability and implementation of a "fail-safe" tracking system for adherence to all study visit requirements and interventions appears crucial for fulfillment of a trial protocol in any clinical center (Sackett, 1979) that has more than 100 trial participants, and perhaps in those with even less. Appointment keeping and records of attendance to clinic visits become a major effort, with ample opportunity for unintentional omissions. An integral part of the surveillance system requires that a series of reports be generated locally and automatically at regular intervals so that the current status of adherence to various aspects of the protocol are kept squarely in front of clinical center staff.

The system developed for this program required that a master file of participant demographic data be established. Further, an input file was necessary that had all records for each visit made by the participant to the clinic. After each visit the data in the input file were made current so that the date of the visit just completed, the date of the next visit, the study intervention adherence percentage, and any other pertinent data specific to the trial could be entered.

At the B-MC a current visit adherence form was filled out at every visit on each individual and checked with all other study forms for correctness at the end of that clinic day. These forms were then entered into the input file by keypunch operators. Editing facilities were easily available for clinic staff. The semimonthly reports automatically generated were used as working documents in the clinic as part of the routine activities, and in particular were reviewed regularly by key clinic staff as part of the ongoing program for remediation of adherence problems (Table 21.8). The reports focused on these categories of participants in the trial: dropouts, zero adherers, and delinquent participants.

The three types of participants mentioned above were identified as problem participants. Two of these had been specifically defined by the CPPT:

Dropout—any participant who had failed to make a visit to the clinic within 6 months of his last visit.

Zero Adherer—any participant who had not been taking the study medication or any participant who had failed to visit the clinic withhin the last 3 months.

These two definitions represent different degrees of adherence on the same continuum. For our purposes at the B-MC we saw it as useful to identify another set of individuals on the same continuum, the delinquent participants.

TABLE 21.8 Format of Computer Printout for Delinquent Participants, Zero Adherers, and Dropouts

Name	Last visit no.	Last date in clinic	Latest date in next clinic visit window	Last visit adherence

Delinquent participant—any participant who had failed to make a regular clinic visit within 70 days of his last visit.

The identification of this third category of participants allowed for planning an organized counseling approach and an early intensified effort where necessary for those with other than satisfactory reasons for delinquency before the 90-day criterion had been achieved and a potentially more serious state of nonadherence reached.

While this computer-based surveillance system was essential to the recovery program, it would have been insufficient by itself to correct the dropout problem described below. Although one could potentially use a card-sort system for this surveillance type of recordkeeping, the ease of use and accessibility of computer facilities at most institutions would appear to obviate that approach.

The Sequence of Operational Activities and Procedures

While the study protocol was being reinstituted for a dropout participant, a standardized stepwise sequence was used. Generically this meant dividing the protocol into a series of small progressive steps that could, if necessary, be implemented singly or a few at a time (the counseling technique of successive approximation; Freedman & Fraser, 1966). This allowed the wary participant to progress at his own comfortable pace.

In every protocol there will be points of resistance to increased participation. In this protocol, divided into 13 specific operational activities and procedures (Table 21.9), the two points of resistance were identified by tabulated experience as the first face-to-face visit of any sort (clinic, home, or office) and adequate resolution of the adherence problems (adverse effects, somatic, psychosocial).

In the CPPT the study medication was seen as at least inconvenient and was thought by some to be aversive. Despite this, the reinstitution of the study medication (operational activity 11) was not difficult in most cases if the adherence problems were first resolved (operational activity 10). Staff members were urged to avoid reinstitution of medication even in those dropouts who asked for it unless substantial resolution of the abovementioned adherence problems was evident. The sequence of 13 operational activities and procedures is described in detail elsewhere, and the reader is referred to that source for more information (Probstfield et al., 1986).

Zero adherers at the BM-C were virtually always at step 10 of the Sequence of Operational Activities and Procedures. Attempts were made to deal with their adherence problems before medication was reinstituted. For this reason the category of zero adherers had the greatest influx and efflux during the trial of any of the adherence categories by deciles. The same principles and goals for adherence counseling used for dropouts was used for zero adherers or any other

TABLE 21.9 Sequence of Operations and Achievement Levels of 36 Dropouts in the Dropout Recovery Program at 55 Months

Sequence of operational activities and procedures	Participants[†] per achievement level
1. Reassign dropout to physician	36
2. Establish and maintain contact	36
*3. Achieve clinic attendance	35
4. Obtain physical and lab data	35
5. Obtain medical information	35
6. Discuss general health problems	35
7. Facilitate solution of health care problems	35
8. Obtain diet information (Trial Protocol)	35
9. Obtain information about study medication taking	35
*10. Solve adherence problems	34
11. Reinstitute the study medication	24
12. Reinstitute constant care by adherence counselor	24
13. Continue problem solving and reinforce achievement	24

*Sequence items at which resistance is experienced.
†Includes one recovered dropout who died of trauma after 18 months and achieving item 13 in the recovery program.
Reprinted with permission. From J. L. Probstfield et al. (1986). © *American Journal of Medicine*.

category of reduced adherence. Further, in the B-MC Recovery Program a diary record was kept on each zero adherer for additional ease in planning and recording progress.

Recovery Program Results

The dropout problem, its development, and its subsequent resolution at the B-MC are shown in Figure 21.1. Since dropouts and zero adherers have similar effects on study power, it was appropriate to track both. If the number of dropouts would decrease only to have the number of zero adherers increase either commensurately or even substantially, there would be little if any benefit for study power.

There were 36 dropouts at the beginning of the Recovery Program at the B-MC. The proportion of dropouts and zero adherers at the B-MC during the first 2 years after randomization was somewhat higher than but paralleled that seen in other CPPT clinics. During the third year, however, the number of participants in both categories increased dramatically. The substantive increase in the slope of both curves just prior to the inception of the recovery program was not

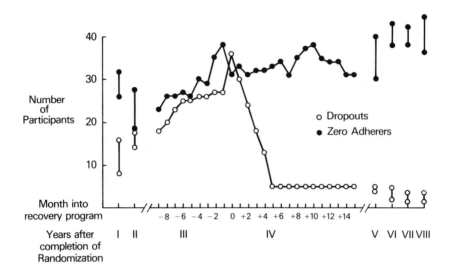

FIGURE 21.1   Development, successful recovery, and long-term status of dropout and zero adherer groups at a single clinic of a clinical trial.

Cumulative record of all dropouts and zero adherers at the Baylor-Methodist Clinic of the Coronary Primary Prevention Trial. It demonstrates the number of participants in each of the two groups. Ranges are indicated for years I, II, V, VI, VII, and VIII after completion of randomization. All points are plotted on a monthly basis for 9 months before and 15 months after institution of the recovery program. The graph represents the totals at the time intervals indicated. There was substantial movement into and out of the zero adherer group. (Reprinted with permission. From J. L. Probstfield et al., 1986, *American Journal of Medicine*).

indicative of true increases in either category at that point. It was only a manifestation of a more accurate assessment obtained by a computerized surveillance system. At the inception of the recovery program (Time 0) the B-MC had the largest number of dropouts in the CPPT.

Table 21.6 shows the percentage of the dropouts at the beginning of the Recovery Program at B-MC who had dropped out at the second week, fourth week, and 7.4-year points in the study. The highest percentage of dropouts at the B-MC during the study was 12%. Approximately one-third of these had done so within the first month of randomization.

The graph shows a precipitous drop in the number of dropouts during the recovery program, with relative stability in the number of zero adherers during the first 14 months after the inception of the recovery program. Many dropouts chose to reinstitute the intervention immediately. There is a relatively modest increase in the number of zero adherers in subsequent years until the termination of the trial. The number of dropouts remained low during the remainder of the trial. Only three new dropouts occurred during the remainder of the study, and one (3%) of the original group recurred. Of these four, three were recovered.

Data presented in Table 21.10 clearly demonstrate that the length of time a participant has been a dropout has little bearing on whether or not he can be recovered to active participation in the study. Further, only modest influence can be demonstrated in the data on whether or not those participants who have been dropouts for extended periods will reinstitute medication. Full participation can be expected of many who are recovered, but this number was particularly difficult to assess in the CPPT, where an aversive medication was the intervention used.

A Suggested Preventive Approach

Dropouts that might occur in a clinical trial may be substantially obviated by the following multifaceted preventive approach.

Sensitive Staff

A keen sense for those who demonstrate less than optimal motivation during screening and recruitment is very useful. Anecdotal and descriptive data (Cramer et al., 1988; Webster, Newnham, & Petrie, 1985) from clinical trials suggest that sensitive trial staff members can identify certain potential nonadherers and target them for special counseling efforts during the maintenance phase of the trial. Potential participants who have difficulty scheduling or keeping appointments

TABLE 21.10 Comparison of Duration of Dropout Status and Recovery from Dropouts Status at 55 Months

Dropout duration	Participants recovered	Participants taking medication	Mean % adherence
< 1 yr.	9	7	62
1 yr.	6	4	16
18 mos.	3*	3*	32*
2 yrs.	5	4	50
30 mos.	4	2	94
3 yrs.	4	2	28
> 4 yrs.	3	1	92
Total	34*	23*	35*

*Does not include one participant who died (traffic accident) after 18 months in the recovery program.

should be regarded with suspicion. Helpful clues may be frequent rescheduling to get through the screening visits and past performance in other behavioral modification programs (e.g., smoking cessation, weight loss, exercise initiation). Despite the undeniable pressures during recruitment to enroll as many as possible, a balanced review of each screenee's long-term adherence performance potential before randomization must occur. Perhaps one should expect that as many as 10 to 15% of those who are otherwise "number eligible" should not be randomized because of their uncertain or predictable poor adherence potential (Hunninghake, 1989).

Run-In and Test-Dosing Periods

If the first month's medication-taking performance in a clinical trial is such a powerful predictor and, further, if the data show that most dropouts occur early in a clinical trial, this information should be used in identifying and subsequently preventing those who will drop out. Some procedures have been developed and can be undertaken to minimize those who will drop out before randomization has taken place.

A run-in period or the "faint of heart test" has been used successfully to eliminate those screenees who have difficulty taking medication. These prerandomization procedures can be used to evaluate medication-taking behavior and can be done with either placebo or active medication. An excellent example of this procedure and its effect on adherence is the U.S. Physicians Trial (Hennekens, 1984). In this trial with a factorial design, a 6-month run-in period was conducted using one active drug (aspirin) and one placebo (beta-carotene). Initially 33,223 physicians volunteered for the program. Only 22,071 met the adherence criteria (consumption of two-thirds of the amount of each medication prescribed for the run-in period). The adherence to prescribed regimens in the subsequent randomized portion of the study was 87.6% consuming at least one medication and 83.0% consuming both medications at an average of 57 months of follow-up (The Steering Committee of the Physicians' Health Study Research Group, 1988).

Protocols frequently allow one repeat attempt of the adherence test if, in the judgment of the clinician, there are extenuating circumstances for failure of performance on the first attempt. A performance level of 75 to 80% medication consumed of the prescribed therapeutic dose is a minimal expectation. This is an arbitrary definition of good adherence used by many trials, although an average adherence of 80% has a profound impact on study power. The run-in procedure is meant to exclude those who are potentially the worst adherers from the randomized portion of the study. While this type of exclusion criteria has raised for some the problem of generalizability of trial results, there is already clear evidence that those who are randomized in clinical trials are different from the population at large (Remington, Taylor, & Buskirk, 1978), and the number eliminated by this procedure is usually small, about 5 to 10%. The amount of staff time saved during the follow-up phase of a trial, however is large. It is crudely estimated from the B-MC CPPT experience that to maintain a low dropout rate without the kind of prerandomization procedures described required an additional full-time staff member in the clinic for a cohort of about 300.

Certain medications are intrinsically more difficult to consume, have a high frequency of adverse effects, or have profoundly adverse effects that will exclude certain individuals. For these special circumstances a "test-dosing" prerandomization period will allow the identification and exclusion of some of those individuals who will not be able to participate before enrollment in the trial and helps to minimize the loss of study power.

A good example of this situation is the one presented by the general class of agents Angiotensin Converting Enzyme Inhibitors, ACE-I. Congestive heart failure patients are sick individuals and usually have a limited prognosis, somewhat dependent upon the severity of their illness (Furberg & Yusuf, 1985). In planning for the Studies of Left Ventricular Dysfunction the ACE-I enalapril was chosen as the active agent. The hypothesis to be tested is: In those with left ventricular dysfunction, would lives be prolonged by producing the physiological phenomenon of peripheral vasodilation (The Studies of Left Ventricular Dysfunction Protocol, 1985)? Enalapril is known to produce severe adverse effects in 3 to 5% of those who take it. Common reactions include severe hypotension, worsening renal failure, neutropenia, and angioedema. While clinical characteristics appear to predict patients at high risk for severe hypotension or worsening renal function (Edwards & Padfield, 1985; Packer, Medina, & Yushak, 1984), there is nothing currently known that will predict accurately who will develop angioedema. The use of small doses of enalapril initially further reduces the number of those who have a severe initial response to the drug (Cleland et al., 1985; Webster et al., 1985). Nonetheless, there remain those who are not able to take enalapril.

The use of a small dose of the active agent for 2 to 7 days prior to enrollment has allowed for the identification of about 3% of the screenees to be excluded who ordinarily would have been randomized but not able to fully participate in the trial and therefore would reduce study power (Table 21.11; Davis, 1990). It is therefore suggested that during any trial protocol development careful consideration for both a test-dosing and a run-in period be given in the light of the interventions to be used.

Signs and Symptoms of Potential Non-Adherence: "Red Flags"

Roth and Caron (1958, 1978) pointed out graphically in a series of studies that physicians, regardless of experience or level of training, are no better than

TABLE 21.11 2-Day Test Dose Experience in Congestive Heart Failure Trials with ACE Inhibitors

Study and Agent	% Withdrawn
CMRG (Captopril)[a]	3%
International Enalapril[b]	3%
Dig/Captopril/placebo[c]	3%

[a]Captopril Multicenter Research Group, 1983.
[b]Long-Term Effects of Enalapril in Patients with Congestive Heart Failure, 1987.
[c]Comparison Effects of Captopril and Digoxin in Patients with Mild to Moderate Heart Failure, 1988.

chance at predicting adherence during studies. However, we have learned to spot some aspects of behavior that are clues that adherence performance in the trial has either already been altered or may be altered soon. These so-called signs and symptoms of potential nonadherence or "red flags" of poor adherence are listed in Table 21.12 and have been compiled by two of us (MLR and JLP) based on our personal experiences with several hundred patients. The entities listed require only a knowledge of the relationship between the phenomenon and the possibility of subsequent poor adherence. Further, they represent everyday activ-

TABLE 21.12 Signs and Symptoms of Potential Nonadherence: "Red Flags"

 1. Missed visits
 2. Difficulty in reaching by phone or failure to return calls
 3. Rescheduling twice for an appointment (change in behavior)
 4. Complaints about office visits
 5. Impatience during clinic visit
 6. Length of time (mandatory) at each visit
 7. "Distance" during interview
 8. Length of time since participation in study was discussed between physician and participant
 9. Humor dealing with negative aspects of the trial or study medication
10. Sarcasm about trial or study medication
11. Any expression by participant that he/she may discontinue study medication
12. Unusual or unexplained change in adherence to study medication
13. Unconcern by participant about adherence rate
14. Reassignment to new primary care manager
15. Reassignment to other new clinic personnel
16. Any illness with increased attention to "trial-related disease"
17. Hospitalization for any reason
18. Any major change in life-style that is imminent (before the next visit)

ities that can be observed by any sensitive staff member with no special behavioral science or psychosocial training. These phenomena of human behavior are frequently exhibited before deterioration of adherence occurs by participants to support staff, rather than to the professional staff, because it is less threatening to do so. Therefore, all clinic staff must be aware of the "red flags" of problem adherence.

One of these signs or symptoms may occur in isolation for a given participant with little subsequent change in adherence performance noted. More important is the appearance of several of these for a single individual who has been performing well in the trial. Most important of all is any profound change; for example, the participant who always reschedules promptly when not able to keep an appointment suddenly does not reschedule. Even with the first failure to reschedule a clinic visit, sensitivity for a change in that participant's performance should be alerted in that participant's primary caretaker or any other person on the trial staff.

Negotiated Adherence Regimens

With the precautions from the first three points of the preventive program fully implemented, the treatment regimen will remain difficult for some. Frustration with their individual performances, a feeling of embarrassment about failure to fulfill real and imagined expectations, and diversion of interest and energies to other life activities will cause some trial participants to wish for and seek discontinuance of trial participation.

The six principles and corresponding goals for participant counseling (Table 21.7) are easily adapted for use in dealing with the participant who has adherence problems but has not as yet dropped out. Depending on the circumstances, any of the last five principles may be crucial to the prevention of a dropout. Perhaps numbers 3 through 5 are especially important. Everyone wants someone to have his or her best interests in mind, everyone wants to do well at whatever they are doing, and everyone likes to be praised. The proactive step of devising a plan of modified protocol adherence, "a negotiated adherence regimen," will be received with gratitude. This is especially true of the participant who expresses concern either about continuing in the clinical trial or generally about "getting everything done" during an upcoming period of intense activity or emotional distress. Modification of the adherence expectations on a temporary basis by identifying the crucial elements (e.g., Table 21.9) will allow for the development of an informal contract between participant and trial staff. This has a high probability of fulfillment and virtually assures that participant's continued participation in the clinical trial. While cessation of any trial activity is not recommended unless specifically asked for by the participant, demonstrating sensitivity to the participant's potential problems may be enough. More importantly, it may allow the reluctant participant to discuss further concerns that he or she would not have felt comfortable discussing if the opportunity had not been offered.

A "Fail-Safe" Surveillance System

Through all periods of clinical trial activity a record system should be maintained of participant performance on visit attendance and adherence to interventions. With the availability of microcomputers, such information is ideally computerized. This allows the staff to be highly aware of adherence performance and helps them to keep these issues in front of the participant, who has so many other demands he considers of higher priority. Although the format of Table 21.8 may be useful generically, the specific trial may require that modifications be made.

Validation for This Preventive Approach

There are two pieces of validation for this preventive system. The first is the low recidivism present in the recovery and follow-up of the LRC-CPPT dropout group reported. The second is from a study done for health promotion and disease prevention in the workplace carried out by one of the authors (MLR) (Bowne, Russell, Morgan, Optenberg, & Clarke, 1984). This study at the worksite had a minimal dropout rate throughout its conduct. No trial with all aspects of dropout prevention instituted has reported the number of dropouts in that trial.

SUMMARY AND CONCLUSIONS

Despite our best efforts at careful screening and enrollment, including the use of prerandomization procedures of the run-in and test-dosing periods, and in spite of special training and sensitivity frequently present in clinical trials staffs, dropouts to study protocol will occur. Calculations regarding the effect of this reduction in adherence demonstrate profound effects on study power if these should occur even at relatively low levels and remain unchanged. Dropouts from RCTs appear to be demographically similar to other participants. Most dropouts occur early in the postrandomization period, and most appear to be preventable. A specific rehabilitative approach to dropouts with over 95% effectiveness during 5 years of follow-up has been described. High adherence to the study protocol with low recidivism is possible. Substantial recovery of study power is the attainable goal. Collaborative and tactful negotiations requiring skill and fortitude are key elements in both the recovery and prevention of dropouts. The best approach to clinical trial dropouts is prevention. Specific recommendations with limited validation using modified portions of the recovery program and other techniques are suggested as a preventive approach.

REFERENCES

A randomized controlled trial of aspirin in persons recovered from myocardial infarction. (1980). *Journal of the American Medical Association, 243,* 661–669.

A randomized trial of propranolol in patients with acute myocardial infarction I. Mortality results. (1982). *Journal of the American Medical Association, 247,* 1707–1714.

Allport, R. H. (1934). The J-curve hypothesis of conforming. *Behavioral Journal of Social Psychology, 134,* 141–183.

Bowne, D. W., Russell, M. L., Morgan, J. L., Optenberg, S. A., & Clarke, A. E. (1984). Reduced disability and health care costs in an industrial fitness program. *Journal of Occupational Medicine, 11,* 807–816.

Caldwell, J. R., Cobb, S., Dowling, M. C., & De Jongh, D. (1970). The dropout problem in antihypertensive treatment. *Journal of Chronic Diseases, 22,* 579–592.

Captopril multicenter research group. A placebo controlled trial of captopril in refractory chronic congestive heart failure. (1983). *Journal of the American College of Cardiology, 2,* 755–763.

Cardiac Arrhythmia Pilot Study. Unpublished data, 1985.

Caron, H. S., & Roth, H. P. (1958). Patients' cooperation with a medical regimen. *Journal of the American Medical Association, 203,* 922–926.

Cialdini, R. B., & Schroeder, D. A. (1976). Increasing compliance by legitimizing paltry contributions: When even a penny helps. *Journal of Personality and Social Psychology, 34,* 599–604.

Cleland, J. G. F., Dargie, H. J., McAlpine, H., Ball, S. G., Morton, J. J., & Robertson, J. I. S., & Ford, I. (1985). Severe hypotension after first dose of enalapril in heart failure. *British Medical Journal, 291,* 1309–1312.

Comparison effects of captopril and digoxin in patients with mild to moderate heart failure, Captopril-Digoxin group. (1988). *Journal of the American Medical Association, 259,* 539–544.

Coronary Drug Project Research Group. (1980). Influences of adherence to treatment and response of cholesterol on mortality in the Coronary Drug Project. *New England Journal of Medicine, 303,* 1038–1041.

Cramer, J. A., Collins, J. F., & Mattson, R. H. (1988). Can categorization of patient background problems be used to determine early termination in a clinical trial. *Controlled Clinical Trials, 9,* 47–63.

Cramer, J. A., & Mattson, R. H. (1980). Central case validation. *Controlled Clinical Trials, 1,* 168.

Davis, C. E. (1990). *Prerandomization compliance screening in clinical trials.* In S. A. Shumaker, E. B. Schron, & J. K. Ockene (Eds.), *Handbook of health behavior change*. New York: Springer Publishing Co.

Dropouts from clinical trials. (1987). *Lancet*, 2, 892–893.

Dunbar, J. (1990). *Predictors of patient adherence*. In S. A. Shumaker, E. B. Schron, & J. K. Ockene (Eds.), *Handbook of health behavior change*. New York: Springer Publishing Co.

Edwards, C. R. W., & Padfield, P. L. (1985). Angiotension-converting enzyme inhibition: Past, present and bright future. *Lancet*, 1, 30–34.

Five-year findings of the hypertension detection and follow-up program. I. Reduction in mortality of persons with high blood pressure including mild hypertension. (1979). *Journal of the American Medical Association*, 242, 2562–2577.

Freedman, J. L., & Fraser, S. C. (1966). Compliance without pressure: The foot-in-the door technique. *Journal of Personality and Social Psychology*, 4, 295–302.

Friedman, L. M., Furberg, C. D., & DeMets, D. L. (1985). *Fundamentals of clinical trials* (2nd ed.). Littleton, MA: PSG Publishing, p. 95, pp. 246–249.

Furberg, C. D., & Yusuf, S. (1985). Effect of vasodilator on survival in chronic congestive heart failure. *American Journal of Cardiology*, 55, 1110–1113.

Gillum, R. F., & Barsky, A. J. (1974). Diagnosis and management of patient noncompliance. *Journal of the American Medical Association*, 228, 1563–1567.

Goldman, A. I., Holcomb, R., Perry, H. M., Jr., Schnaper, H. W., Fitz, A. E., & Frohlich, E. D. (1982). Can dropout and other noncompliance be minimized in a clinical trial. *Controlled Clinical Trials*, 3, 75–89.

Gordis, L., Markowitz, M., & Lilienfeld, A. M. (1969). Studies in the epidemiology and preventability of rheumatic fever IV. A quantitative determination of compliance in children on oral penicillin prophylaxis. *Pediatrics*, 43, 173–182.

Haynes, R. B. (1979). The disease and the mechanics of treatment. In R. B. Haynes, D. W. Taylor, & D. L. Sackett (Eds.), *Compliance in health care* (pp. 49–62). Baltimore: Johns Hopkins University Press.

Haynes, R. B., Sackett, D. L., Gibson, E. S., Taylor, D. W., Hackett, B. C., Roberts, R. S., & Johnson, A. L. (1976). Improvement of medication compliance in uncontrolled hypertension. *Lancet*, 1, 1265–1268.

Hennekens, C. H. (1984). Issues in the design and conduct of clinical trials. *Journal of National Cancer Institute*, 73, 1473–1476.

Hulley, S. B., Furberg, C. D. Gurland, B., McDonald, R., Perry, H. M., Schnaper, H. W., Schoenberger, J. A., Smith, W. M., & Vogt, T. (1985). Systolic hypertension in the elderly program (SHEP). Antihypertensive efficacy of chlorthalidone. *American Journal of Cardiology*, 56, 913–920.

Hunninghake, D. B. (1990). *Recruitment in clinical trials. Impact on adherence*. In S. A. Shumaker, E. B. Schron, & J. K. Ockene (Eds.), *Handbook of health behavior change*. New York: Springer Publishing Co.

Lachin, J. M. (1981). Introduction to sample size determinations and power analysis for clinical trials. *Controlled Clinical Trials*, 1, 13–27.

Lasky, J. J. (1962). The problem of sample attrition in controlled treatment trials. *Journal of New Mental Disease*, 135, 32–337.

Lipid Research Clinics Coronary Primary Prevention Trial results: Participant recruitment to the Coronary Primary Prevention Trial. (1983b). *Journal of Chronic Diseases*, 5, 451–465.

Lipid Research Clinics Coronary Primary Prevention Trial results: I. Reduction in incidence of coronary heart disease. (1984). *Journal of the American Medical Association*, *251*, 351-364.

Lipid Research Clinics Program: Design and implementation. (1979). *Journal of Chronic Diseases*, *32*, 609-631.

Lipman, R. S., Rickels, K., Uhlenhuth, E. H., Park, L. C., & Fisher, S. (1965). Neurotics who fail to take their drugs. *British Journal of Psychiatry*, *3*, 1043-1049.

Long-term effects of enalapril in patients with congestive heart failure. A multicenter, placebo controlled trial. (1987). *Heart Failure*, *3*, 102-107.

Mattson, R. H., Cramer, J. A., Collins, J. F., and the VA Epilepsy Cooperative Study Group. (1985). Comparison of carbamazepine, phenobarbital, phenytoin and primidone in partial and secondary generalized tonic clonic seizures. *New England Journal of Medicine*, *313*, 145-151.

Mattson, R. H., Cramer, J. A., Smith, D. B., Delpado Escueta, A. V., & The VA Epilepsy Cooperative Study Group. (1983). A design for the prospective evaluation of the efficacy and toxicity of antiepileptic drugs. *Neurology*, *33*(Suppl. 1), 26-37.

Meinert, C. L. (1986). *Clinical trials, design conduct and analysis*. New York: Oxford University Press.

Packer, M., Medina, N., & Yushak, M. (1984). Relationship between serum sodium concentration and the hemodynamic and clinical responses to converting enzyme inhibition with captopril in severe heart failure. *Journal of the American College of Cardiology*, *3*, 1035-1043.

Pre-entry characteristics of participants in the Lipid Research Clinics (LRC) Coronary Primary Prevention Trial. (1983a). *Journal of Chronic Diseases*, *36*, 467-479.

Probstfield, J. L., & Russell, M. L. (1983). Unpublished data.

Probstfield, J. L., Russell, M. L., Henske, J. C., Reardon, R. J., & Insull, W., Jr. (1986). Successful program for recovery of dropouts to a clinical trial. *American Journal of Medicine*, *80*, 777-784.

Remington, R. D., Taylor, H. L., & Buskirk, E. R. (1978). A method for assessing volunteer bias and its application to a cardiovascular disease prevention program involving physical activity. *Journal of Epidemiology and Community Health*, *32*, 250-255.

Roth, H. P., & Caron, H. S. (1978). Accuracy of doctors' estimates and patients' statements on adherence to a drug regimen. *Clinical Pharmacology and Therapeutics*, *23*, 361-370.

Sackett, D. L. (1979). A compliance practicum for the busy practitioner. In R. B. Haynes, D. W. Taylor, & D. L. Sackett (Eds.), *Compliance in health care* (pp. 286-294). Baltimore: Johns Hopkins University Press.

Sackett, D. L., & Snow, J. C. (1979). The magnitude of compliance and noncompliance. In R. B. Haynes, D. W. Taylor, & D. L. Sackett (Eds.), *Compliance in health care* (pp. 11-22). Baltimore: Johns Hopkins University Press.

Steering Committee of the Physicians' Health Study Research Group. (1988). Preliminary report: Findings from the aspirin component of the ongoing physicians health study. *New England Journal of Medicine*, *318*, 262-264.

Studies of Left Ventricular Dysfunction Protocol. (1985).

Webster, J., Newnham, D. M., & Petrie, J. C. (1985). Initial dose of enalapril in hypertension. *British Medical Journal*, *290*, 1623-1624.

Wilcox, R. G., Hampton, J. R., Rowley, J. M., Mitchell, J. R. A., Roland, J. M., & Banks, D. C. (1980). Randomized placebo-controlled trial comparing oxyprenol with disopyramide phosphate in immediate treatment of suspected myocardial infarction. *Lancet, 2,* 765-769.

Wilcox, R. G., Roland, J. M., Banks, D. C., Hampton, J. R., & Mitchell, J. R. A. (1980). Randomized trial comparing propranolol with atenolol in immediate treatment of suspected myocardial infarction. *British Medical Journal, 1,* 885-888.

Wu, M., Fisher, M., & DeMets, D. (1980). Sample sizes for long term medical trials with time dependent dropout and event rates. *Controlled Clinical Trials, 1,* 109-121.

Commentary: Adherence Issues in Clinical Trials

Graham W. Ward

It is clear, from the range and depth of the well-considered presentations in this section, that clinical trials represent a very special form of health care. In many respects, such trials are far more difficult and demanding to operate than is the provision of routine clinical care or preventive services in the community. In a few respects, clinical trials are easier. Because this volume has examined such a broad range of issues and settings, I believe that some perspective is needed.

The needs and issues in clinical trials, patient care, and community-based prevention measures are not wholly interchangeable. Nor is a solution or a useful insight in one of these arenas necessarily applicable to another. One way to understand the issues better is to contrast some of the behavioral issues in both clinical trials and clinical practice.

The major consideration driving most decisions regarding clinical trials is the believability of the results. Above all, what we, society, look for in a clinical trial is proof. A clinical trial is virtually a trial of a capital offense—the life of an idea is at stake. Looming largest among the credibility factors is numbers. How many people were in the trial? How many observed the trial protocol? The statistician's measures of trial power and significance of differences are sharp goads for those engaged in clinical trials. Were resources (time, money, trained personnel) infinite—or at least, substantially larger than they are now—the pressures would be less piercing. But they are not. Therefore, heavy emphasis must be placed upon effective means for achieving trial recruitment and regimen adherence goals.

Although these issues are scarcely unimportant in clinical practice, they are less acutely pressing. Society makes little to no attempt to *believe* the result of clinical practice. Society asks physicians, nurses, pharmacists, nutritionists, health educators—all care providers—to produce results, not proof.

As to the significance of numbers, in many settings discouraging overutilization is a far larger problem than recruitment. And, from a societal perspective, small increments of success can have an appreciable impact due to the multiplier of a large national population. If, for example, community practitioners individually increased their success at controlling hypertension by only four patients, the nation would have 200,000 or more additional controlled hypertensives. Clinical trials have no such mammoth effect multipliers to lean upon. As much as we must impress investigators of the need for the greatest possible numbers, we must exert even more effort to persuade care providers of the high value of limited numbers of successes. Commercial competitors will spend millions to achieve a 5% increase in their marketing success. The health care and health promotion markets are subject to the same arithmetic if only we will allow, even encourage, it.

Predicting, measuring, and modifying regimen adherence are further issues. In either case, clinical trial or practice, predicting regimen adherence is a tricky and undependable undertaking. Many of the predictors just described are unmodifiable or very difficult to modify (e.g., smoking). Furthermore, even those that can be altered may not, if changed, result in a differing adherence pattern. A predictor is not necessarily a causal agent.

Whether the question is changing a predictor or simply attempting to use such state-of-the-art as we possess to influence health behaviors, clinical trials are sharply limited in capability. An ever-present issue is available resources, but even more important in the special case of trials is the risk of diluting or confounding the anticipated trial outcome. Community efforts can (although too few do so effectively) use a full array of marketing tools. These strategies include pricing, product development or modification, distribution (place), and promotion (education) — the four p's of marketing. There are no methodological barriers to full use of mass media, worksite reinforcement, regulatory or policing action, or a host of other imperfect but still result-producing actions.

This is not so for the perpetrators of clinical trials. Such actions can rarely be limited to reaching only the experimental population. If they reach and influence actions of the control population, outcome differences may be so reduced that even a trial with a large sample size may lack sufficient power to detect significant differences. Under usual circumstances, the risk is too great even to consider such approaches.

A further limitation of trials is the scientific method. To achieve control of as many variables as possible, investigators have little choice but to create a highly contrived, artificial situation. Sometimes severe compromises must be made between an ability to generalize the findings and an ability to prove the hypothesis. In this gamble for improving knowledge, most often the hypothesis, like the casino operator, wins any ties. Generically, hypothesis testing requires use of a fixed protocol leading to suspected, but as yet unproved, outcomes. Investigators must swing their prespecified ax in a prescribed manner and for a fixed number of times, then let the chips fall where they may. Conductors of a clinical trial are not free to modify their product to meet better the needs of their population. A trial cannot be altered very much in progress without destroying its integrity. The only major modification alternative is to stop the trial—and this is done if the sought effect is significant early on or if unanticipated dangers are detected.

Community programs use an almost reverse paradigm. Desired outcomes are stated at the outset, and the protocol used is changed as necessary to achieve those outcomes. If the ax doesn't work, the community clinician may switch (resources, ethics, and politics permitting) to a pocket knife, a chain saw, a bulldozer, or dynamite—or simply take more time. The danger in community-based efforts is that the objectives and means may become too fixed. Some failures arise, not from lack of objectives (although this is a high-prevalence condition), but from failure to adapt goals or product to changing social conditions or fast-moving technology.

An important resource—time—is limited in clinical trials. Schedule is often an important protocol element, and certainly timely completion of a $10 to $15 million per year experiment is a highly sought-after goal. Community practitioners most often work under an openended or at least highly flexible time frame.

There are some strengths in clinical trials, some opportunities less or not available in typical community practice, that make things easier. High on that list is the usually single focus of a clinical trial. A clinical trial does not—by deliberate design may not—address every human affliction that walks through the door. This passing of the buck, of sending unwanted problems elsewhere, is considered quite ethical in a trial situation. Elsewhere, this luxury for trial conductors bears the epithet "dumping" and is a source of both high dudgeon and conflict.

Akin to selective focus is selection of subjects. Potential trial subjects may be excluded for a variety of reasons—the presence of conditions confounding to the study, of excessive risk to the subject, or simply a high potential for uncooperativeness. Reduction of any of these or other factors can make a clinical trial more manageable and interpretable. Exclusionary practices are not so readily accepted in other circumstances. In community practice nowadays, exclusion is becoming more risky for the practitioner than for the patient.

Small numbers in the treated population, the bane of the statistical staff, may be a boon to the clinical staff. Often these smaller numbers permit an intensity of rapport, of personal reinforcement opportunity, of tracking and recontact well beyond that practical in a community program.

Similarly, trial staff often have measures and information-processing methods for monitoring variables that cannot be economically adopted community-wide. To the extent that improved information equates with increased control, trial staff have substantially more control over their situation than community practitioners.

The trial situation also results in a stronger subject–provider contract, in part but not wholly arising from the informed consent process of research. The roles of subject and experimenter are more likely better understood by all parties in the clinical trial than in usual practice. The term "compliance"—bothersome to many health professionals (myself included)—is perhaps most aptly used in a clinical trial situation, provided it applies *equally* to subject and experimenter.

CONCLUSIONS

If one accepts the suggestion that clinical trials are, indeed, very special situations, a clear research need is investigations that are clinical-trial-specific to address the specialized recruiting and regimen adherence needs of clinical trials. Behavior prediction tools can aid subject selection and exclusion decisions. Behavior-influencing methods can reduce the impact of adherence as a study confounder in some study design cases.

Sponsors of clinical trials may find it useful to seek, prior to issuing a solicitation, a consensus among experienced investigators, study analysis experts, and behavioral scientists on the advisability of using prerandomization screening for adherence behavior in a given trial. And sponsors must recognize that adherence applies also to investigative staff as well as subjects. Sponsor management should include training programs for trial investigators prior to population recruiting on overall study management methods and anticipated problems of recruitment and subject regimen adherence. In the discussions presented in this section, there is abundant evidence and logic suggesting that rigorous application of some relatively straightforward management methods and principles will do much to alleviate some of the clinical trial problems experienced in the past.

SECTION VI

Life-Style Change and Adherence: The Broader Context

Sally A. Shumaker, Editor

A simple health behavior, such as the daily use of medication, rarely meets with perfect adherence. Yet, today's consumers are not asked to adopt "simple" behaviors; rather, they are asked to make multiple behavior changes to prevent disease or decrease the impact of an existing disease. Recommendations for healthier lifestyles often entail the acquisition of new habits *and* the elimination of old ones. To reduce the *probability* of developing heart disease, for example, the asymptomatic hypertensive patient might be asked to eat less salt, exercise more frequently, stop smoking, practice relaxation techniques, and take medications. Consistent compliance with all of these recommendations is an herculean task. As discussed throughout this book, obstacles to adherence may arise due to a number of factors, including the complexity of a particular regimen; behavioral or biological disincentives; poor communication between the patient and health practitioner; public policies and social contexts that reinforce negative health behaviors; and the complex needs of specific populations. Furthermore, accurate and reliable assessments of adherence are difficult to obtain. In spite of these problems, however, there is an implicit assumption throughout this book that better adherence is almost always worth pursuing. Thus, our focus has been on developing methods to enhance adherence.

In the final section of this book, the authors step back from the assumption that adherence is primae facie good and should be relentlessly pursued by both consumers and health care providers. These authors consider the possibly unintended consequences of "good" adherence, the reliability of data upon which health promotion is based, who in society is ultimately responsible for health behavior changes, and the underlying ethical issues inherent in the contracts between health providers and their patients.

In chapter 22, Czajkowski and Chesney discuss the potential consequences of adherence in experimental studies which include placebo and treatment groups. These authors consider how various factors, including one's belief in the efficacy of treatment, can produce treatment-like effects in the placebo condition. Further, this "placebo effect" is strengthened by adherence. These authors suggest that as long as the "placebo effect" is treated as a nuisance variable rather than as a phenomenon worthy of study in its own right, differences in adherence between treatment and placebo groups may lead to incorrect interpretations of data. Czajkowski and Chesney describe several models to explain the placebo effect and discuss its implications for clinical research and for assumptions regarding treatment efficacy.

In Chapter 23, Rosenstock makes a distinction between disease *prevention* or that which government and organizations do for people, and health *promotion* or that which people do for themselves. He further considers the issue of blame for having a problem versus responsibility for resolving it. Rosenstock discusses the concept of adherence within the context of several dialectics, including: social policy versus personal autonomy, cost-effectiveness versus cost-saving, and individual rights versus the "social good." In his provocative consideration of *what* constitutes health behavior, Rosenstock challenges the consistency and clarity of health knowledge and health behavior recommendations, as well as the degree to which "knowledge" changes over time as data or the interpretations of existing data change.

In Chapter 24, Faden highlights the key moral issues relevant to the question of adherence to lifestyle changes. She discusses the differences implied in normative and applied ethics when considering adherence in three very different contractual relationships: the clinician and the patient, the researcher and the subject, and the government and its citizenry.

In these three concluding chapters, the authors discuss adherence within the broader social context and challenge health providers to look more carefully at the implications of adherence to health behavior interventions for the individual and society. In her concluding remarks, Mullen underscores the importance of this broader perspective for effective health care.

22

Adherence and
the Placebo Effect

Susan M. Czajkowski, Margaret A. Chesney

Traditionally, adherence has been viewed as a critical element in the success of a treatment or health regimen, for without it patients may not receive the full benefit of treatment. Given the importance of adherence to treatment success, other chapters in this volume focus on factors that predict or influence adherence to a specific treatment and on strategies for increasing adherence. In contrast, in this chapter we consider adherence from another perspective: the potential consequences of adherence that could lead to incorrect conclusions about treatment efficacy. That is, in addition to its role in maximizing the *active, specific* effects of the treatment, adherence may also increase treatment effectiveness by activating *nonspecific or placebo* effects that influence treatment success. Thus the mere act of adherence to a treatment regimen may in itself produce positive health outcomes, regardless of the actual efficacy of the intervention, due to a placebo effect.

We begin by outlining a hypothetical model of the role adherence may play in enhancing the nonspecific effects of an intervention and thus in affecting treatment outcome. Then a brief overview of placebo effects is presented, including a discussion of possible mechanisms through which placebos exert their influence. Applying the model, we then suggest an explanation for why adherence to a treatment may enhance a placebo response. Finally we present an example from the clinical trial literature that illustrates aspects of this perspective and discuss implications of the model for both clinical applications and research.

MODEL: THE NONSPECIFIC EFFECTS OF ADHERENCE

The model (see Figure 22.1) proposed here is one in which adherence to an intervention is seen as enhancing not only the effects of active treatment components, but also the effects of nonspecific components of that intervention as well. Specifically, the model suggests that adherence enhances the following nonspecific components that can influence intervention outcomes: (1) patient and provider *expectancies* of the intervention's success, and (2) the *social support* available to the patient from the provider and others in the patient's environment.

In several chapters in this volume (e.g., Chapters 3, 9, and 16), expectancies and social support have been described as predictors of adherence. The model presented here suggests that these factors may also be "effects" of adherence. Adherence influences the expectancy of treatment success to the extent that patients who follow an intervention develop the expectation that they will experience positive health outcomes. Conversely, patients who *do not* adhere should have a diminished expectancy of positive outcomes from the intervention. Patient adherence also impacts provider expectancies regarding the outcome of the intervention. For example, a physician is more likely to expect lower serum cholesterol levels in a patient who is adhering to a prescribed low-fat diet than a patient who continues to eat the typically high-fat American diet. Similarly, patient adherence may influence the amount of social support extended to patients by providers and others in the patient's social network, since adhering to a prescribed medical regimen is likely to be rewarded by positive responses from family, friends, and caretakers.

As portrayed in the model, the relationship between adherence and the nonspecific components of treatment is a reciprocal one. Expectancies and social support are affected by adherence and, in turn, influence subsequent adherence. For example, the patient who adheres to the low-fat diet, and meets with a physician who expresses a positive expectancy for lower cholesterol levels and praises the patient for adhering, is more likely to continue adhering to the prescribed diet.

In the model, expectancy and social support are considered not only in terms of their relationship to adherence but in terms of their roles as nonspecific factors influencing treatment outcomes. This aspect of the model is based on evidence that these two variables are important in influencing health outcomes (Agras, Horne, & Taylor, 1982; Hovell et al., 1986). Thus the perspective added by this model is that the expectancies and social support fostered by adherence may

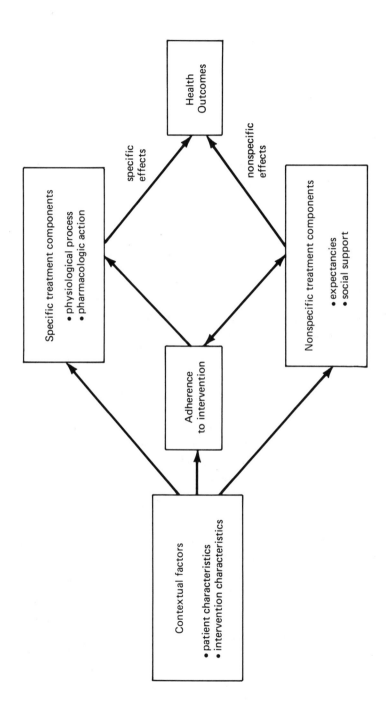

FIGURE 22.1 The effects of adherence on health outcomes

411

have an affect on health that is independent of any active treatment the patient may receive.

Finally, the literature indicates that nonspecific effects are influenced by some of the same factors known to influence adherence. These factors include *patient characteristics* (e.g., health beliefs, severity of disease, and attitudes toward providers) and *intervention characteristics* (e.g., therapeutic setting, provider characteristics, treatment cost and method of treatment delivery). Figure 22.1 shows these characteristics as having effects on adherence and on nonspecific treatment components; in addition, patient characteristics can directly influence specific treatment effects (e.g., due to individual differences in sensitivity to the therapeutic agent).

OVERVIEW OF THE PLACEBO EFFECT

Shapiro and Shapiro (1984, p. 372) define a placebo as "any therapy or component of therapy that is deliberately used for its nonspecific, psychological, or psychophysiological effect, or that is used for its presumed specific effect but is without specific activity for the condition being treated." A placebo effect is defined as "the psychological or psychophysiological effect produced by placebos" (Shapiro & Shapiro, 1984, p. 372). This definition implies that active treatments may have placebo components and that the effects of specific therapies (i.e., nonplacebos) are often due to both placebo and nonplacebo effects (Shapiro & Shapiro, 1984).

Historically, the term "placebo" has referred to inactive pills or tablets given to control subjects in drug trials. Over time, however, the term "placebo effect" has come to refer to a variety of nonspecific effects on health outcomes that are integrally related to the delivery and monitoring of treatment but that are not attributable to the specific therapeutic agent under study. In this chapter, the terms "placebo" and "nonspecific" will be used interchangeably.

The nonspecific effects of treatments are well documented in the literature on medical and behavioral interventions. More recently, these effects are receiving increased attention in clinical trials that have found greater than expected improvements in the health of subjects in placebo control groups, in some cases equivalent to or greater than those observed in patients receiving active tretment. In the area of hypertension control, for instance, a number of studies, including the Multiple Risk Factor Intervention Trial (Multiple Risk Factor Intervention Trial Research Group, 1982), the Hypertension Detection and Follow-up Program (Hypertension Detection and Follow-up Program Cooperative Group, 1979), and the Australian National Blood Pressure Study (Management Committee, 1980) have found significant and persistent reductions in blood pressure for usual care or placebo control groups. Similar results have been reported for several other studies that compared the effects of behavioral treatments for hypertension (e.g., relaxation training, biofeedback, cognitive restructuring) with the effects of placebo treatment (e.g., flexibility training) or blood pressure monitoring alone (Agras, Taylor, Kraemer, Southam, & Schneider, 1987; Chesney, Black, Swan, & Ward, 1987; Jacob et al., 1986; Ward, Swan, & Chesney, 1987). The results of these studies have stimulated inquiry into possible explanations for the significant improvements or changes found for control groups and have focused attention on the impact of nonspecific and behavioral factors on control groups in clinical trial research (Kramer & Shapiro, 1984).

It is important to note that in the clinical trials mentioned above as well as in other studies, nonspecific effects have been demonstrated to involve not only improvements in subjective symptoms, but also objectively measured cardiovascular risk factor and end organ changes as well (Gould, Davies, Mann, Altman, & Raftery, 1981). Indeed, the physiological effects of placebos are acknowledged as being very powerful: Placebos can induce addiction and have been reported to be more effective than, or even to reverse the effects of, some pharmacologic agents (Shapiro & Shapiro, 1984). In addition, the range of physiological processes that have been shown to exhibit placebo effects are very broad and include inhibited gastric acid secretion, reduced adrenocortical activity, and decreased serum lipoproteins (Bush, 1974).

MECHANISMS OF THE PLACEBO EFFECT

The recognition that nonspecific treatment components may influence health outcomes raises questions regarding the mechanisms underlying these effects. Placebos are thought to exert their effects through both *psychological* and *biological* mechanisms (Wilkins, 1985).

Psychological Mechanisms

Models that focus on the psychological mechanisms underlying the placebo effect fall into two categories: (1) *learning theory* models, which explain placebo effects as classical conditioning phenomena; and (2) *cognitively oriented* models, which emphasize the role of mental processes, such as expectancy.

Learning Theory Models

Models based on a learning theory approach focus on the placebo effect as a *conditioned response*. According to this explanation, the complex of stimuli surrounding the administration of a drug (e.g., taking a pill) become conditioned stimuli because of their repeated association with drug administration and relief from suffering during the person's developmental history (Wickramasekera, 1985). Support for the learning theory model involves mostly animal research, which has confirmed the conditioning of physiologic and pharmocologic responses as an important element in placebo phenomena (Ader, 1985). This model is useful in explaining placebo effects associated with the administration of drugs; however, it is less applicable to situations involving nonpharmacologic treatment, such as behavioral or life-style interventions.

Cognitive Models

Currently the most widely accepted cognitively based explanation for the placebo effect is that it is based on people's expectations of therapeutic benefit or success. The expectancy model of placebo effects is similar to an earlier cognitively based hypothesis that postulates a relationship between an individual's response to placebo and his or her suggestibility. However, although it is commonly believed that individuals who score high on measures of suggestibility are more prone to the placebo response, no consistent relationship has been found between this response and either suggestibility or hypnotizability (Evans, 1985).

Another early cognitive model of placebo effects involved *anxiety reduction*, resulting from an individual's belief in the pain-reducing effects of a treatment. According to this model, placebo effects are attributable to decreased perceptions of pain and distress associated with anxiety reduction. This hypothesis was supported by studies showing that for chronically anxious individuals, feelings of reduced anxiety following placebo ingestion lead to a significant increase in pain tolerance (Evans, 1985). While the anxiety-reduction hypothesis addresses the effects of placebos on pain, it does not generalize easily to the many other physiological processes affected by placebos.

More recently, a number of studies have shown that responses to treatment are mediated by patient *expectancies* generated within the therapeutic relationship. One study found that students who expected a relaxation training procedure to produce an immediate lowering of blood pressure had significantly lower systolic blood pressures immediately following the procedure than did a group of subjects who were led to believe that the relaxation training would produce a delayed effect (Agras et al., 1982). In contrast, Wadden (1984) found no differences in blood pressure reduction between subjects assigned to a cognitive therapy condition, which involved a positive expectancy of blood pressure change, and those assigned to relaxation therapy. Several other studies have also suggested that the effects of relaxation therapy may be primarily due to nonspecific factors, such as positive expectancy or social support (Brauer, Horlick, Nelson, Farquhar, & Angras, 1979; Luborsky et al., 1982).

Evidence also suggests that the placebo effect is influenced not only by patient expectancies but by doctor or experimenter expectations. For example, when the physician believes a powerful drug is being used in a double-blind study, the placebo effect is stronger than if he or she believes the medication is less effective (Evans, 1985). Thus the physician's belief about a drug's efficacy may be communicated to the patient and appears to mediate treatment effectiveness.

An individual's expectations about treatment success may be influenced by a variety of factors. For example, the *social support* received from family, friends, and health providers may enhance patients' beliefs or expectations about the efficacy of therapy. When a spouse is supportive of the patient receiving a specific form of therapy, the patient may come to believe such therapy will be beneficial. The effect of social support from members of a patient's network can be especially powerful when those others are seen as credible sources of information and when the patient has a great deal of faith in them. Plotkin (1985) emphasizes the impact of the patients' faith in the therapist as an important condition for behavioral change to occur in therapy.

Evidence for the influence of social support on health outcomes is provided in a study of the effects of personalized care, operationalized as greater personal attention and warmth shown to the patient, on blood pressure reduction in hypertensives (Hovell et al., 1986). In this study, patients receiving personalized care differed significantly in the magnitude of their blood pressure reductions from those receiving usual care. Several other studies have documented similar effects for personalized versus usual care, although the mechanisms for such effects remain unknown (Dunbar, Marshall, & Hovell, 1979; Finnerty, Mattie, & Finnerty, 1973). Hovell et al. (1986) speculate that personalized care may evoke a generalized relaxation response and suggest that future research is needed to determine the mechanisms underlying the effects of social support on blood pressure reduction.

Biologically Based Models

There have been few attempts to investigate the ways in which psychological processes, such as expectancy, translate into the physiological changes observed in placebo phenomena. Levine, Gordon, and Fields (1978) hypothesize that placebo effects are based on biochemical processes that produce psychological and somatic changes. According to their model, placebo expectancies activate the endorphin system, which reduces pain. Evidence supporting this model includes several studies showing that with dental postoperative pain, naloxone (an opiate antagonist that blocks the release of endorphins) counteracts placebo-induced analgesia (Levine, Gordon, & Fields, 1979; Levine, Gordon, Jones, & Fields, 1978). Further research is needed on the biological bases of the placebo effect, using both pain and nonpain paradigms, since the existing literature in this area has been criticized for methodological problems and failure to replicate (Gracely, Wolshee, Deeter, & Dubner, 1982; Grevert & Goldstein, 1977, 1978; Mihic & Binkert, 1978).

ADHERENCE AND THE PLACEBO EFFECT

Returning to the original thesis that adherence activates or enhances placebo effects, how might adherence influence these effects? There are two leading explanations: (1) adherence per se activates nonspecific components of treatment; or (2) certain characteristics of individuals who adhere to a treatment enhance the nonspecific components of treatment.

With the first explanation, given the hypothesis discussed in the previous section that expectancies of therapeutic benefit or success activate placebo effects, then any factor in a therapeutic situation that enhances such expectancies would indirectly influence placebo effects as well. Adherence to treatment may be one such factor, since adherence is integrally related to patient expectancies in a therapeutic situation.

Patient adherence to treatment is influenced by the expectation that the treatment will produce the desired effect (e.g., lower cholesterol, reduce weight). For example, individuals will be more likely to adhere to a low-calorie diet if they believe that doing so will be effective in producing weight loss *and* if they see themselves as capable of adhering to the diet. Bandura (1977) refers to the former belief as an outcome expectancy (the belief that a given behavior will lead to a particular outcome) and the latter as an efficacy expectation (the belief that "one can successfully execute the behavior required to produce outcomes"). According to Bandura (1977), success in a therapeutic situation is based on the acquisition of expectancies of increased personal effectiveness, or efficacy expectancies. High-efficacy expectancies are related to perseverence of effort at a task (e.g., adherence) and thus to maintenance of therapeutic improvement.

Thus expectations about treatment effectiveness and one's ability to comply to a treatment are important determinants of actual adherence to treatment. However, as noted earlier, the relationship is reciprocal, since expectancies of success can also be a *consequence* of complying with treatment: The more one adheres to the treatment regimen, the more likely one is to expect treatment success. By complying with treatment, the patient enhances the expectation that the treatment will work. Expectancies of change and improvement are therefore important as both antecedents and consequences of adherence.

If this is true, then efforts to increase adherence (especially by enhancing expectancies of treatment success) may increase treatment effectiveness not only because they maximize the extent to which the patient receives active treatment, but also because these adherence-induced expectancies activate placebo responses to treatment. In the same way, social support may influence patients' beliefs or expectations about the efficacy of treatment and thus influence nonspecific treatment responses.

The second explanation of how adherence influences placebo effects, that there are certain characteristics of adherers that activate nonspecific components of treatment, may also be based on an expectancy effect. For example, if adherers are more likely to have an enhanced sense of control over events in their lives, and therefore to believe that they can affect their health positively by complying to treatment, then treatment effectiveness may be due primarily to the greater expectancies for treatment success held by these individuals, rather than to the treatment itself. Other characteristics that differentiate adherers from nonadherers (e.g., "hardiness" or greater resiliency under stress; less depression and anxiety) may also be important determinants of treatment success to the extent that they influence patient expectancies regarding treatment outcomes.

EVIDENCE FOR ADHERENCE-INDUCED PLACEBO EFFECTS

There has been no research to date that adequately tests the model proposed in this chapter concerning the role that adherence may play in enhancing nonspecific treatment effects. This is partly due to the lack of attention paid to nonspecific treatment components in health research. Although placebo effects are acknowledged as being of sufficient importance to necessitate the inclusion of placebo controls in most studies of medical or behavioral interventions, biomedical researchers have not made use of the placebo condition as an opportunity to examine and better understand the nonspecific effects of treatment. Instead, placebos have traditionally been viewed as nuisance variables to be controlled for, rather than as variables that are important for study in their own right or as important adjuncts to active treatment (Evans, 1985). This is in contrast to the current emphasis on nonspecific factors in psychotherapy outcome studies (Frank, 1971; Garfield, 1980, 1982; Smith, Glass, & Miller, 1980; Stone, Imber, & Frank, 1966). In this literature, psychotherapy researchers have identified a number of nonspecific factors, or "common ingredients," as being important contributors to positive therapy outcomes, regardless of the particular mode of therapy used (Garfield, 1982). The nonspecific factor thought to be most central to therapeutic outcome is the patient's expectation of benefit (Frank, 1961, 1983; Garfield, 1982; Goldstein, 1962), which has also been implicated as an important mechanism underlying placebo effects.

An example of a study utilizing physical health outcomes that suggests the potential importance of adherence to treatment in the evaluation of treatment efficacy is the Coronary Drug Project (The Coronary Drug Project Research

Group, 1980). The Coronary Drug Project was designed to evaluate the efficacy and safety of several lipid-influencing drugs, such as clofibrate, in the treatment of coronary heart disease. In this study, male patients who had experienced a myocardial infarction within 3 months of entry were randomly assigned to either a condition in which they received clofibrate or to a placebo control group. The results showed no significant difference in 5-year mortality between the two groups. (For the 1103 men treated with clofibrate, 5-year mortality was 20%; for the 2789 men given placebo, it was 20.9%.)

Further analyses performed to determine whether adherence to clofibrate influenced 5-year mortality showed that good adherers (defined as patients who took 80% or more of the drug during the 5-year follow-up period) had a significantly lower 5-year mortality (15%) than did poor adherers (24.6%). However, this was true for those receiving the placebo as well; good adherers to placebo had significantly lower mortality than nonadherers to placebo (15.1% for good adherers versus 28.2% for poor adherers) and in fact had *lower* mortality rates than poor adherers to clofibrate. Furthermore, this effect held even when multivariate statistical methods were used to adjust for baseline differences between the two groups on 40 variables that were related to 5-year mortality (e.g., indices of disease severity, use of hypertensive medication; see Table 22.1).

These results appear to show an effect of adherence on mortality, since patients who received no active drug but who adhered to the treatment regimen had lower mortality than those who did not adhere. Unfortunately, several confounds in this study limit the ability to make this interpretation. First, the retrospective design means that assignment to adherence subgroups involved self-selection rather than random assignment to condition. Thus, an explanation for the adherence results is that those individuals who adhered to the placebo or drug treatments differed from nonadherers on some health-related variable or variables that also caused differences in mortality and that were not adjusted for in the multivariate statistical analyses. For example, the nonadherers may have

TABLE 22.1 Influence of Adherence on Mortality Rates* in the Coronary Drug Project

Adherence	Treatment group	
	Clofibrate	Placebo
Good adherers (> 80% adherence)	15.0% (15.7)**	15.1% (16.4)
Poor adherers (< 80% adherence)	24.6% (22.5)	28.2% (25.8)

*Percentages are 5-year mortality rates.
**The figures in parentheses are adjusted for 40 baseline characteristics.
From The Coronary Drug Project Research Group. Influence of adherence to treatment and response of cholesterol on mortality in the Coronary Drug Project. *The New England Journal of Medicine*, 1980, *18*, 1038-1041.

been individuals who abused drugs or alcohol and who were therefore negligent about taking their medication. If these individuals were also less healthy than adherers, as would be expected, their survival rates over the 5-year follow-up period would be lower than those in the "high-adherence" group. In this case, both adherence and mortality would result from a third, unmeasured variable—alcohol/drug abuse—and would actually be unrelated to each other when that variable was controlled for.

There were also problems with the measurement of adherence in the Coronary Drug Project that may have resulted in a selection bias. Adherence was determined by physician estimates of the number of pills taken by patients each day. These estimates were based on the number of pills returned by patients at their clinic visits and on interviews in which patients were questioned about problems with the medication, including side effects, that may have affected adherence to the regimen. Because of the subjective nature of this measure of adherence, it is likely that physicians' assessments of patient adherence were determined to a large extent by their assessments of the health of individual patients. Thus the healthier patients may have been assigned to the high-adherence group, and their lower mortality rate simply reflects this bias in assignment to adherence condition.

Although these problems with the study make it impossible to interpret the results as indicating an adherence-induced placebo effect, it is clear that some nonspecific factor (that is, something *not related* to the active treatment, but associated with adherence) was related to reduced mortality. It is possible that at least some of the variance in mortality attributed to adherence was due to increased patient expectancies or social support generated by adherence to treatment. However, research is needed to delineate the role of adherence in enhancing nonspecific treatment effects. In the next section, we discuss some of the ways future research can lead to a better understanding of this phenomenon.

IMPLICATIONS AND RESEARCH DIRECTIONS

The model presented in this chapter suggests that adherence to treatment may affect health outcomes by enhancing or activating nonspecific effects of treatment (e.g., expectancies, social support). This has important implications for clinical trials and other research studies involving interventions, since there are several situations in which such adherence-induced placebo effects could lead to inaccurate conclusions about treatment efficacy.

While placebo control conditions are commonly used in studies involving the evaluation of drug therapies, studies evaluating other types of interventions (especially behavioral or life-style interventions) often do not use placebo conditions or use inadequate placebo controls. This is due to the difficulty in designing a placebo control condition when the treatment is behavioral in nature. When the treatment is pharmacological, it is possible to manufacture a pill that is identical in every respect (e.g., in appearance) to the pharmacological agent being used. But it is often difficult to devise a placebo for a behavioral treatment that is identical to the treatment itself in every way except that it has no active component (Buck & Donner, 1982). Clearly, given the possibility that adherence to an intervention may affect the evaluation of a treatment's effectiveness, care must be taken in selecting placebo conditions for all studies involving patient adherence to some intervention, whether behavioral or pharmacological in nature.

Problems may arise even when adequate placebo controls are used if adherence rates differ between the treatment and control groups. One reason for different adherence rates that could influence patient expectancies regarding treatment success (and therefore affect treatment effectiveness via those expectancies) is that some patients receiving treatment who are particularly sensitive to physiological cues and sensations might interpret the presence or absence of such sensations to indicate whether they are receiving the active treatment (Wilkins, 1985). Because patients in the active treatment group would be more likely to become "unblinded" in this way, and therefore more likely to adhere to treatment and to expect a successful outcome, it would be difficult to pull apart the actual treatment effect from an expectancy-induced effect. In this case, a more positive outcome for the treatment group could be inaccurately attributed to treatment efficacy when it was actually due to increased expectations of treatment success. This suggests that adherence rates between the treatment and placebo conditions should always be assessed to rule out the possibility that adherence-induced placebo effects are responsible for any effects found.

The model presented in this chapter has implications not only for the internal validity of studies that involve adherence to interventions, but also for the generalizability of such studies. For example, one disadvantage of prerandomization screening (as discussed in Chapter 18 of this volume) is that by screening out nonadherers, any effects found for a particular treatment can only be generalized to those individuals who are likely to adhere to a treatment regimen. Since these individuals may have certain psychosocial characteristics that affect their adherence behavior (e.g., high self-efficacy) and that may also affect treatment success, the finding of a treatment effect would be applicable only to a narrow subgroup of patients, thus calling into question the usefulness of the study for a broader range of individuals.

There is no research that currently tests the effects of adherence on treatment outcome. Therefore, future research should attempt to: (1) determine whether adherence-induced expectancies do in fact activate placebo effects; and (2) identify and evaluate aspects of the act of adherence or characteristics of those that comply that may enhance placebo effects. Furthermore, clinical trials and other studies that evaluate the effects of interventions should use designs that allow researchers to partial out or control for these effects. Rosenthal (1985) and Ross and Buckalew (1985) suggest experimental designs that can be used to better understand how nonspecific effects may impact on evaluations of treatment effectiveness. Additionally, an approach that may help clarify whether patient expectancies are mediating the effects of adherence on mortality and morbidity is a causal modeling approach that tests the effect of adherence on health outcomes directly and indirectly (via expectancy as a mediating variable). Aspects of the model presented in this chapter can also be tested experimentally. Examples of this approach include laboratory studies in which subjects' expectations about the effects of a particular treatment are manipulated (see Agras et al., 1982).

Finally, more attention should be focused on the role of nonspecific factors in health-related research, similar to the increased focus being given to such factors in psychotherapy outcome research (Garfield, 1982). Perhaps certain components of health care interventions, such as enhanced expectation of benefit or the perceived social support available from the health care provider, are "common ingredients" that enhance health-related outcomes regardless of the treatment or disease process involved. Future research should focus on identifying such common ingredients and using them to increase the effectiveness of health-related interventions.

In summary, both experimental and nonexperimental methodologies should be used to determine the role adherence may play in enhancing the nonspecific effects of an intervention. This knowledge can be used in the design of clinical trials and other intervention-based research studies, and in the enhancement of treatment effectiveness in the clinical setting through the manipulation of those nonspecific factors known to affect treatment efficacy.

REFERENCES

Ader, R. (1985). Conditioned immunopharmacological effects in animals: Implications for a conditioning model of pharmacotherapy. In I. L. White, B. Tursky, & G. E. Schwartz (Eds.) *Placebo: Theory, research and mechanisms* pp. 306-331. New York: Guilford Press.

Agras, W. S., Horne, M., & Taylor, C. B. (1982). Expectation and blood pressure lowering effects of relaxation. *Psychosomatic Medicine, 44*, 389-395.

Agras, W. S., Taylor, C. B., Kraemer, H. C., Southam, M. A., & Schneider, J. A. (1987). Relaxation training for essential hypertension at the worksite: II. The poorly controlled hypertensive. *Psychosomatic Medicine, 49*, 264-273.

Bandura, A. (1977). Self-efficacy: Toward a unifying theory of behavior change. *Psychological Review, 84*, 191-215.

Brauer, A. P., Horlick, L., Nelson, E., Farquhar, J. W., & Agras, W. S. (1979). Relaxation therapy for essential hypertension. *Journal of Behavioral Medicine, 2*, 21-29.

Buck, C., & Donner, A. (1982). The design of controlled experiments in the evaluation of non-therapeutic interventions. *Journal of Chronic Diseases, 35,* 531-538.

Bush, P. J. (1974). The placebo effect. *Journal of the American Pharmaceutical Association, NS14,* 671-672.

Chesney, M. A., Black, G. W., Swan, G. E., & Ward, M. M. (1987). Relaxation training for essential hypertension at the worksite: I. The untreated mild hypertensive. *Psychosomatic Medicine, 49,* 250-263.

Coronary Drug Project Research Group. (1980). Inlfuence of adherence to treatment and response of cholesterol on mortality in the Coronary Drug Project. *New England Journal of Medicine, 18,* 1038-1041.

Dunbar, J., Marshall, G., & Hovell, M. (1979). Behavioral interventions in compliance. In R. B. Haynes, D. W. Taylor, & D. L. Sackett (Eds.), *Compliance with therapeutic and preventive regimens* pp. 174-190. Baltimore, MD: The Johns Hopkins University Press.

Evans, F. J. (1985). Expectancy, therapeutic instructions and the placebo response. In L. White, B. Tursky, & G. E. Schwartz (eds.), *Placebo: Theory, research and mechanisms* pp. 215-278. New York: The Guilford Press.

Finnerty, F. A., Jr., Mattie, E. C., & Finnerty, F. A., III. (1973). Hypertension in the inner city I: Analysis of clinic dropouts. *Circulation, 47,* 73-75.

Frank, J. D. (1961). *Persuasion and healing: A comparative study of psychotherapy.* Baltimore, MD: Johns Hopkins University Press.

Frank, J. D. (1971). Therapeutic factors in psychotherapy. *American Journal of Psychotherapy, 25,* 350-361.

Frank, J. D. (1983). The placebo is psychotherapy. *Behavioral and Brain Sciences, 6,* 291-292.

Garfield, S. L. (1980). *Psychotherapy: An eclectic approach.* New York: Wiley.

Garfield, S. L. (1982). Eclecticism and integration in psychotherapy. *Behavior Therapy, 13,* 610-623.

Goldstein, A. P. (1962). *Therapist-patient expectancies in psychotherapy.* New York: Macmillan.

Gould, B. A., Davies, A. B., Mann, S., Altman, D. G., & Raftery, E. B. (1981) Does placebo lower blood pressure? *Lancet, ii,* 1377-1381.

Grevert, P., & Goldstein, A. (1977). Effects of naloxone on experimentally produced ischemic pain and on mood in human subjects. *Proceedings of the National Academy of Sciences USA, 74,* 1291-1294.

Grevert, P., & Goldstein, A. (1978) Endorphins: Naloxone fails to alter experimental pain or mood in humans. *Science, 199,* 1093-1095.

Hovell, M. F., Black, D. R., Mewborn, C. R., Geary, D., Agras, W. S., Kamachi, K., Kirk, R., Walton, C., & Dawson, S. (1986). Personalized versus usual care of previously uncontrolled hypertensive patients: An exploratory analysis. *Preventive Medicine, 15,* 673-684.

Hypertension Detection and Follow-up Program Cooperative Group. (1979). Five year findings of the Hypertension Detection and Follow-up Program: I. Reduction in mortality of persons with high blood pressure, including mild hypertension. *Journal of the American Medical Association, 242,* 2562-2571.

Jacob, R. G., Shapiro, A. P., Reeves, R. A., Johnsen, A. M., McDonald, R. H., & Coburn, P. C. (1986). Relaxation therapy for hypertension: Comparison of effects with concomitant placebo, diuretic and beta blocker. *Archives of Internal Medicine, 146,* 2335-2340.

Kramer, M. S., & Shapiro, S. H. (1984). Scientific challenges in the application of randomized trials. *Journal of the American Medical Association, 252,* 2739-2745.

Levine, J. D., Gordon, M. C., & Fields, H. L. (1978). The mechanism of placebo analgesia. *Lancet, 2,* 654-657.

Levine, J. D., Gordon, N. C., & Fields, H. L. (1979). Naloxone dose dependently produces analgesia and hyperalgesia in postoperative pain. *Nature, 278,* 740-741.

Levine, J. D., Gordon, N. C., Jones, R. T., & Fields, H. L. (1978). The narcotic antagonist naloxone enhances clinical pain. *Nature, 272,* 826-827.

Luborsky, L., Crits-Christoph, P., Brady, J. P., Kron, R. E., Weiss, T., Cohen, M., & Levy, L. (1982). Behavioral versus pharmacological treatments for essential hypertension—A needed comparison. *Psychosomatic Medicine, 44,* 203-213.

Management Committee. (1980). The Australian therapeutic trial in mild hypertension. *Lancet,* 1261-1267.

Mihic, D., & Binkert, E. (1978). *Is placebo analgesia mediated by endorphine?* Paper presented at the Second World Congress on Pain, Montreal, Quebec, Canada.

Multiple Risk Factor Intervention Trial Research Group. (1982). Multiple Risk Factor Intervention Trial: Risk factor changes and mortality results. *Journal of the American Medical Association, 248,* 1465-1477.

Plotkin, E. B. (1985). A psychological approach to placebo: The role of faith in therapy and treatment. In L. White, B. Tursky, & G. E. Schwartz (Eds.), *Placebo: Theory, research and mechanisms* pp. 237-254. New York: The Guilford Press.

Rosenthal, R. (1985). Designing, analyzing, interpreting and summarizing placebo studies. In L. White, B. Tursky, & G. E. Schwartz (Eds.), *Placebo: Theory, research and mechanisms* pp. 110-136. New York: The Guilford Press.

Ross, S., & Buckalew, L. W. (1985). Placebo agentry: Assessment of drug and placebo effects. In L. White, B. Tursky, & G. E. Schwartz (Eds.), *Placebo: Theory, research and mechanisms* pp. 67-82. New York: The Guilford Press.

Shapiro, A. K., & Shapiro, E. (1984). Patient–provider relationships and the placebo effect. In J. D. Matarazzo, S. M. Weiss, J. A. Herd, N. E. Miller, & S. M. Weiss (Eds.), *Behavioral health: A handbook of health enhancement and disease prevention* pp. 371-383. New York: Wiley.

Smith, M. L., Glass, E. V., & Miller, T. I. (1980). *The benefits of psychotherapy.* Baltimore, MD: Johns Hopkins University Press.

Stone, A. R., Imber, S. D., & Frank, J. D. (1966). The role of non-specific factors in short-term psychotherapy. *Australian Journal of Psychology, 18,* 210-217.

Wadden, T. (1984). Relaxation therapy for essential hypertension: Specific or nonspecific effects? *Journal of Psychosomatic Research, 28,* 53-61.

Ward, M. M., Swan, G. E., & Chesney, M. A. (1987). Arousal reduction treatments for mild hypertension: A meta-analysis of recent studies. In S. Julius (E.), *Handbook of hypertension. Volume 10: Behavioral factors in hypertension* pp. 285-302. New York: Elsevier.

Wickramasekera, I. (1985). A conditioned response model of the placebo effect: Predictions from the model. In L. White, B. Tursky, & G. E. Schwartz (Eds.), *Placebo: Theory, research and mechanisms,* pp. 255-287. New York: The Guilford Press.

Wilkins, W. (1985). Placebo controls and concepts in chemotherapy and psychotherapy research. In L. White, B. Tursky, & G. E. Schwartz (Eds.), *Placebo: Theory, research and mechanisms* pp. 83-109. New York: The Guilford Press.

23

Personal Responsibility and Public Policy in Health Promotion

I. M. Rosenstock

The modern concept of responsibility for health has its roots in two major social developments of the twentieth century: the transition from infectious to chronic diseases as leading causes of morbidity and mortality and the development of reasonably effective disease preventives and treatments. With the increasing importance of the chronic diseases, questions began to be raised about the role of life-style in disease causation, whereas such questions had not been crucial to an analysis of the causes of infectious diseases. Concern over issues of responsibility for health also awaited the development of effective treatments. Only within the past 50 years have we developed confidence that planned interventions can prevent, delay, or control disease. And it is still more recently—perhaps within the decades beginning in the 1970s—that we have begun to pay serious attention to the issue of personal responsibility for health.

The Surgeon General's report *Healthy People* (DHEW, 1979) has drawn a sharp distinction between disease prevention and health promotion, which begins to imply some critical issues concerning responsibility for health. The report indicates that "Disease prevention begins with a threat to health—a disease or environmental hazard—and seeks to protect as many people as possible from the harmful consequences of that threat" (p. 119). In contrast, "health promotion begins with people who are basically healthy and seeks the development of community and individual measures which can help them to develop lifestyles that can maintain and enhance the state of well-being" (p. 119). Preventive and protective services include those that "can be delivered to people by health providers . . . and measures which can be used by governmental and other agencies, as well as by industry, to protect people from harm" (p. 81). Health promotion, on the other hand, consists of "activities which individuals and communities can use to promote healthy lifestyles . . ." (p. 81). Thus preventive and protective activities include things that government and industry can do to and for people, while health promotion includes things that people and communities can do for themselves. This distinction concerning the locus of responsibility is important because it implies quite different approaches to coping and helping.

CONCEPTS OF RESPONSIBILITY

Because of our increasing conviction that life-styles influence health, we have been increasingly exhorted to take responsibility for our own health. Knowles (1977) authored the well-known statement that "over 99% of us are born healthy and made sick as a result of personal misbehavior and environmental conditions. The solution to the problems of ill-health in modern American society involves individual responsibility . . ." (p. 58). Two years later Joseph Califano, then Secretary of Health, Education and Welfare, wrote that "You the individual can do more for your own health and well-being than any doctor, any hospital, any drug, any exotic medical device" (DHEW, 1979, pp. viii–ix).

How responsible should individuals be for their own health, how responsible should practitioners be for the health of their patients, and how responsible should government be for the health of its residents?

In a recent paper, Daniel Wikler (1987) summarizes a number of rationales that have been used to justify policies that single out individuals for special treatments or that justify coercion to adopt new life-styles. Three frequently used rationales are paternalism, general utility, and fairness. The *paternalistic* argument is straightforward: individuals can be required to take good care of themselves to avoid needless suffering and expense; coercion is justified by concern with individuals' welfare. The *general utility* argument is basically an economic one; the need to contain costs requires that people adopt healthy life-styles that will delay or prevent costly treatment for later chronic illness and disability. An amalgam of the first two arguments is the *communitarian* rationale, which holds that the public health is valued as something more than the sum of the health status of individuals and that community needs should always take precedence over the needs and desires of individuals. This rationale is paternalistic and utilitarian in encouraging the total community to decide what is good for people and what actions will serve the general, societal good. These rationales do not assign fault or blame to individuals; indeed, they seem to imply that people are not free agents and therefore need society's help.

The third argument described by Wikler is that of *fairness*, which rests squarely on fault. Those who engage in unhealthy life-styles are potentially incurring costs that may have to be borne by others. These risk takers should therefore be required to pay the costs of their risky life-styles through various mechanisms.

These rationales have served as the basis for policy proposals, but they are themselves based on a number of assumptions whose truth is far from certain. For example, it is sometimes argued that those who take risks with their health unfairly burden others, but there are problems with this argument. Life is unfair. Even the most health-conscious of us may have genetic predispositions that doom us to lose life or to become burdens on society long before our biblical promise of 70 years of life has been fulfilled. Shall we punish the cigarette smoker but not the person with genetic disease? Do we want to argue that the smoker has free choice while the victim of Huntington's Disease does not? Could the parents of the victim have chosen not to have children? Does the smoker have free choice? The issue of free will versus determinism is, of course, far from settled.

Even if we allow for freedom of choice, we must still ask whether any person's behavior might not have potentially adverse effects on others. Joggers may be protecting their own health, but if they spent their jogging time in taking up a second job, their additional taxes would reduce the tax burden on others. At the extreme, this line of argument would suggest that all people should choose the most lucrative possible careers, live in the highest-paying regions, and devote as little time as possible to nonremunerative leisure activities. This is clearly an unattractive policy endorsed by no one, but it is not easy to find a legitimate reason for resisting this generalization if we really believe that we should not be forced to pay for the unhealthy behavior of others.

Those who could prescribe behavior for the individual should be obliged to demonstrate that their prescription will accomplish a desirable end and that the clients they are prescribing for are more in need of behavior modification than those writing the prescriptions.

MODELS OF HELPING AND COPING

While Wikler's discussion contributes to our understanding of the arguments underlying various policy alternatives, it is insufficient in several ways. For one, it does not separate out the issues of fault or blame for having a potential problem from the issue of responsibility for solving the problem. The role of the provider of health care is also omitted. Nor does Wikler's analysis clarify issues of how the public good may be better served by different rationales under different conditions.

To address such questions more systematically, it is useful to consider disease prevention and health promotion in a new perspective that sharpens views of the proper roles of providers in working with clients. This new perspective is drawn from work on models of helping and coping with a problem (Brickman et al., 1982). In these models, two critical questions are asked about responsibility for a problem (whether it concerns health, education, criminal justice, or any other problem in social welfare): Who is to blame for causing the problem, and who is responsible for solving the problem? Posing these questions permits us to derive the four models portrayed in Figure 23.1. The horizontal axis reflects the issue of how to attribute blame for the problem: Is the victim personally responsible for having caused the problem, or is the cause of the problem attributed to a source outside the victim? The vertical axis allocates responsibility for the

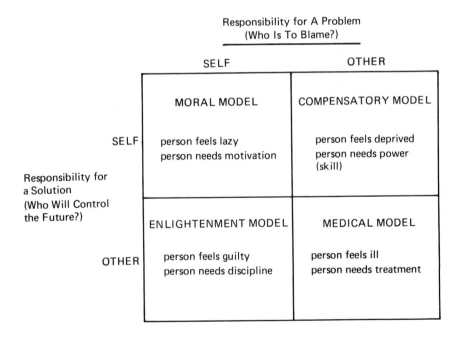

FIGURE 23.1   Four models of helping and coping.

Adapted from Brickman et al., 1982.

solution to the problem: Is the victim expected to take responsibility for solving the problem, or is the solution beyond the victim's capability to solve?

Most people are familiar with the moral model, wherein persons are held responsible both for problems and solutions; they are believed to require only the proper level of motivation to solve their problem. The prototypic view is "you got yourself into this—now get yourself out." Others are not obligated to help, since people's problems are of their own making and they must therefore find their own solutions. In this model, substance abuse, smoking, obesity, and sedentary life-styles are signs of weak character, and only willpower can help. This orientation often leads to blaming the victim; in its extreme form, sick people chose to be sick, rape victims chose to be raped. When victims themselves adopt this model, they come to feel guilty and to develop self-perceptions as individuals who lack moral fiber.

One is reminded of a policital cartoon in the *Washington Post* during the 1964 Goldwater campaign for the presidency. An obviously cold, ill-clad, ill-fed mother and two children are sitting on a street curb in the winter, while a well-to-do middle-aged man wearing a top hat and an expensive outer coat with a fur collar is striding by and exhorting the woman, "Don't just sit there. Why don't you go out and inherit a department store or something?" Turning to the enlightenment model, so named because persons are "enlightened" as to the cause of their problem, they are themselves seen as the cause. As is the case in the moral model, these "enlightened" individuals must learn that their impulses to drink, smoke, gamble, or overeat are due to their own weakness and are out of control; but, unlike the moral model, they believe that help can only come by submitting to the discipline of authority. Alcoholics Anonymous is one of the most successful examples of an enlightenment model. Alcoholics both take responsibility for their own past drinking and admit that it is beyond their power to control by themselves; they need the help of God and the community of ex-alcoholics. The treatment is believed to be effective only so long as one maintains the relationship with the agents of authority.

In the medical model, people are not held responsible for the origin of their problems, nor are they expected to solve them. A typical example might be a bacterial ear infection: We would not attribute the cause to the affected patients, nor would we ordinarily expect them to recover by acts of will or by putting their faith in a higher power or in others with similar conditions. Instead, a course of antibiotics would be prescribed. The individual is not blamed for having the condition, and we expect prompt recovery if the condition is diagnosed and treated by an expert. The only responsibility of the victim or the victim's guardian is to comply with the doctor's advice; responsibility for providing the solution rests with the expert. Parsons's (1951) conceptualization of the "sick role" exemplifies this model. Note also that the medical model is not restricted to disease and the practice of medicine but can include all cases where people are thought to be subject to forces beyond their control. Radical behaviorism exemplifies this model: Human behavior is viewed as determined by rewards and punishments over which people have no personal control (Skinner, 1976).

Finally, in the compensatory model, people are not blamed for causing their problems but are supposed to compensate for their handicaps by acquiring the power or skills needed to overcome these problems. They see themselves as suffering from the failure of the environment to provide needed resources for them to solve their problems. Thus individuals who smoke or overeat or abuse substances are not blamed for their problems, nor is energy devoted to searching for original causes. They are, however, expected to acquire the skills necessary to control their urges. In acquiring these skills they may enlist the aid of experts, but responsibility for the solution rests upon the person with the problem. An application of the compensatory model may be found in the often-quoted statement by the Reverend Jesse Jackson: "You are not responsible for being down, but you are responsible for getting up." The critical distinction between compensatory and medical models is that in the medical model the therapist advises, "Do as I say," while in the compensatory model the therapist asks, "How can I help you?" The mutual participation model developed by Szasz and Hollender (1956) to describe a desirable provider–client relationship reflects a compensatory model.

APPLICATIONS TO HEALTH PROMOTION AND COMPLIANCE

Consider how a problem such as obesity might be viewed and treated under each set of assumptions. In the moral model, obese persons would be told (and would believe) that they have only themselves to blame for their obesity. If they wish to lose weight they must become motivated and use willpower. In the enlightenment model, obesity would be blamed on the victims, who would then be instructed that their problem could be managed only by relying for support on other victims and perhaps on some higher power, possibly for the remainder of their lives. Were they to give up that support, they would be judged likely to revert to their obese condition. In the medical model, obese individuals would not be blamed for their condition, but medical or surgical procedures would be used to control weight. Traditional (noncognitive) behavior modification techniques such as those derived from operant conditioning might also be used, all under the strict control of the therapist. In the compensatory model (as in the medical model), the behavioral causes of obesity would not be sought—but unlike the medical model, the overweight victims would now be expected to acquire skills to enable them to control their urges to overeat. The therapist here would not be in charge, but rather would serve more as an expert consultant to the client, with the client maintaining control.

What does compliance mean in each of these models? In the moral model it means picking oneself up by one's bootstraps—simply giving up the unwanted behavior by an act of will. Any failure is a sign of weakness of character. In the enlightenment model compliance means continual submission to the discipline of the authoritative force. In the medical model compliance is "the extent to which the patients' behavior . . . coincides with the clinical prescription" (Sackett & Haynes, 1976, p. 1). This of course is our traditional definition of compliance. Finally, in the compensatory model compliance loses much of its traditional meaning and refers to a partnership—a therapeutic alliance between client and provider in which clients adhere to goals they have set using skills they have acquired.

How is a healthful life-style to be attained according to the precepts of each approach? In the moral model, it can only be achieved through self-determination, a personal commitment to discarding undesirable behaviors and the acquisition of desirable ones; any failure to do this is an indication of character weakness. In the enlightenment model, it can only be acquired by admission of personal weaknesses, and then through continual submission to the discipline of authoritative forces. In the medical model, the road to healthful life-styles is reliance on the expert and subsequent compliance with the professional's advice. Finally, in the compensatory model, healthful life-styles are achieved by clients' acceptance of responsibility for their own solution and by their acquisition of requisite behavioral skills through a therapeutic alliance with a consultant. Clients adhere to goals they themselves have set using skills they have learned. A slip in the application of their skills is an occasion not for guilt, but for finding ways of avoiding future slips.

The compensatory model is probably the approach best suited to efforts at effecting life-style modification—that is, situations in which clients must learn new behavioral skills and relinquish old, often longstanding habits. Physicians and other health care providers who can learn to view life-style practices within the framework of a "compensatory" rather than a "medical" model will be better able to assist clients in achieving their own goals, at their own pace, in their own priority order. The relapse prevention program of Marlatt and Gordon (1985) represents a most promising application of the compensatory model, and it seems applicable to initial life-style modification as well as to prevention of relapses.

True patient–provider contracting (Janz, Becker, & Hartman, 1984) may reflect the best use of the compensatory model. In this approach, the client and professional agree on a specific, written treatment goal (however modest) with a time limit for its accomplishment, and both sign the document. This technique is effective when properly used because the patient and provider are in a true therapeutic alliance, with both involved in goal-setting and in selecting goals for which the client has a high degree of self-efficacy (i.e., the conviction that he or she can successfully undertake the needed behaviors within the time limit) (Bandura, 1977; Strecher, DeVellis, Becker, & Rosenstock, 1986). When a client does achieve the goal, self-efficacy is enhanced and the client is ready to contract for a newer, more difficult goal.

While the compensatory model is recommended as providing the best single model for health promotion, it clearly cannot always be the sole method of choice. Certain health conditions, particularly those of an emergency nature, require prompt application of a medical model. Moreover, some individuals may not be able to accept the responsibility imposed by the compensatory model, preferring instead the security of the enlightenment or medical models. Individual differences must always be considered in developing health promotion policy.

An additional factor that should influence health promotion policy concerns the accuracy of our knowledge about what individuals can do to stay healthy. Most of our beliefs about behavioral risk factors derive from epidemiological applications to individuals. And this is very dangerous because personal practices account for so little variance in disease and longevity, a realization that undermines many current applications of Health Risk Appraisals (Wagner, Beery, Schoenbach, & Graham, 1982). While it is true that a healthy white 44-year-old married male cigarette smoker has 1.9 times the risk of dying of lung cancer in the next 10 years as his nonsmoking counterpart, the fact is that neither of them is likely to die of lung cancer in the next 10 years and most smokers will never die of lung cancer. When we consider other risk factors such as eating high-fat foods, overweight (however that may be defined), and drinking more than 45 alcoholic beverages per month, our knowledge is still less certain. We simply do not know very much about how life-style affects the health and longevity of a given individual, even though we may be able to make accurate actuarial predictions for groups of 100,000. We must therefore temper our policy recommendations by our level of knowledge or ignorance.

LOCUS OF INTERVENTIONS

The discussion has thus far focused on the individual as the locus of responsibility for health, and the tendency of the contemporary health promotion movement is to locate responsibility for the cause and the cure of health problems in the *individual* (Becker, 1986). A number of problems may result from such a narrow, "life-style" approach: (1) we may tend to ignore the influence of the social environment on health and health behavior; (2) as was indicated in discussing the "moral model," it becomes easy to "blame the victim," stigmatizing those who continue to engage in risky behaviors as "having no willpower"; and (3) being healthy may become an end in itself, rather than a means to achieving still broader life goals.

Life-style interventions directed at individuals have undoubtedly achieved some measure of success (Matarazzo, Weiss, Herd, Miller, & Weiss, 1984). It is equally clear, however, that interventions at the individual level are sometimes not longlasting (Marlatt & Gordon, 1985). It therefore becomes important to examine possibilities for promoting health through interventions at the level of the social and physical environment. Green (1984) draws a useful distinction between health education and health promotion, defining health education as "any combination of learning methods designed to facilitate voluntary adaptation of behavior conducive to health" (p. 186) and health promotion as "any combination of health education and related organizational, economic, and environmental supports for behavior conducive to health" (p. 190). Health promotion thus includes both educational and environmental interventions.

It has long been understood that the public's health is sometimes better protected by modifications of the physical environment than by direct education of individuals. We may note here the unquestioned benefits of sewage treatment, chlorination and fluoridation of public water supplies, pasteurization of milk, legal restrictions regarding disposal of hazardous wastes, restrictions on smoking in public (to protect the nonsmoker), and safety equipment requirements in automobiles. Of course, even in cases of environmental intervention, prior educational interventions are always required to enlist the support of key decision makers—legislators, administrators, employers, judges, and sometimes the general public.

Health and health-relevant behaviors are also strongly influenced by the social environment (Levine, 1981; Syme & Guralnik, 1987). Vast changes over the past 20 years in behavior and attitudes toward smoking clearly illustrate the influence of social factors; other examples might include attitudes and behaviors concerning drinking, diet, and exercise. Social legislation impinges on the social environment and often modifies it. It would be unthinkable for the United States to abolish our Social Security retirement system. Even Medicare, only 20 years old, has so permeated and affected our notions of social justice that it has become part of the fabric of American social values. Working with the social environment provides an important locus for interventions to modify health behaviors to promote health.

An interesting ongoing attempt to alter the social environment with the aim of improving health is reported by Syme (1986). His team is attempting to solve certain health problems observed among San Francisco bus drivers, including high prevalence of hypertension, musculoskeletal system problems, and diseases of the gastrointestinal tract. A traditional medical model approach to this problem might have focused on teaching drivers more healthful eating habits, better posture, and effective ways of coping with job stress. Syme's team, however, is also looking at the bus drivers' social environment; they have observed the "tyranny of the schedule" (Syme, 1986, p. 503), in which the company sets schedules that are virtually impossible to keep. Long shifts and social isolation of the drivers have also been noted. Because of these factors, drivers tend not to go home immediately after work; instead they remain in the bus yard for several hours after work in order to wind down. By the time the drivers arrive home, it is so late that they usually go directly to bed, thus limiting interactions with spouses, children, and friends. This combination of circumstances is probably an important contributing factor in observed hostile or impatient behavior by the drivers.

The research team is attempting to introduce interventions not only among the drivers but directly on those factors associated with the job. For example, if schedules were arranged to be more realistic and rest stops were located in or near central cities to permit drivers to meet other drivers from time to time, the bus company might be able to increase revenues by reducing absenteeism, accidents, and sickness. Because this investigation is still in progress, its success cannot yet be evaluated; however, it is hardly debatable that working conditions can affect emotional and physical health, and that therefore efforts to optimize working conditions are worthy of attention. Permanent modifications of life-style are most likely to be accomplished by strategies whose focus encompasses the physical/social environment and the individual.

THE ETHICS OF INTERVENTION

In addition to considerations of the relative effectiveness of both passive and active interventions, one must also consider the ethics of intervention at each level. A number of ethicists have emphasized the immorality of intervening at the individual level where there is good reason to believe that governmental interventions at the societal level would be more effective. In summarizing this argument, Faden (1987) alludes to health campaigns that "are morally suspect . . . [if they] are directed toward health problems for which there exist technological, regulatory, or engineering solutions; but the government is avoiding these solutions, perhaps for political or economic reasons" (Faden, 1987, p. 35).

She also reviews the argument made by many ethicists that "if the government is convinced that an industry is marketing an unhealthful product . . . the government should ban all promotional advertising of the product. Better yet, the government should either set standards that make the product healthful or . . . make the product illegal" (Faden, 1987, p. 35). Yet questions also arise as to ". . . whether the government ought to be in the business of promoting certain life-styles above others, in the first place" (Faden, 1987, p. 30).

When ethicists criticize government policy for promoting solutions to social problems that are known to be ineffective, they do in fact call attention to possible duplicity in social policy. When, however, they also call for effective governmental intervention that would certainly reduce people's autonomy and then question the right of government to promote life-styles at all, they reveal values that seem to be internally inconsistent. Would we reduce people's autonomy more by using informational campaigns to persuade them not to smoke than by laws with penalties that prohibit the manufacture and sale of tobacco products? It certainly would appear that legal prohibitions would reduce autonomy more than the most successful educational campaigns. Moreover, governmental policy concerning smoking, for example, may not be deceitful but may reflect political and economic realities and the need to satisfy the desires of differing constituencies. One could thus argue that educational campaigns maximize individual autonomy. It has always seemed puzzling that public health workers are generally opposed to limiting individual rights to smoke, overeat, and drink to excess, provided such behavior does not adversely affect others, while at the same time endorsing plans to levy prohibitive taxes on cigarettes and alcohol and plans to require processors of food to label their products more completely. Are not the two approaches intended to have the same effect? And if so, why is one preferred over the other? The answer seems to be that the passive approach—the social engineering approach—is more distantly related to the behavior we are trying to shape, though no less effective, and perhaps even more effective, as Levine (1981), Syme (1986), and others (DHHS, 1986) suggest.

The potential adverse side effects of health promotion should always be considered in planning programs. Millions of people in our society now possess a fear of obesity that may be worse than the disease—people are spending hundreds of millions of dollars each year to lose weight and are perhaps worrying or dieting themselves into avoidable illness. In 1985, 53% of *all* American women 18 years and older considered themselves overweight (compared to 37% of all men), and 44% of all women reported that they were "now trying to lose weight" [National Center for Health Statistics (NCHS), 1986, p. 3], while only 25% of men gave that response. When one considers that these are probably underestimates of concern with weight because they include persons above 75 years of age, who are generally not trying to lose weight, the pervasiveness of the problem seems even greater. As some wag has noted, practically every middle-class American woman feels either hungry or guilty. For all the people whose dietary practices are damaging their health, there may be an equal number whose fears about diet are equally damaging. While techniques of behavior modification and relapse prevention are being developed for the benefit of those who want them, we must guard against imposing an arbitrary set of values on those who do not. Adopting a compensatory model for guiding interventions will help avoid the temptation to be experts in all matters.

CONCLUSIONS AND IMPLICATIONS

There can be no reasonable doubt that certain life-style practices influence the length and quality of life. Although additional epidemiological study is needed to specify more precisely the relationships between behavior and health, it seems entirely appropriate to allocate additional resources to the promotion of more healthful life-styles based on what is already known. Thus, at a minimum, we ought to continue efforts to eliminate smoking, to encourage moderation in drinking, and to educate for increased levels of physical activity and acceptance of "healthy" diets. As more light is thrown on the effects of stress and coping on health, additional pertinent recommendations will likely emerge. Resources should also be devoted to improving ways of preventing relapse among those who have begun to adopt more healthful life-styles. There is every reason to believe that widespread adoption of recommended practices for smoking, drinking, exercise, and dietary excesses would prolong lives and improve quality of living in the population.

As a matter of public policy, it is important to seek the most cost-effective means of controlling these problems. And it is important to distinguish cost-effectiveness from cost-saving (Warner, 1987). To the extent that health is a desired societal goal we should be prepared to spend in order to attain it, but we should always seek the most efficient means of attaining that goal. The search for cost-effective interventions is the subject of a recent monograph, *Integration of Risk Factor Interventions* (DHHS, 1986), which clarifies some of the key issues needing resolution before proper choices may be made. Substantial evidence supports the conclusion that a focus on fewer than 10 risk factors could prevent 40% to 70% of all premature deaths, one third of acute disability, and two thirds of chronic disability. However, attempts to target interventions to so-called "high-risk" subpopulations should be avoided, since the population does not for the most part sort into high- and low-risk groups, and even where it does, the majority of disease, though not the rate, occurs in the low-risk group. Moreover, there is no reason to believe that efforts to change norms and values underlying life-styles would be more easily accomplished in subgroups of the population than in the entire population.

Would it be better to address one risk factor at a time, or should a "menu" of alternative life-style interventions be offered? Few risk factors are present in the entire population; for example, for cardiovascular risk factors, fewer than one third of the population are smokers, only one quarter are hypertensive, and about half the population have serum cholesterol levels in the accepted optimal range. Yet, "more than half the population has a cardiac risk factor in the top quartile of the risk distribution" (DHHS, 1986, p. 5). When one adds to these data the risk factors for other major causes of morbidity and mortality, it would appear that nearly everyone could contribute to lower morbidity and mortality rates and probably reduce the cost of health care by altering one or more behavioral risk factors. Individuals vary, however, in their preferences and self-efficacy regarding behavior change; some may wish to work on smoking rather than on diet (or before diet), others may wish to develop physical fitness first, and so on.

Based on these considerations, it would seem appropriate to develop coordinated, multiple-risk-factor national and regional programs to promote healthier life-styles concerning smoking, drinking, exercise, and diet. These programs should include both active interventions (requiring voluntary behavior change by the individual) and passive interventions (which emphasize social and physical changes in the environment to alter the probability of behavior without conscious resolve by the individual). Active interventions may be undertaken by individuals and public and private sector groups, while passive interventions frequently require the involvement of industry and government. Passive interventions, including laws and economic incentives, have proven useful in reducing incidence and prevalence of smoking, reductions in alcohol-related traffic deaths, and (probably) changes in attitudes and behavior concerning diet and exercise (Syme, 1986; U.S. DHHS, 1986). Passive intervention alone, however, will not be sufficient. At a minimum, education is required to persuade decision makers of the need for such passive interventions as legal requirements to increase automobile safety or to raise minimum drinking ages. Such education may be targeted directly at the decision makers or at their constituents (or both). Moreover, even when laws have been passed, their effectiveness depends greatly on the willingness of the governed to be governed—on their agreement with the goals of the law. Thus most Americans are now ready to accept severe restrictions on smoking but are not yet prepared to accept legislative enforced seat belt use. The continuing interplay of active and passive interventions will yield better results than will reliance on either approach alone.

Still another justification for promoting active as well as passive interventions is the ethical one—the nearly universal acceptance in our culture of the rights of freedom of choice and voluntariness. We hold dear peoples' rights to be let alone—to do as they wish as long as their behavior does not infringe upon our rights (including our right to health). Accordingly, we feel that individuals must be free to reject our educational efforts. There will always remain considerable numbers of individuals who are not motivated to modify their behavior (and consequently will not do so)—people with full knowledge of the risks associated with their particular life-styles who nonetheless *prefer* those life-styles. Our objectives should therefore emphasize encouraging people to make voluntary but informed decisions.

REFERENCES

Bandura, A. (1977). Self-efficacy: Toward a unifying theory of behavioral change. *Psychological Review, 34*(2), 191–215.

Becker, M. H. (1986). The tyranny of health promotion. *Public Health Reviews, 14*, 15–25.

Brickman, P., Rabinowitz, V. C., Karuza, J., Jr., Coates, D., Cohn, E., & Kidder, L. (1982). Models of helping and coping. *American Psychologist, 37*(4), 368–384.

Faden, R. R. (1987). Ethical issues in government sponsored health campaigns. *Health Education Quarterly, 14*, 27–37.

Green, L. W. (1984). Health education models. In J. D. Matarazzo, S. M. Weiss, J. A. Herd, N. E. Miller, & S. M. Weiss (Eds.), *Behavioral Health* (pp. 181–198). New York: Wiley.

Janz, N. K., Becker, M. H., & Hartman, P. E. (1984). Contingency contracting to enhance patient compliance: A review. *Patient Education and Counseling, 5*, 165–178.

Knowles, J. H. (1977). The responsibility of the individual. In J. H. Knowles (Ed.), *Doing better and feeling worse: Health in the United States* (pp. 57–80). New York: Norton.

Levine, S. (1981). Preventive health behavior. In H. Wechsler, R. W. Lamont-Havers, & G. F. Cahill (Eds.), *The social context of medical research*. Cambridge, MA: Ballinger.

Marlatt, G. A., & Gordon, J. R. (1985). *Relapse prevention*. New York: Guilford.

Matarazzo, J. D., Weiss, S. M., Herd, J. A., Miller, N. E., & Weiss, S. M. (1984). *Behavioral Health*. New York: Wiley.

National Center for Health Statistics (NCHS). (1986). *Health promotion data for the 1990 objectives: Estimates from the National Health Interview Survey of health promotion and disease prevention: U.S. 1985* (DHHS Publication No. (PHS) 86-1250). Hyattsville, MD: U.S. Government Printing Office.

Parsons, T. (1951). Illness and the role of the physician: A sociological perspective. *American Journal of Orthopsychiatry, 21*, 452–460.

Sackett, D. L., & Haynes, R. B. (1976). *Compliance with therapeutic regimens*. Baltimore, MD: Johns Hopkins University Press.

Skinner, B. F. (1974). About behaviorism. New York: Knopf.

Strecher, V. J., deVellis, B. M., Becker, M. H., & Rosenstock, I. M. (1986). The role of self-efficacy in achieving health behavior change. *Health Education Quarterly, 13*, 73–91.

Syme, S. L. (1986). Strategies for health promotion. *Preventive Medicine, 15*, 492–507.

Syme, S. L., & Guralnik, J. M. (1987). Epidemiology and health policy: Coronary heart disease. In S. Levine & A. Lilienfeld (Eds.), *Epidemiology and health policy*. London: Travistock.

Szasz, T., & Hollander, M. H. (1956). A contribution to the philosophy of medicine: The basic models of the doctor–patient relationship. *American Sociological Review, 97*, 585–592.

U.S. Department of Health, Education, and Welfare (DHEW). (1979). *Healthy People: The Surgeon-General's Report on Health Promotion and Disease Prevention* (DHEW Publication No. 79-55071). Washington, DC: U.S. Government Printing Office.

U.S. Department of Health and Human Services (DHHS), Office of Health Promotion and Disease Prevention, Public Health Service. (1986, November). *Integration of risk factor interventions*. Washington, DC: U.S. Government Printing Office.

Wagner, E. H., Beery, W., Schoenbach, V. J., & Graham, R. M. (1982). An assessment of health hazard health risk appraisal. *American Journal of Public Health, 72*(4), 347–352.

Warner, K. E. (1987). Selling health promotion to corporate America: Uses and abuses of the economic argument. *Health Education Quarterly, 14*, 39–55.

Wikler, D. (1987). Who should be blamed for being sick? *Health Education Quarterly, 14*, 11–25.

24

Ethical Issues
in Life-Style Change
and Adherence

Ruth Faden

In this chapter I examine issues in life-style change and adherence from the perspective of normative ethics. Central to frameworks of ethical analysis in normative ethics is the notion that moral deliberation and justification ordinarily rest on principles, rule, and rights, understood as abstract action guides. These action guides, the choice and analysis of which are inherently controversial, together with questions of their relationship with one another and their relationship to a theory of virtues, constitute the heart of modern ethical theory.

Structures of principles and rules, rights, and virtues can be used to analyze questions of morality, in particular concrete situations and arenas of social life. Often such analysis is referred to as "applied ethics." Numerous areas of applied ethics have been identified, such as business ethics and journalism ethics.

Three areas of applied ethics of particular relevance to the themes of this volume are the ethics of the healing professions, research ethics, and ethics and public policy. For our purposes, these fields can be understood as the ethics of the professional-patient relationship, the ethics of the researcher-subject relationship, and the ethics of the government-citizenry relationship, respectively.

In this chapter I highlight the origins and characteristics of some of the key moral issues related to life-style and adherence in each of these areas: clinician-patient, researcher-subject, and government-citizenry. Relevant principles and rules emerge as each area is discussed.

Before proceeding, however, one caveat is in order having to do with the difficulty of treating together questions of adherence in a clinical context and questions of life-style for the general public. The ethical issues raised by adherence with prescribed medical regimens for the clinically ill can be substantively different from the issues raised in relation to adoption of recommendations of the Surgeon General or the American Heart Association regarding healthy life-styles. While it is beyond the scope of this chapter to take these differences systematically into account, the sections that follow vary in the extent to which they focus on adherence versus general life-style issues.

THE CLINICIAN-PATIENT RELATIONSHIP

Most of the chapters in this volume have focused specifically on adherence and life-style issues in health care services and the clinical encounter. In Freidman's chapter (Chapter 4), reference is made to how different models of the physician-patient relationship affect issues of adherence. Medical ethics also operate with models of the doctor-patient relationship. One such approach argues that the doctor-patient relationship in particular, and all health professional-patient relationships generally, are dominated by two competing models of moral responsibility—the beneficence model and the autonomy model (Beauchamp & McCullough, 1985).

Under the beneficence model, the *primary* obligation of clinicians is to seek the best balance of good over harm for their patients. Goods and harms are understood in strictly medical terms, such that the chief goods are health, the prevention or elimination of disease and injury, relief from pain and suffering, the amelioration of disabilities, and the prolongation of life. The principal harms at issue are death, disease, disability, pain, and suffering.

By contrast, under the autonomy model the values and beliefs of the patient become the primary moral consideration. If the patient's values conflict with the values of medicine, the clinician's primary moral obligation is to respect and facilitate the patient's perferences.

Both models speak to important moral truths about the professional-patient relationship. However, occasionally the requirements of these models can come into conflict. A central moral task is fixing the limits of each of these two models, in light of the demands of the other, in particular contexts.

The perspective of the beneficence model provides strong moral support for adherence interventions in clinical settings. Under this model, clinicians have a moral obligation, an affirmative duty, to take actions that will preserve the health of their patients and prevent them from disease and injury. Thus, insofar as clinicians are not taking seriously their obligations to secure the adherence of their patients to medically indicated regimens, clinicians are morally blame-worthy. This moral obligation has been given legal force in a California case in which a physician was held liable for not adequately informing his patient of the risks of failing to have a Pap test (*Truman v. Thomas*, 1980).

There are, of course, limits under the beneficence model to the clinician's obligation to be proactive in securing patient adherence. It is a fundamental maxim of ethics that "ought implies can." Insofar as it is not possible for clinicians to implement adherence interventions or otherwise secure adherence, they have no obligation to do so. Whether or not it is possible for physicians to secure adherence raises a host of issues discussed in earlier chapters, including the amount of time and the kinds of skills needed to be successful in promoting adherence in clinical contexts.

A related point is the relative moral priority of competing clinical duties in a context of limited resources. When the amount of time and dollars to be spent on clinical encounters is limited, what priority is to be placed on activities that cure disease, as compared with those that allay suffering, prevent deterioration, or promote health? Although clinicians may have a prima facie obligation to seek adherence to medical regimens and life-style recommendations, these obliga-tions may necessarily be less weighty than other duties competing for the clinician's attention.

In contrast to the beneficence model, the autonomy model does not provide clinicians with a direct moral warrant for securing adherence to medical recom-mendations. Under the autonomy model, if the patient's values do not include improving his or her health prospects by altering life-style or adhering to medications, then the clinician is obligated to respect that value preference.

This is not to say, however, that the autonomy model releases clinicians from any obligation in relation to adherence and life-style. At minimum, respect for the patient's autonomy requires the clinician to ascertain the basis for the patient's position and, in particular, to establish whether the patient's rejection of the clinician's recommendation is based on an adequate understanding of what is at stake. As Andrew Baum pointed out earlier in this volume (Commentary, Section I), one cannot assume that naive theories of disease conform to medical theories of disease and thus that lay persons and clinicians will necessarily share an understanding of the importance of certain recommended behaviors in prevent-ing or curing disease.

What if the clinician ascertains that the patient has a correct understanding of what is at stake in refusing to adhere to medical recommendations and still wishes to ignore them? In my view, the clinician's beneficence-based obligations require the clinician to attempt to persuade the patient to change his or her position. I have argued elsewhere that persuasive interventions, properly constrained, do not violate obligations to respect patient autonomy (Faden & Beauchamp, 1986). However, if, after reasonable attempts at persuasion, the patient's values remain fixed, these must be respected.

The ascendence of the autonomy model in thinking about the ethics of the physician–patient relationship has been reflected in the adherence literature. What was once referred to as the problem of "compliance with doctor's orders" has become the problem of "adherence to the recommendations of professionals." Even this second adherence formulation is not wholly satisfactory. In line with the autonomy model, a more desirable formulation would entail something like the following: "assisting individuals to make informed and reflective choices about whether to adopt or reject professional recommendations."

Contrasting the beneficence model of professional–patient relationships with the autonomy model helps highlight the central moral issues raised by adherence and life-style interventions in clinical settings. However, in isolation this approach draws too stark a contrast between competing moral principles and fails to capture much of the textual richness of the clinician–patient relation. An alternative approach in moral theory, frequently referred to as the care perspective, draws attention to issues of responsiveness and compassion in the moral life, including the need to respond to that which is unique and particular about the other in a moral relationship (Areen, 1988; Hanen & Nielsen, 1987). The care perspective reminds us to refrain from being formulaic in our approach to moral issues. In clinical encounters, each patient brings a unique history and life experience. From the care perspective, assisting "individuals to make informed and reflective choices" about medical regimens or life-style changes requires compassionate attention to the needs of the patient as a unique individual.

In providing such assistance, professionals should recognize that there exist genuine epistemic challenges to the validity of medical knowledge and thus to the force of medical opinion and recommendation. Earlier I made reference to the recognition that naive theories of disease are not always isomorphic with medical theories and thus that patients may be basing their decisions to reject medical recommendations on false beliefs and incomplete understanding. It is also the case, however, that naive theories of disease are not always so naive. That is, patients' beliefs about the etiology and treatment of disease can be more correct than the opposing beliefs of medical experts. As Rosenstock notes in Chapter 23, the medical community has a notable history of being wrong in its predictions and recommendations regarding both health risks and protective behaviors. Patients of the past who refused to increase their consumption of eggs and who refused to take swine flue shots were all at the time considered to be "noncompliers" who held "false beliefs" by contemporary medical standards. To a significant extent, this sort of disagreement between patient and physician is an epistemic problem about the nature of medical knowledge and its evidentiary base, in a context of ever-evolving scientific theories of disease and illness. At stake is whether physicians can offer anything stronger than medical opinions, a far cry from the tradition of the "doctor's order."

THE RESEARCHER–SUBJECT RELATIONSHIP

The ethics of the researcher–subject relationship has a different tradition and a different social imperative from that of the physician–patient relationship. In the clinical context, ethics is guided, at least in part, by the assumption that both clinician and patient share the goal of seeking to improve the patient's welfare. By contrast, in research the primary goal is not to benefit the subject but to produce generalizable, "scientific" knowledge. Because the welfare of the subject is not central to the research enterprise, there is no beneficence model in research ethics corresponding to that in clinical ethics. As a result, obligations to respect the autonomy of research subjects are generally difficult to validly override, even by appeal to arguments grounded in beneficence or conceptions of the public good.

The implications of this understanding of the ethics of the researcher–subject relationship for adherence issues in research are straightforward. In general, it is not morally permissible for researchers to overlook their obligations to seek valid informed consent from their subjects and respect potential subjects' decisions to refuse to participate or to drop out of studies, even when honoring these obligations threatens or compromises the scientific integrity of their research. When tensions arise between respecting the refusals of subjects and promoting the cooperation of subjects, the interventions of researchers should be restricted to persuasion and to inducements that do not substantially undermine the voluntariness of the subjects' decisions.

THE GOVERNMENT–CITIZENRY RELATIONSHIP

That government has both the obligation and the right to protect the public health is clear. What is less clear is the scope of this government obligation. What kinds of threats to health are covered under this government obligation? What means should the government use to control these threats?

The answers to these questions turn on a complex of principles and values, including, most prominently, respect for autonomy, justice, public welfare, and utility. How the demands of these principles are to be balanced or blended depends critically on one's theory of the state, in our case, on one's theory of the liberal state in a democratic society.

In Chapter 23, Dr. Rosenstock suggests that I and other writers on this subject have been internally inconsistent in our position on government-sponsored health campaigns. I have expressed concerns about autonomy issues in health education efforts while calling for restrictive government regulatory action (Faden, 1987). However, Rosenstock's criticism is a misreading of my analysis. There is no inconsistency involved; rather, there is an application of the principles to different cases, cases that differ in the extent to which the different principles come into play.

Strong state action is most clearly morally demanded when the health of innocent parties is placed at risk by the actions of others and there is a feasible way to remove the risk through regulation or environmental control. Classic examples here include asbestos and lead exposures in the workplace or the home, unsafe appliances, and carcinogenic food additives.

State action is demanded in such cases by a complex of principles including justice and utility. It should be noted that these cases do not raise relevant autonomy issues. That is, there is no substantive conflict between the demands of justice and obligations to respect autonomy. To be facetious, one rarely asserts a liberty right to be exposed to lead or asbestos.

Note also that the lead and asbestos cases are classic examples of what has been referred to in the literature as victim-blaming situations. Health education interventions to promote the wearing of respiratory protective gear among workers in inadequately ventilated plants or to promote more vigilant behavior among tenants in lead-contaminated apartments are indeed morally suspect, and in many circumstances morally unconscionable.

The moral issues are somewhat more complicated when we move to cases where there are plausibly some autonomy interests at issue, but the autonomy interests do not involve weighty liberty values. The classic example here is the seat belt and air bag controversy.

Those outside the automobile industry opposed to compulsory seat belt legislation claim, among other things, a liberty right to drive unharnessed. Those opposed to mandatory air bags claim, among other things, a liberty right to decide whether they wish to pay the additional costs of air bag installation, which will be passed on to consumers.

The position one takes in relation to this controversy depends to a significant extent on the value one places on these particular liberty interests, in comparison to values placed on the other principles. Whether media campaigns or other forms of behavioral interventions as alternatives to regulation are morally preferable or morally questionable turns on a complex balancing of these competing values and principles.

Not all health issues entail strong arguments for coercive state action—either because the autonomy interests outweigh any other consideration, or because effective technological or regulatory solutions do not exist or are by themselves insufficient. Here, interventions directed at individuals are particularly fitting. I have in mind such health issues as oral hygiene, breast self-exam, safer sexual practices, and exercise.

In many of these instances, where the autonomy interests are strong it is important to evaluate behavioral interventions in terms of their effect on autonomous choice. There is not, however, always consensus about which health issues entail strong autonomy interests, at least in part because of fundamental disagreements about the causal determinants of behavior. Nevertheless, at least for some people, many of the classic life-style issues of diet and exercise fall into this area. More paradigmatically, reproductive behaviors—abortion in the instance of fetuses who would be disabled, contraceptive use, and so on—are recognized by many to entail strong autonomy interests such that any intervention, behavioral or otherwise, must be carefully scrutinized for its impact on autonomous choice.

The discussion thus far has focused on ethics, to the exclusion of politics. However, any evaluation of the ethics of government life-style and adherence interventions must recognize that there are instances in which regulatory or environmental intervention is morally preferable but politically impossible, at least at the moment. How government officials and researchers ought to proceed under such circumstances is difficult to stipulate in the abstract. Consider, for example, Altman's discussion about smoking behavior and advertising in Chapter 13. Under such circumstances, there will certainly be situations in which interventions directed at individuals are morally permissible as the only available strategy for dealing with a health problem.

SUMMARY

This chapter focuses on traditional issues of justice and autonomy as they relate to adherence and life-style issues. One variant of the justice and autonomy themes not discussed is the morality of promoting healthier life-styles in a context in which millions of Americans are denied access to basic health services. Any thorough examination of the ethics of life-style change and adherence must address not only whether the characteristics of specific interventions conform with obligations to respect autonomy, but also whether the resources needed to mount these interventions have been justly allocated.

A thorough examination of the ethics of life-style change and adherence must also address how our ethics affect our evaluation designs. To the extent that we claim that our objective is merely to encourage people to make informed voluntary decisions regarding their health, then should not our primary evaluation criterion be the quality of the choice made by those to which our interventions are aimed, rather than the choices themselves? If this is true, then our evaluation criterion is not how many subjects stayed in the trial, but how well they understood what was involved in participating in the trial, regardless of whether they consented or refused, stayed in or dropped out. The issue becomes not how many hypertensives took their medications according to directions, but how many made an informed reflective decision about whether they wanted to take the medication as recommended. Whether we are willing to have our evaluations conform with our ethics remains a challenge for the field.

REFERENCES

Areen, J. (1988). A need for caring. *Michigan Law Review, 86*, 967–1082.

Beauchamp, T. L., & McCullough, L. B. (1984). *Medical ethics.* Englewood Cliffs, NJ: Prentice-Hall.

Faden, R. R., & Beauchamp, T. L. (1986). *A history and theory of informed consent.* New York: Oxford University Press.

Hanen, M., & Nielsen, K. (Eds.). (1987). Science, morality and feminist theory. *Canadian Journal of Philosophy, 13* (Supplement).

Truman v. Thomas, 165 Cal. Rptr. 308, 611 P.2d 902 (Cal. 1980).

Commentary: Life-Style Change and Adherence: The Broader Context

Patricia D. Mullen

The earlier chapters in this book provide a review of models of patient behavior. Such models tend to be made explicit—at least in written representations of the project or program. The chapters in this final section remind us that we have implicit models of *responsibility*—for the problem and the solution—that profoundly influence the direction of our research and program activity. The notion that social problems arise in social contexts and are always subject to particular and limited constructions of reality means that the behavior of the one who defines the problem is as problematic as that of the patient–client.

Rosenstock notes our timidity in seeking change in providers and in environmental conditions, and he speculates on the reasons for our preference for solutions at the individual level. Faden provides us with a framework for assessing the tradeoffs involved in various types of solutions. Czajkowski and Chesney challenge another of our models in suggesting that adherence is a *correlate* of health status improvement, rather than a predictor. That is, adherence can be a consequence of health status improvement. Furthermore, Czajkowski and Chesney suggest that if adherence is a predictor of improvement, it may exert a direct affect through nonspecific or placebo factors and not just through the therapeutic treatment. These authors describe several mechanisms by which the alternative effects might operate, and they provide evidence from a clinical trial for this adherence-related placebo effect.

These three chapters remind us of the need to assess our degree of certainty that the treatment or other behavioral recommendation is effective and that it produces net benefits for individuals or society. Rosenstock presents examples of life-style change recommendations that may turn out to be unfounded, Faden highlights relevant ethical issues, and Czajkowski and Chesney point out the difficulties of designing clinical trials to rule out confounding placebo effects.

Faden elaborates and challenges several of Rosenstock's themes, and she offers us a broad range of concepts from applied ethics with which to assess the models and ethical assumptions that guide our everyday behavior as researchers, professionals interacting with clients, and participants in the process of forming public policy. Her presentation also points out the relative absence in our professional vocabularies of the concepts of ethical discourse. Analyses such as Faden's and the assessment of public and professional opinion would be productive avenues for research.

Rosenstock mentions the idea of informed decision making as an outcome measure—an idea that bears some similarity to the individual-level cost-benefit analysis described earlier in this book by Kaplan. The chapters in this book, coupled with other current work in the field of health behavior, support the perspective that the sources, functions, and consequences over time of behavior models can give us an understanding of why our focus in formulating models of health improvement should not only be on health but also on other areas that fit into patients' equations. Additionally, nonadherence can best be viewed as a behavior and not as a personal attribute. People can walk in and out of that behavior over time with respect to the same recommendation, or they can select across recommendations. This may explain the relative paucity of conclusions in the elusive search for the profile of the "noncomplier" or even for predictors of noncompliance that are rooted in a preoccupation with health rather than larger issues of social functioning. Thus, this final collection of chapters broadens our perspective on life-style change and adherence and should make us self-conscious about certain biases of perspectives and methods that, if left unexamined, may limit the solutions open to us.

Index

Author/Subject Index